In the Hands of Doctors

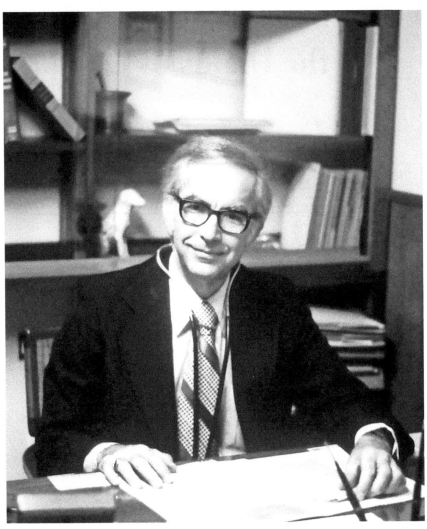

William Stepansky, M.D.
the author's father

In the Hands of Doctors

Touch and Trust in Medical Care

PAUL E. STEPANSKY

Keynote Books, LLC   *   Montclair, NJ   *   2017

for
Deane
who makes me whole

Where there is love of one's fellow man, there is love of the Art.
Hippocrates, *Precepts, 3*

Contents

Preface to the Paperback Edition

Medical Freedom, Then and Now

In our time, political speech and writing are largely the defense of the indefensible.

— George Orwell, *Politics and the English Language* (1946)

A nation's liberties seem to depend upon headier and heartier attributes than the liberty to die without medical care.

— Milton Mayer, *The Dogged Retreat of the Doctors* (1949)

N ow, less than a year after publication of *In the Hands of Doctors,* the Patient Protection and Affordable Care Act of 2010 (aka Obamacare), which I roundly endorse in this book, is gravely imperiled. Congressional Republican legislators have joined a Republican President in a commitment to repeal the bill that has provided health insurance to over 20 million previously uninsured Americans. The legislation thus far presented to replace it by the U.S. Senate (the "Better Care Reconciliation Act of 2017") would, according to the Congressional Budget Office, leave 15 million Americans uninsured in 2018 and 22 million by 2026. Proposed cuts and caps to the Medicaid budget, which are part of the legislation, would, according to the CBO, decrease enrollment in the program by 16% over the next decade. In brief, these cuts and caps would jeopardize the health and well-being of the one in five Americans and one in three American children dependent on the support provided by Medicaid. Disabled and other special-needs children as well as elderly nursing home residents would suffer the most. A Congressional vote simply to repeal Obamacare absent new legislation would have even more catastrophic consequences.

Congressional opponents of the Affordable Care Act, no less than President Donald Trump, appear to live in a hermetically sealed bubble that makes only grazing contact with the socioeconomic ground below. They share space in the bubble with colliding political abstractions that they grasp, one after the other, and radio back down to earth. The political bubble dwellers offer us yet again the palliatives of context-free "medical choice" and "medical freedom" as remedies for the real-world suffering addressed by Obamacare.

But these terms, as used by politicians, do not speak to the realties of American health care in 2017. Rather, they hearken back to the era of the Founding Fathers, when issues of health, illness, freedom, and tyranny were much simpler. Freedom, as the founders understood it, operated only in the intertwined realms of politics and religion. How could it be otherwise? Medical intervention did not affect the course of illness; it did not enable people to feel better and live longer and more productive lives. With the exception of smallpox inoculation, which George Washington wisely made mandatory among colonial troops in the winter of 1777, governmental intrusion into the health of its citizenry was nonexistent, even non-sensical.

Until roughly the eighth decade of the nineteenth century, you got sick, you recovered (often despite doctoring), you lingered on in sickness, or you died. They were the options. Medical freedom, enshrined during the Jacksonian era, meant being free to pick and choose your doctor without any state interference. So liberty-loving Americans picked and chose among mercury-dosing, bloodletting "regulars," homeopaths, herbalists, botanical practitioners, eclectics, hydropaths, phrenologists, Christian Scientists, folk healers, and faith healers. State legislatures stood on the sidelines, rescinding or gutting medical licensing laws and applauding the new pluralism. It was anarchy, but anarchy in the service of medical freedom of choice.

Now, mercifully, our notion of medical freedom has been reconfigured by two centuries of medical progress. We don't just get sick and die. We get sick and get medical help, and, *mirabile dictu,* the help actually helps. In antebellum America, deaths of young people under 20 accounted for half the national death rate, which was more than three times the death rate today. Now our children don't die of small pox, cholera, yellow fever, dysentery, typhoid, and pulmonary and respiratory infections before they reach maturity. When they get sick in early life, their parents take them to the doctor and they almost always get better. Their parents, on the other hand, especially after reaching middle age, don't always get better. So they get ongoing medical attention to help them live longer and more comfortably with chronic conditions such as diabetes, coronary heart disease, inflammatory bowel disease, Parkinson's, and many forms of cancer.

When our framers drafted the Constitution, the idea of being free to live a productive and relatively comfortable life with long-term illness did not compute. You died from diabetes, cancer, bowel obstruction, neurodegenerative disease, and major infections. Among young women, such infections included the uterine infection that routinely followed childbirth. A major heart attack simply killed you. You didn't receive dialysis and possibly a kidney transplant when you entered kidney failure. Major surgery, performed on the kitchen table if you were of means or in a bacteria-infested public hospital if you were not, was rarely attempted because it invariably resulted in massive blood loss, infection, and death.

So, yes, our framers intended our citizenry to be free of government interference, including the Obamacare "mandate" that impinges on Americans who choose to opt out of the program. But then, with the arguable exception of Benjamin Franklin, the framers never envisioned a world in which freedom could be extended by access to expert medical care that relieves suffering, often effects cure, and prolongs life. But then, neither could they envision the enfranchisement of former slaves and women, the progressive income tax, compulsory vaccination, publicly supported health clinics, mass screening for TB, diabetes, and syphilis, or Medicare and Medicaid. Throughout the antebellum era, when physicians were reviled by the public and when neither regular medicine nor the rival alternative sects could stem the periodic waves of cholera, yellow fever, and malaria that decimated local populations, it mattered little who provided one's doctoring. Many, like the thousands who paid $20.00 for the right to practice Samuel Thomson's do-it-yourself botanical system, chose to doctor themselves.

Those who seek repeal of Obamacare without a credible legislative alternative that provides equal, preferably greater, health benefits to all Americans seem challenged by the very idea of medical progress. Their use of terms like "choice" and "freedom" invokes an eighteenth-century political frame of reference to deprive Americans of a *kind* of freedom associated with a paradigm-shift that arose only in the final quarter of the nineteenth century. It was only then that American medicine began its transition to what we think of as modern medicine. Listerian antisepsis and asepsis; laboratory research in bacteriology, immunology, and pharmacology; laboratory development of specific remedies for specific illnesses; implementation of public health measures informed by bacteriology; modern medical education; and, yes, government regulation to safeguard the public from incompetent practitioners and toxic medications – all were part of the transition. The Jacksonian impulse persisted into the early twentieth century, flaring up in organized opposition to compulsory childhood vaccination, and finally petering out in the 1930s, by which time it was universally accepted that scientific medicine was, well, scientific, and, as such, something more than one medical sect among many.

"We hold these truths to be self-evident," Thomas Jefferson began the second paragraph of the Declaration of Independence, "that all men are created equal, that they are endowed by their Creator with certain unalienable Rights, that among these are Life, Liberty and the pursuit of Happiness." What Jefferson did not stipulate, indeed what he *could* not stipulate in his time and place, were the hierarchical relationships among these rights. Now, in the twenty-first century, we are able to go beyond an eighteenth-century mindset in which "Life, Liberty, and the pursuit of Happiness" functioned as a noun phrase whose unitary import derived from the political tyrannies of King George III and the British parliament. Now we can place life at the base of the pyramid and declare that *quality* of life is indelibly linked to liberty and the pursuit of happiness. To the extent that quality of life is diminished through disease, liberty and the pursuit of happiness are necessarily compromised. In the twenty-first century, health is life; it is life poised to exercise liberty and pursue happiness to the fullest.

Why, then, is it wrong to require all citizens to participate in a national health plan, either directly or through a mandate (i.e., a tax on those who opt out), that safeguards the right of people to effica-cious health care regardless of their financial circumstances, their employment status, and their preexisting medical conditions? What is it about the Obamacare mandate that has proven so troubling to our legislators? When you buy a house in this country, you pay local prop-erty taxes that support the local public schools. These taxes function like the mandate: They have a differential financial impact on people depending on whether they directly benefit from the system sustained by the tax. To wit, you pay the tax whether or not you choose to send your children to the public schools, indeed, whether or not you have children at all. You are obligated to subsidize the public educa-tion of children other than your own because public education has been declared a public good by the polity of which you are a part. The same goes for that portion of local taxes that provides police and fire protection. We accept a mandate to support policemen and firefighters whether or not we will ever need them, in the knowledge that other members of the community assuredly will. Similarly, those who opt out of Obamacare *should* pay a price, because they remain part of a society committed to health as a superordinate value without which liberty and the pursuit of happiness are enfeebled.

It is inconceivable that the Founding Fathers would have found unconstitutional or unfair or governmentally oppressive a law that provided life-promoting health care that enabled more Americans to discharge the duties of citizenship and live more freely and produc-tively in pursuit of happiness. They declared that citizens – all of whom, be it noted, were white, propertied males – were entitled to life consistent with the demands and entitlements of representative democracy. Their pledge, their declaration, was not in support of a compromised life that limited the ability to fulfill those demands and enjoy those entitlements.

When, in our own time, the word "choice," as used by Republican politicians, means that millions of Americans who rely on Obamacare will end up leading compromised lives, the word becomes semantically contorted and ethically bankrupt. The absence of Obamacare does not, ipso facto, empower lower-income, assistance-dependent Americans to buy the comprehensive health insurance they need, especially when the tax credits under legislation proposed thus far provide far less support than the subsidization lower-income families now receive. Freeing insurers from Obamacare regulations so that they can offer inadequate policies that lower-income Americans can afford to buy does nothing but maximize the medical risks of these financially choice-less Americans. Here is a fact: Economic circumstances wipe out the prerogative to make prudent choices in one's own best interest. For lower-income Americans, a panoply of inadequate choices is not the pathway to right-minded decision making. With the Senate's "Better Care Reconciliation Act," unveiled in June and updated in July, 2017, millions of low-income Americans, especially those dependent on Obamacare subsidies and Medicaid, would have had an absence of credible and affordable choices for obtaining health care adequate to their needs. The call simply to repeal the Affordable Care Act, which the Senate has rejected as of this writing, would take us back to a status quo ante when millions of Americans were either priced out of, or completely denied, health coverage.

Of course, *adult* citizens may repudiate mainstream health care altogether on the basis of philosophical or religious predilections. Christian Scientists and Jehovah's Witnesses, for example, hold theological beliefs that often lead them to refuse medical treatment. Certainly, they are free to pursue health through spiritual healing or, in the manner of medieval Christians, to disavow corporeal health and earth-bound life altogether. But by law they cannot deny their children, who deserve to live to maturity and make their own choices, the healing power of modern medicine, whether it comes in the form of insulin, antibiotics, blood transfusions, or surgery. Nor should they be allowed to undermine social and political arrangements, codified in law, that support everyone else's right to pursue life and happiness through twenty-first century medicine. Those who, prior to the Affordable Care Act, had inadequate insurance or no insurance at all are not struggling to free themselves from the clutches of federal regulation; they are not crying out for new free market health plans through which they can exercise freedom of choice. Rather, they are struggling to put food on the table and keep themselves and their families healthy. To this end, they need to be free to avail themselves of what modern medicine has to offer, unencumbered by politically debased notions of freedom and choice.

At this moment in history, in a fractionated society represented by a President and Congressional leaders whose daily missives bear out George Orwell's acute observation about the corruption of language brought on by political orthodoxies, *In the Hands of Doctors* may have a wistful ring. I hope not. I am addressing the personal side of health care – the reality of a doctor and patient, alone in a consulting room, often surrounded by high-tech diagnostic aids but always containing those vital low-tech instruments with which one person reaches out to the other: the physician's eyes and hands and voice. The human face of doctoring, which now includes the doctoring of nurse practitioners and physician assistants, remains essential to the success of any doctor-patient relationship, whatever the institutional arrangements that bring together this doctor and this patient, the former to help the latter.

Endeavoring to understand the several aspects – and possibilities – of the doctor-patient relationship, I write about the nature of clinical caring; the relation between caring and patient trust; the need to recruit and train physicians who can bring this caring sensibility to their patients; the role of empathy in medical caring; and the obligation of medical educators to revivify primary care medicine to meet the critical shortage of frontline physicians within underserved American communities. These issues will not go away, whatever the fate of Obamacare.

When federal legislation, through the practical assistance it provides, extends the reach of trusting doctor-patient relationships to the most vulnerable groups in society, it has a function that is both binding and enabling. It fortifies the webbing that underlies the increasingly disparate parts of our national mosaic. Obamacare, the Children's Health Insurance Program, Medicaid – these programs do not "bring us together" in a feel good way. They do, however, prevent a free fall in which the subcommunities and interest groups into which society has decomposed land so far apart they are no longer in hailing distance of one another. As to the enabling function, a comprehensive medical safety net for all Americans – let's call it what it is: universal health care – revitalizes political democracy by extending to all Americans a greater possibility of life, liberty, and the pursuit of happiness. In the everyday world, this pursuit boils down to the ability of more people to stay on the job or to work from home rather than not work at all. Society benefits, since chronically ill people pursuing happiness under the umbrella of universal health care will better resist the complications and collateral illnesses that follow from their primary illness or illnesses. Society also benefits by enabling healthier happiness-pursuers to avoid hospitalization and, among the elderly, to push back the time when nursing home care is required. And finally, society benefits by seeing to it that all children, especially those who are disabled, receive every medical advantage as they traverse their own challenging paths to productive, choice-wielding citizenship.

Obamacare is a far cry from universal health care, but for all its limitations and current financial straits, it has provided these binding and enabling functions for millions of Americans previously without a medical safety net. Woe to politicians who shred it in the name of choice, a pleasing vacuity that evades the reality of disease and pain among many who are relieved to have a single avenue of subsidized care where none was previously available.

Health care should be a national trust; everyone deserves what twenty-first century medicine has to offer, regardless of how much or how little choice can be worked into the offering. Politicians who feel otherwise are enemies of the polity. Jefferson, who as president helped set up the first smallpox vaccination clinics in the south and then, in retirement, planned a state-supported clinic to provide free medical care to those who could not afford it, would not have brooked the empty insistence that medical freedom and medical choice, unhinged from socioeconomic reality, trump access to medical care per se. Nor, for that matter, does choice, whatever it may or may not mean, obviate our moral obligation as a society to see to it that best available treatment, whatever the pathway that leads to it, means treatment rendered by caring doctors willing to know their patients as people.

PES

August 2017

Preface

W hen it comes to doctoring in America, there is a long-established and growing rift between being well treated and feeling
well cared for. On the one hand, patients want doctors who know
them and are caring of them. They are frustrated with the kind of
care dispensed in very brief office visits. They are unhappy having
their bodies parsed into organs and systems that elicit matter-of-fact
diagnoses and impersonally rendered treatments. They may want the
"facts," but they want them conveyed by a human being who understands their apprehension, uncertainty, and confusion in the face of
them. The facts are never neutral in their psychological impact on
the patient's sense of self. They establish that the patient is in some
manner and to some degree damaged, and therefore in need of a physician able to bring expert knowledge to bear in helping the patient
overcome his illness and dis-ease and regain his peace of mind and
wholeness. This means that patients expect their physicians to be able
and willing to give them enough time to come to know them as persons
whose apprehension, uncertainty, and confusion are deeply personal.
To the extent that the doctor humanizes the encounter by providing
the patient with sympathy and support, perhaps even empathy, the
patient feels he is in the hands of a knowing and caring doctor. This is
the viewpoint of the bioethicist Edmund Pellegrino.

On the other hand, patients expect their doctors to respect their
right to make their own medical decisions. And they want doctors

who not only grant them autonomy in principle but cede autonomy in action. In order to make informed decisions about their bodies, they need the facts, all of them. And so patients expect to be told directly, perhaps even collegially, what may ensue if they accept or reject one or another of the treatment recommendations that follow from the facts. But that is where medical care ends. The patient alone must decide what to do with the facts of the matter, the facts of his or her *bodily* matter as the doctor has scientifically arrived at them. Armed with information, explanation, and expert risk assessment, the patient will choose a course of treatment, which the physician and/or his colleagues will then implement to the best of their ability. To the extent the physician implements the patient's treatment plan absent any intrusion of his or her own preferences and values, he or she treats the patient well and truly and leaves the patient, in turn, feeling well treated and well cared for. This is the perspective of the bioethicist Robert Veatch.

Between these polar viewpoints on what it means to be a doctor and a patient, respectively, I interpose the notion of medical caring, which is less simple than it appears. Medical caring can humanize the doctor-patient relationship without imposing values and goals that are antithetical to the patient. At its best, medical caring is a reaching out to the patient that transcends the banalities (and uncertainties) of diagnosis and treatment in ways that patients throughout history have welcomed, and this because patienthood often compromises the patient's personhood. Here I side with Pellegrino: In some primal way, we call on doctors when we feel not fully ourselves, or less than ourselves, or anxious about our ability to remain ourselves, and we look to doctors to return us to the normal selves we want to be.

In the chapters to follow, I argue that the notion of medical caring has its own historical trajectory, though I focus on only a small part of it. Medical caring, that is, is responsive not only to the medical knowledge of a given time and place, but also to the cultural and political arrangements through which a society provides for the coming together of patients and doctors. It is from these arrangements that the mindsets of patients and doctors arise and, with varying degrees of success, arrive at a concordant notion of what it means for the former to be in the care of the latter.

In a society that increasingly *commands* patient empowerment in the service of unilateral decision making, a focal concern with medical caring adds the cautionary reminder that we deprive physicians of their own right to counsel, admonish, and persuade at our peril. At a certain point, however indistinct and wavy, however variable among different patients and different doctors, the legal assertion of rights begins to undermine the doctor's prerogative to doctor in ways responsive to the patient's needs and expectations. Doctors, after all, are also moral agents with a Hippocratic obligation to draw on their humanity, however flawed, in ministering to their patients. And patients, for their part, have the right to rely on a physician in ways that are human but not strictly factual as to diagnosis and treatment. To relinquish voluntarily a measure of autonomy to a trusted physician *is* an act of autonomy.

The notion of medical caring captures the sense that doctors are not just doctors in some timeless generic sense, any more than patients are just generic purchasers of medical treatment as a commodity. The same doctors who, mindful of patient rights, seek to make contact with their patients in more than bland informational ways are themselves the patients of other doctors, as are their loved ones, so the *predicament* of the patient, whose decision-making autonomy is often compromised, will not be so alien to the doctor as proponents of value-free medicine believe. Doctors are all patients, at least patients in potentia. And patients for their part come in all shapes and sizes, maturationally, temperamentally, characterologically, and otherwise. Some will neither want nor possess the ability to be autonomous decision makers. In a caring relationship, doctor and patient together, with or without participation of the patient's significant others, make the determination, person to person.

A historical perspective on medical caring is cautionary in another respect. It reminds us that concepts such as "paternalism" and "autonomy" are themselves historical constructs, not timeless Platonic forms. Bioethicists who use these terms in essentialist ways overlook the historical and cultural location of doctor-patient relationships. The paternalism of physicians in ancient Rome, in Renaissance Florence, in seventeenth-century Paris, in nineteenth-century London, in postbellum America, in America of the mid- twentieth century – these are not the same thing. And none of them is tantamount to what paternalism – or maternalism, or avuncular regard, or brotherly or sisterly concern – may still mean in an age of digital medicine, the Internet, and patient rights.

It bears remembering, finally, that the *feeling* of being well cared for by a doctor is responsive not only to the treatment options of a given time and place, but also to cultural assumptions that enter into doctor-patient relationships. Different norms of caring typify different periods in the history of medicine. Patients in the eighteenth century who were bled to syncope (fainting) felt well cared for. Several decades into the nineteenth century, many insisted on being bled, and some would seek out new doctors when their own refused to drain them further. Antebellum physicians who purged the bowels of dehydrated cholera patients with toxic mercury compounds were caring physicians within the framework of Galenic medicine; they were doing their best to restore their patients' humoral balance. Plenty of caring surgeons of the late nineteenth century applied vaginal leeches and performed ovariotomy on women who, without signs of serious gynecological disease, demanded that doctors recognize their complaints and do something to relieve their suffering. Within a medical paradigm in which even minor pelvic abnormalities explained symptoms of depression and nervous exhaustion (neurasthenia), surgery counted as a caring intervention and was widely understood as such. Similarly, obstetricians of the late nineteenth century who treated postpartum women suffering from exhaustion and agitated depression ("puerperal insanity") by legitimating their symptoms and ordering compulsory "time outs" from stifling domestic obligations were caring physicians within the gendered constraints of Victorian society. Prefrontal lobotomy was widely considered a caring intervention for schizophrenics from the late 1930s through the mid-1950s. The surgery, for its many proponents, restored a measure of function, however compromised, to patients who would otherwise have ossified in the chronic wards of mental hospitals. Now the care of schizophrenic patients is far different and, from a twenty-first century vantage point, far more humane.

But this is beside the point. It is easy to dismiss bleeding to syncope, heroic dosing with the remedies of the day, vaginal leeching, prefrontal lobotomy, and innumerable other treatments as relics of the past – misguided, unscientific, often harmful. But such judgments, such exercises in presentism, do not negate the caring intent with which such treatments were administered by doctors and received by patients. There is much to be learned by putting aside the triumphal march of medical treatment in the nineteenth and twentieth centuries and focusing instead on the history of caring and feeling cared for. It is with respect to these intertwined dimensions of doctoring that the past is more than past. The period in American history covered in this book, roughly from the end of the American Civil War through the 1960s, guides us to a deeper understanding of what patients of our own time want and expect from doctors and what, if anything, doctors can do for them beyond diagnose and treat.

By mining the vagaries of caring and feeling cared for over time, then, we gain historical perspective and edge closer to comprehending all that it has meant, and continues to mean, to be a doctor and to place oneself in a doctor's hands. What we discern can be unsettling, as the examples above suggest. But taken together, they provide a luminous counterpoise to the progressively depersonalized, cost-driven, productivity-obsessed medicine of the past 40 years. I offer my work as an example of how thinking with history broadens the ground of Francis Peabody's oft-cited insistence that "the secret of the care of the patient is in caring for the patient."

I am grateful to those who have provided assistance in my research and writing. John Burnham and Howard Kushner encouraged my late-career transition to history of medicine and provided sound advice and encouragement along the way. I am grateful to the DeWitt Wallace Institute for the History of Psychiatry of Weill Cornell Medical College for giving me a forum for presenting my ideas about psychiatry and medicine over the past 35 years. My friends Lou Breger and David Newman have provided unwavering support, both of this project and of my work in general. John Kerr, my brilliant colleague at The Analytic Press, has once again given me the benefit of a critical reading of great acuity and understanding. Kathie Bischoff and Dawn Harley of Becton, Dickinson and Company; Emily Yates of The Mütter Museum in Philadelphia; Mara Scheelings of Museum Boerhaave in Leiden; and Laurie Slater, owner of phisick.com, could not have been more helpful in directing me to relevant objects from their collections and aiding me in securing permission to include images of them in the book.

I am grateful to my brothers, David Stepansky, Robert Stepansky, and Alan Stepansky, and my sons, Michael Stepansky and Jonathan Stepansky, for ongoing support of my work in ways too numerous to mention. Special thanks to Dave, an internist with ranging insights about healthcare in America, for many stimulating conversations about some of the issues explored in the book. My late father, William Stepansky, M.D., true physician and healer, illuminates this work and shares in whatever merit resides in it. My debt to him and to my mother, Selma Brill Stepansky, is incalculable.

I am fortunate to have physicians of my own who bear out my claim that generalists and specialists alike can give patients the time, attention, and support they need. I have been well cared for over the years by Dr. Naomi Grobstein, Dr. Eugene Chiappetta, and Dr. Lloyd Zbar, and I thank them for their availability, concern, and reassurance. My retinologist, Dr. Francis Cangemi, has demonstrated to me time and again that outstanding clinical care, with its reliance on state-of-the-art diagnostics and treatment technologies, can coexist with the deeply human and humane values of the caring physician. He has my deepest gratitude, as do the members of his excellent staff, who have helped me through difficult times. They exemplified all that is meant by the "patient-centered medical home" long before the concept came into vogue.

I wish I had the words to thank my wife, Deane Rand Stepansky, for all she means to me and all she has given me. But, alas, I do not. She has been intimately involved with every aspect of this project as confidante, sounding board, critic, grammarian, Latinist, and proofreader par excellence. She has urged me on when my resolve flagged. She knows, I hope, that I could not have set out on the path that led to this book without her, that I could not have completed it without her, and that my wordless gratitude yields only to Virgil's simple declaration: *Omnia vincit amor.*

In the Hands of Doctors

CHAPTER 1

Introduction: Medical Caring, Past and Present

In the Hands of Doctors: Touch and Trust in Medical Care. Sometimes it's all in the title. We are all in the hands of doctors. We come to them unwell, uncomfortable, in pain, often anxious, sometimes panicky. We come to them, as the bioethicist Edmund Pellegrino insists, as petitioners; we bring them our "wounded humanity" and petition them for reassurance, remediation, restoration, cure.[1] At the same time, it is literally through the hands of doctors that we hope to achieve these things, to feel better and get better. It is all quite circular: Our doctors do things to us with their hands, and we welcome their hands because we have placed ourselves in their hands. And it is the doctor's touch, which can be either direct or, as we shall see, mediated through instruments and even exotic technologies, that justifies our initial leap of faith and provides one important basis for a trusting doctor-patient relationship. Allowing for the variegated meanings of touching and being touched—by doctors' hands, by nurses' hands, by instruments, as an aspect of medical procedures, as an expression of human connection—it is all about the touch. We seek through touch of one kind or another reassurance that our doctors have everything in hand, that we are, as it were, in good and caring hands.[2]

The everyday reality of being in the hands of doctors and looking to them for treatment that is not only competent but caring persists in the face of labyrinthic bureaucracy, third-party intrusions, excrescences of paperwork, and, for patients, abbreviated and dissatisfying office visits. It likewise persists in the new age of medical informatics, where doctors' hands are pulled away from their patients' bodies to keyboards, where they do endless, often infuriating, battle with the "clunky, confusing, and complex" software of electronic health records (EHRs). In an era of diagnostic checklists, data entry, and protocol-driven ordering of laboratory and imaging studies, physicians' ability to touch their patients increasingly yields to the most summary sensory inspection.[3]

And yet we remain in their hands. Our physicians bring us not only their expertise in diagnosis and treatment but, so we hope, their commitment to our health and well-being. And such commitment is an outgrowth of the human side of medical caregiving; it falls back on our doctors' ability and willingness to care for us in all our neediness and vulnerability. In this existential sense, EHR checklists or not, we come to them as damaged and, per Pellegrino, look to them to regain our bodily integrity, our wholeness, and our freedom. We wait for their hands to turn away from their keyboards and return to our bodies, and not just for purposes of visual inspection, palpation, and procedural intervention. A 1996 survey of 376 patients from 20 urban and rural family practices across Ontario found that a majority of patients (66.3%), male and female alike, welcomed their physician's *comforting* touch; indeed a majority of them (57%) believed that the physician's touch could be *healing*.[4] To be sure, one can hardly generalize from a single small-scale study, but I am aware of no other patient survey like it, and the results are, at the least, highly suggestive.

In the Hands of Doctors revisits the meanings and actualities of medical caring, glancing back at medical practice in the nineteenth and early twentieth centuries but focusing on the seven decades since the end of World War II. More pointedly, it provides a contrast between the manner in which physicians were able to care for us through the two decades that followed the war and the manner in which, increasingly and for a variety of reasons, they are consigned to care for us now. The book is not a narrative history of care and caring in medicine. Rather, it is an exercise in comparative history that gathers its subject matter into chapters that encircle the caring dimension of doctoring through a series of topical studies. They address, inter alia, the role of procedural medicine in caring; the nature and goals of medical training; the cultivation of "empathy" in doctors; the meaning of friendship between doctor and patient in the postwar decades and now in the "friending" era of social media; and the human dimension of medical technologies, old and new. In the concluding chapters, I turn to the rise and fall of family medicine as a medical specialty and the role of physician assistants and nurse practitioners in contemporary health care.

I write neither as an aggrieved patient with a story to tell nor as a frustrated doctor burdened by lost ideals and pondering whether the doctor-patient relationship can survive and "Why Doctors Are Sick of Their Profession."[5] This is not another jeremiad about the ill health of contemporary American medicine. It is not a cautionary recital of the various "cognitive errors" to which all-too-human physicians are prone, in the face of which they must learn to withhold premature judgment even as their patients learn to push them to think outside the diagnostic box.[6] Nor, finally, is it an effort to mobilize physicians themselves to "stand up together" and revivify American medicine through a patient-centered activism that seeks out innovative "front-line best practices" in provider groups and hospitals throughout the country and then applies them to everyone's "home organization."[7]

So what kind of book have I written and, more to the point, why should anyone care what I have to say about dilemmas, frustrations, malaises, and challenges that so many others have spoken to so eloquently and well? I am not a physician, and I cannot bring to these reflections the wealth of clinical experience, typically refracted through cases studies, vignettes, and anecdotes, of popular physician-writers such as Atul Gawande, Sherwin Nuland, Jerome Groopman, and Oliver Sacks. Nor am I a medical economist who can analyze health care delivery systems in order to illuminate the underlying inefficiencies, redundancies, disparities, and inequalities that, sadly, are a hallmark of contemporary American medicine.

What then do I bring to the table? I am a European intellectual historian by training, and I cut my eyeteeth on the foundational movements of nineteenth- and early twentieth-century Europe—utilitarianism, romanticism, socialism, Darwinism, modernism, psychoanalysis—and thinkers like Hegel, Marx, Nietzsche, and Freud. I moved on to a scholarly career as a historian of Freud and his movement, a turn facilitated by a 27-year career as an editor and publisher of psychoanalytic and psychiatric books and journals. Beginning in the mid-1990s, I began a return to my roots and segued from history of psychiatry and psychoanalysis to history of medicine, with a special interest in the evolution of primary care medicine in America.[8]

Given my academic background and lengthy sojourn in the land of psychoanalysis, what are the "roots" that pulled me back to history of medicine? Here matters become personal. Long before I studied intellectual and cultural history, I was my father's son. And my father, William Stepansky, whose fascinating story I recount elsewhere,[9] was one of those remarkable battle-tested general practitioners who trained immediately after World War II. A Jewish émigré from Russian Kiev, born in Rumania in 1922 during his parents' flight from the post-World War I Kievan pogroms, my father grew up in modest circumstances in the Jewish enclave in South Philadelphia. A surgical tech in a medical battalion attached to the 80th Infantry Division of Patton's Third Army, a licensed pharmacist, and a gifted violinist who studied with Emmanuel Zetlin of the Curtis String Quartet, he began medical training in 1948 at Philadelphia's Jefferson Medical College and followed medical school with a one-year rotating internship at Montgomery Hospital in the outlying town of Norristown.

Then, in 1953, two years after my birth, he hung his shingle in the tiny borough of Trappe, Pennsylvania. A rural farming town 30 miles west of Philadelphia, Trappe had a population of about 1,000, but, counting the adjoining borough of Collegeville, home to the post office and shops, and adjacent towns, my father's practice served an immediate population of perhaps 5,000. There he practiced general medicine until his retirement at the end of 1990, after which he continued to counsel and comfort his patients until his death in 2008. General medicine in Trappe in the 1950s and '60s really was multispecialty *family* medicine: my father practiced pediatrics, internal medicine, cardiology, allergy, ENT, dermatology, gynecology, obstetrics (for the first 12 years of practice), urology, office surgery, and psychiatry. If he was deeply understanding of the scientific advantages of specialism, he was no less committed to a modern generalism that could access those advantages and use them to its own advantage.[10]

I write as a historian of the nineteenth and twentieth centuries; the great exemplars of late-nineteenth-century medicine—Jackson, Putnam, Jacobi, Osler, Welch, Halsted, Kelly, Cushing, Thayer, Collins—matter to me, and they occasionally make an appearance in these pages. There is still much to learn from the coterie of physicians who, following study in Germany and Austria, brought scientific medicine to Johns Hopkins University in the last decade of the nineteenth century and then developed a curriculum and clinical training program to pass it on to the next generation. From Osler and his cohort, especially, there are lessons about bedside observation, patient care, and the art of medicine that bear rediscovery and reappraisal over a century later.[11]

But mainly my use of history is informed, and I hope enriched, by my own life experience in the 1950s and '60s. For my father was in the strong sense of the term a "Compleat Physician,"[12] and from him I learned about medicine as art, science, craft, and calling. Working in his office as a "pharmacist's apprentice," getting to know many of his patients, riding shotgun during the daily round of house calls and hospital rounds—these things shaped my sense of what medicine, especially generalist medicine, was in the 1950s and '60s.

To be sure, we cannot return to an earlier period of medical history, nor should we want to—time, technology, treatments, pharmaceuticals, delivery systems, and patient sensibilities have all moved on, far on. But amid the dilemmas and challenges before us—as individuals and as a society and as members of the human race—we still have the opportunity of "thinking with history," to borrow the title of Carl Schorske's collection of essays. Like Schorske, whose courses in European intellectual history helped me grasp the strength of comparative historical analysis as a Princeton undergraduate in the early 1970s, I understand thinking with history as employing "the materials of the past and the configurations in which we organize and comprehend them to orient ourselves in the living present."[13] In this volume, I want to think with history about the living present of American medical care. More specifically, I want to explore a constellation of topics that bears on the nature of *true doctoring* and the manner in which this nature has been refashioned, for better and for worse, over the seven decades that have elapsed since the end of World War II.

What makes the decades of the 1950s and '60s especially interesting is that the true doctoring of the era took place within a world of recognizably modern medicine. And it is the coexistence of this modernity with the true doctoring of GPs like my father that makes these decades both intriguing and edifying; we have much to learn about medical care from the mid-twentieth century. This may seem a surprising, even far-fetched, claim given the enormous diagnostic and treatment advances of the past seven decades. Hopefully, the chapters to follow will bear out the claim, but let me expatiate just a bit on how I understand mid-twentieth-century medical modernity.

In many ways it was a modernity that looked backwards: It was the coming to fruition of the stunning medical and surgical advances made during World War II. Among the most significant were major improvements in the prevention and treatment of 10 of the 28 vaccine-preventable diseases identified in the twentieth century.[14] New vaccines for influenza, pneumococcal pneumonia, and plague were developed and used. There were also new treatments for malaria and the mass production of penicillin in time for D-Day in 1944. Penicillin was not the only miracle drug that grew out of wartime research. Cortisone, the adrenal hormone whose powerful anti-inflammatory properties liberated thousands crippled by rheumatoid arthritis beginning in 1949, was simply "Compound E," whose military potential as a stress-relieving energizer was investigated by the U.S. military in 1942 and 1943.[15]

It was during World War II that American scientists learned to separate blood plasma into its constituents (albumin, globulins, and clotting factors), an essential advance in the treatment of shock and control of bleeding. The German medical scientist Paul Ehrlich coined the term "chemotherapy" early in the twentieth century to characterize any experimental chemical treatment of infectious disease. But chemotherapy in its modern anticancer "cytotoxic" (i.e., cell killing) sense arose from classified wartime research on nitrogen mustards by a group of Yale scientists led by Louis Goodman and Alfred Gilman in 1942.[16] In the psychiatric realm, wartime medicine developed a basically modern understanding of stress under extreme conditions—its triggers, its physiological and psychological characteristics, and its remediation. This approach to what we now term posttraumatic stress culminated in Roy Grinker and John Spiegel's imposing compendium, *Men Under Stress*, published in 1945.

At the outbreak of World War II, the psychiatric drug arsenal was limited to deadening sedatives long available—the bromides and phenobarbital—and amphetamine, which, marketed by Smith, Kline, and French (now GlaxoSmithKline) as Benzedrine Sulfate, was widely prescribed for minor depressions in the late 1930s.[17] But modern psychopharmacology as we know it today grew out of war-related research. In 1945 Frank Berger, a Czechoslovakian bacteriologist working in London, developed a penicillin preservative that, it turned out, also produced deep muscle relaxation, a sleep-like state that Berger characterized a year later as "tranquillization."[18] The drug was mephenesin, and a stronger, longer-acting version of it, meprobamate, became the world's first minor tranquilizer. In 1952, while Berger was observing the "tranquillization" of small rodents injected with meprobamate, Henri-Marie Laborit, a French naval surgeon working at the Val de Grâce military hospital outside Paris, published his first article on the usefulness of chlorpromazine—a chlorinated form of the antihistamine promazine—in calming patients before surgery and preventing them from lapsing into shock during and after their operations. In 1954, Smith, Kline, and French released the drug in America as Thorazine, the first major tranquilizer.

In the surgical realm, World War II medicine developed a panoply of new surgical techniques and rehabilitative procedures; major advances in fracture and wound care; dramatic progress in reconstructive surgery; and the development of vascular surgery, initially an experimental procedure. It was during the war that the San Francisco surgeon Sterling Bunnell created the surgical specialty of hand surgery, which he directed at 10 U.S. Army Hand Centers established in 1944.[19] All these advances, medical and surgical, were the legacy of massive government spending through the Office of Scientific Research and Development, as channeled through a Committee on Medical Research that supervised some 5,500 researchers.[20] They were all part of the war effort.

What do these developments share in common? They pertain largely to the realm of infectious disease (including its prevention); the use of talking therapy, abetted by medication and support, to understand anxiety and depression; and the refinement and expansion of surgery, including postsurgical management.

The breakthroughs of the late 1940s and '50s built on the legacy of wartime medicine in forward-looking ways. In 1948 the isolation of vitamin B-12 as the "anti-pernicious anemia factor" found in raw beef liver rapidly brought one of the most deadly vitamin deficiency diseases under simple control. Left untouched by wartime research was a vaccine for poliomyelitis, the dreaded infantile paralysis that, nationwide, claimed 42,000 new victims in 1949 and another 57,000 in 1952. The field trials of the Salk polio vaccine in the spring of 1954, in which over 1.3 million American school children participated, initiated the era of modern vaccine testing. The Salk killed-virus vaccine, proved effective by the trial, became available to the public before the summertime "plague season" of 1955. It was followed by introduction of the attenuated live-virus Sabin vaccine in 1960. Together, they all but eradicated infantile paralysis in the United States.

In 1955 Wallace Laboratories brought to market Miltown (meprobamate) and thereby initiated the era of office psychopharmacology. In 1956 modern blood-pressure-lowering medication, in the form of the thiazide diuretics, was developed; Paul Zoll reported the first successful defibrillation of the heart; and the National Institutes of Health (NIH) reached a budget of $100 million. C. Walton Lillehei and his team at the University of Minnesota developed the first wearable transistorized pacemaker in 1957, the same year John Crofton and his colleagues at Edinburgh University demonstrated that with triple-drug therapy, tuberculosis was at last 100% curable. Nineteen fifty-eight saw the release of isoniazid, the first of the monoamine oxidase inhibitors (MAOIs), potent antidepressants still used, albeit infrequently, to treat "atypical" depressions that do not respond to other drugs. As the decade drew to a close, the drug company Searle asked the FDA to allow it to market Enovid, available since 1957 to treat menstrual disorders, as a contraceptive; Senator Estes Kefauver launched his historic Senate hearings on overpricing and price-fixing in the drug industry; and the pacemaker became implantable.

By the mid-1960s, then, we had a safe and effective vaccine for polio and curative treatment for TB. We had synthetic corticosteroids like prednisone that lacked the side effects of cortisone but were equally effective in treating rheumatoid arthritis, lupus, asthma, allergies, and inflammatory bowel disease. We had an arsenal of post-penicillin antibiotics isolated in the early '50s (Nystatin, Ilosone [erythromycin]) and mid-'50s (Novobiocin, Vancomycin, Kanamycin). We had sedatives that enabled patients with major psychiatric illness to return to their homes and minor tranquilizers (Miltown, Librium, Valium) and antidepressants (Elavil) for the stress and strain of daily living. We also had safe and effective medication for lowering blood pressure; long-acting insulin and single-use insulin syringes for diabetics; oral contraceptives; implantable pacemakers; ultrasound cardiography; open-heart surgery utilizing the heart-lung machine; long-term kidney dialysis; and Congressional oversight of the drug industry. This, for all intents and purposes, is modern medicine.

General practice in the 1950s and '60s grew out of these discoveries: it was largely medicinal, manual, and mentalistic, which is to say psychiatric. Its modernity resided in things like childhood vaccination; routine obstetrics; the management of infectious disease; wound management and the setting of fractures; the pharmacological and psychotherapeutic management of anxiety and depression; and referrals for a broad range of abdominal, gynecologic, orthopedic, and reconstructive surgeries. It followed that a highly motivated family doctor—a family doctor who, like my father, was both academically oriented and mechanically gifted—could acquire broad competence across a range of specialties simply by reading the journal literature, taking procedurally oriented postgraduate courses, and receiving hands-on instruction by surgical specialists in various office-based procedures. A year-long postgraduate course on "minor surgery" in the postwar era, the kind of course my father took at Philadelphia's Einstein Medical Center in 1959, would have covered basic procedures that, in their contemporary variants, usually require visits to dermatologists, otolaryngologists, urologists, gynecologists, and general surgeons.

II.

To underscore the modernity of American medicine in the postwar decades is hardly to deny its distance from contemporary medicine. In the 1950s and '60s there were no CT scans or PET scans or MRIs to order; no laparoscopic or laser-assisted or computer-guided or micro surgeries. Potent analgesics—codeine, morphine, oxycodone—were available long before midcentury, but the idea of a multidisciplinary pain clinic only emerged in 1953, when John Bonica published *The Management of Pain*. Transplant surgery was in its infancy, with the first kidney transplant performed in 1963 and the first heart transplant in 1967. Cancer treatment was, by contemporary standards, primitive. Understanding of the human immune system, including the cellular nature of acquired immunity, was more primitive still. Most heart disease was managed with bed rest and a limited number of standard drugs, and laboratory studies were fewer and more basic in nature.

True enough. We can do vastly more now for patients with serious illnesses and in serious pain than our mid-twentieth-century predecessors. And we can do vastly more to improve the quality of life of patients with major pain, the pain associated, for example, with neurodegenerative disease, cancer, and end-stage illness. But for the vast majority of mid-twentieth-century patients with routine and manageable aches and pains, and for patients with chronic conditions such as diabetes, hypertension, and arthritis, the modernity of midcentury medicine is still impressive. The experience of making an appointment to see the doctor and then seeing him or her for examination, evaluation, and treatment was similar to what it is more than half a century later. The physician, aglow in postwar science, greeted the patient and asked about the reason for the visit. Blood pressure was checked; heart and lungs listened to with stethoscope; ears inspected with otoscope; bodily orifices probed for abnormalities; the site of the lesion or dysfunction inspected; lab tests ordered; diagnoses made; prescriptions written; and various office- and hospital-based treatments recommended and undertaken. A broad range of procedures, many surgical in nature, would be performed safely and effectively in the doctor's office.

Is this all there was to it? No, not at all. General medicine, apart from the diagnostic studies, drugs, and treatments available to practitioners, was simply different in tone and tenor and caring impulse from the general medicine of today. And it is by examining these differences, by thinking with history about protocol-less issues like the nature of the bond between physician and patient (and the patient's family) and its relation to procedural interventions, ameliorative touch, and the like, that we can learn something new about health care and its discontents seven decades after the end of World War II.

I am *not* suggesting that contemporary physicians, especially primary care physicians, do not care about their patients. Of course they do. But the world of contemporary medicine has made the *kind* of caring associated with true doctoring much harder than it was in the quarter century that followed World War II. The tributaries that flowed into the hands-on, procedurally driven caring of generalist physicians that blossomed after the war and began to taper off in the late 1960s have narrowed and in many locales and contexts all but dried up. In learning with history, we can better grasp the roots of our contemporary discontent with our doctors, and, in turn, their own frustration with the kind of medicine they practice. We also understand better why so few medical students are drawn to the primary care specialties. With an enlarged historical understanding of what has happened and why it has happened, we are better positioned to widen old tributaries and cultivate new ones in the effort to revitalize the caring dimension of medical treatment.

It is with this conceptual apparatus—the mindset, resources, and comparative sensibility of a working historian—that I approach a cluster of intertwined topics. I begin with the simple notions of "care" and "caring," not to make, yet again, the tired claim that what was once intrinsic to doctoring is now irretrievably lost. Rather, I suggest that notions of "care" and "caring" are themselves historical constructs that change over time. We all want caring doctors, but caring medicine, no less than scientific medicine, is subject to the march of progress—a march that brings in its wake new instrumentalities of care, new kinds of health professionals, new cultural values and political agendas, and new patient expectations. I suggest, as noted, that postwar general practice was fortified by a range of procedural interventions. That is, general practitioners through the 1960s and into the '70s simply did things to their patients' bodies that the vast majority of contemporary generalists do not. This laying on of hands, with all it entails, made midcentury generalists *feel* like caregivers, not conduits into the health care system. The diminished role of hands-on physician time with patients, along with the procedural interventions that occurred during this time, has had a devitalizing effect on primary care. The laying on of hands continues to matter, for doctors and patients alike.[21]

Consideration of the procedural medicine of the postwar generation leads to more expansive consideration of "touch" in medicine. It likewise opens to a different perspective on therapeutic "empathy" and how—and even whether—we should train physicians to "be" empathic in the conventional sense of empathy. To this end, it helps to look backwards and examine how early modern physicians became compassionate healers long before medical educators perceived the absence of empathy as a problem and developed curricular innovations to address it.

The cultivation of patient-centered/relationship-centered care, another curricular project of recent decades, also benefits from thinking with history. Now, of course, medical educators find it necessary to "teach" medical students and residents to be patient-centered. In the postwar era, on the other hand, intergenerational family-based care was a fact of medical life; general practice, so much less reliant on third-party provisos and evidence-based protocols, was ipso facto patient-centered. And this patient-centeredness was abetted by house calls, which brought the physician, both concretely and figuratively, into the very heart of the patient's familial and relational world.

Critiques of depersonalized contemporary medicine from all sides and directions have long trained their sights on a common target: technology. Medicine's reliance on technology, which is so centrally involved in the clinical training of medical students, has contributed mightily to the impersonality, even dehumanization, of the treatment experience. We are less with our doctors than with the imposing machinery of screening, diagnosis, and treatment. A chorus of voices, bioethicists, health policy analysts, and medical economists among them, sing in unison: Do we really need all this exotic technology, and do we need to use it as routinely as we do? Do the costs justify the benefits, both for the system and for the patient? What is the point of diminishing returns and, from the patient's standpoint, diminished well-being?

Here again, thinking with history encourages a more nuanced reading of the matter. By considering how physicians and patients reacted to the "high technology" of the past, we can understand that debates about the usefulness and desirability of medical technology are as old as medicine itself. EKG machines, X-ray machines, blood pressure meters (sphygmomanometers), hypodermic syringes, even the humble stethoscope—all were once high technologies that elicited deep ambivalence among physicians and anxiety and displeasure among the patients first subjected to them. Now, when our family physician, variously, listens to our heart and lungs, checks our blood pressure, taps our patellar tendon with a reflex hammer, and gives us an injection, we are content that we have received unmediated hands-on care. What were once newfangled instruments of questionable value have become aspects of personalized, technology-free doctoring. This fact occurs repeatedly in medical history: New tools that at the time of their introduction were discomfiting to physician and patient alike proved their worth over time and were integrated into the physician's armamentarium. Over a span of years, they ceased to be alienating tools interposed between doctor and patient and became tools of a different kind, perhaps not tools at all but simple extenders of the physician's person.

To be sure, as critics will point out, there is a world of difference between hand-held instruments and the imposing machinery of, for example, contemporary scanners and radiation therapy systems. But there is also, I suggest, a historical basis for imputing similarity. Looking back at the manner in which the high-tech instruments of yesteryear were conventionalized over time suggests strategies for rendering less alienating the technologies of today. There may be no possibility of "humanizing" massive machinery brought to bear on our bodies impersonally by task-oriented technicians. Nonetheless, history guides us to the possibility of understanding medical machinery as "caring technology," if only our physicians would understand our need to have their own caring interposed between the machines and us. Patients need not be alone in managing what Pellegrino, four decades ago, termed "the threats of unrestrained technological imperatives." This simple insight is often lost amid the concurrent celebration of technology as instrument of diagnosis and treatment and denunciation of technology as dissipater of humanistic caregiving.

III.

The shortage of generalist physicians (traditionally, general practitioners, aka family doctors), now gathered under the rubric of primary care physicians, has been a mainstay of concern for well over a century. Now, however, the claim is bolstered by sophisticated fore-casting along with statistical analysis of the distribution of providers across the country. Heightened of late by the 33 million Americans in the process of receiving health insurance through the Patient Protec-tion and Affordable Care Act of 2010, the chronic shortage of primary care physicians is seen as a looming crisis capable of dragging us back into the medical dark ages. Where are we to find the 51,880 addi-tional primary care physicians that, according to recent projections,[22] we will need by 2025 to keep up with an expanding, aging, and more universally insured American population?

In the concluding chapters, I think with history about the fall and rise and fall of generalist medicine since the 1940s. In chapter 9, I trace the rise and fall of the American Academy of General Practice, which was established in 1947, followed by the rise and fall, two decades later, of the American Board of Family Practice. The fate of the American generalist—both the "general practitioner" of the post-war decades and the residency-trained "family practice" specialist of the 1970s and thereafter—brings into its compass a range of issues, including the growth of the specialties after World War II; the pub-lic's expectation of specialty care; the development of hospital-based technologies available only to specialists; and the dramatic increase of health insurance among working Americans to pay for hospital-based specialty care. These interlacing developments, gathered around the history of generalist medicine, set the stage for the current crisis of primary care medicine.

How has this crisis been addressed? In chapter 10, I consider recent efforts to draw medical students into primary care, especially family medicine, all of which have proven inadequate to the challenge before us. Then, throwing politics to the wind, I offer a series of recommen-dations that culminate in an immodestly "modest proposal," to invoke Jonathan Swift, that we replace family medicine altogether with a new primary care specialty that emphasizes procedural caregiving. Medi-cal readers may well demur from my belief that the era of the "family medicine" specialty as conceived by its founders in the mid-1960s has come and gone, and that it is time to train a new kind of primary care physician to replace the aging cohort of family physicians. But even skeptics, I trust, will appreciate the spirit of my proposals: There is an urgent need to develop more substantial strategies for pulling medical students into the dwindling ranks of primary care and to channel this care to the underserved communities where it is urgently needed. I hope to be concrete where others have been either exhortative or plangent. There is a future for primary care—indeed, primary care *is* the future—but only if we are willing to consider more consequential strategies of medical student recruitment and a new specialty alignment that strengthens the role and augments the treatment prerogatives of those we will continue to refer to as "family doctors."

My recommendations endorse the team approach to primary care, which revolves around the expanded role of nonphysician providers, especially physician assistants and nurse practitioners. I am equally aware that the nature and extent of this expansion is not self-evident; the "scope of practice" of nonphysician providers remains contested and subject to polemics among the several professional groups involved. In turning to the status of the nurse practitioner (NP) in chapter 11, I again summon history to understand better the quandary of advanced training nurses who become first-line medical providers under the aegis of nursing training and a nursing identity. I also seek to mediate between the expansive claims of nurse practitioner advocates about the range of NPs' diagnostic and treatment prerogatives and the corresponding claims of physician critics intent on restricting their role, often unduly and at the public's expense. The epilogue continues my commentary on the team approach to primary care by returning to the Patient-Centered Medical Home, an innovative approach to health care "delivery" supported by the Affordable Care Act. I invite readers to reflect with me on what exactly it means to consider the site of our medical care a "home," with all the meanings and emotions that this iconic word conjures up. Here, as in preceding chapters, I let my personal experience serve as a window to larger issues about reaching out to doctors in times of need via the telephone or, now, the Internet.

It follows from these interlocking chapters that thinking with history takes us in different directions. It can help us contextualize contemporary discontent with doctors, the treatments they give us, and the physical and human environments in which these treatments are provided. At the level of national policy, such contextualization can, somewhat paradoxically, be a source of comfort, as we come to see the challenges before us now as recycled versions of challenges that earlier generations confronted and dealt with. Thinking with history can also guide us in developing solutions to contemporary problems that have historical analogues; strategies that appear bold and innovative or, alternatively, reckless and ill-conceived, perhaps become less so in the light of history. But alongside these constructive uses of historical thinking, there is a destructive use as well: Thinking with history helps us clear away the rubbish of rhetoric, especially misguided political rhetoric that deforms popular discourse about health care policy, including our perceptions of, and reactions to, proposals for fundamental changes in the delivery and financing of medical care that promote equity. If the reader understands the preceding as a none-too-subtle reference to the Patient Protection and Affordable Care Act of 2010 (Obamacare), then the reader is right.

CHAPTER 2

Does Your Doctor Care?

A friend to all is a friend to none.   —Aristotle

Who cares? Everyone cares. Politicians care. Oil and gas companies care. Banks, drug companies, food manufacturers, political action groups—they all care. Insurance companies cup us in nurturing hands and want to be our good neighbors. Tobacco companies care that we lead healthy, cancer-free lives. Alcoholic beverage manufacturers care that we drink in moderation and drive responsibly. Fast-food chains care that we eat nutritional meals. Automakers care about our safety behind the wheel. Investment houses only want us to reach our goals, provide for our children, and retire in comfort. Professional athletes, uniforms studded with pink, care about finding a cure for breast cancer. Everyone cares about world peace, world hunger, AIDS, illicit drug use, the unemployed, the disadvantaged, the mentally and physically challenged, profiling cops, corrupt politicians, neglected veterans, exploitative landlords, and of course abusive spouses, parents, caregivers, teachers, coaches, and classmates (bullies). Professing to care has been in rhetorical overdrive for so long in America that it has become gestural and empty and, as such, uncaring. And this glut of counterfeit caring makes me sick.

So I turn to those who, we want to believe, are among the last bastions of authentic caring: our doctors. They, after all, enter a profession that, as far back as 2000 BCE,[1] has been dedicated to caring for the sick and restoring them to health. The Greek myth of the archetypal physician (and later physician-god) Asklepius, first related by Homer around 800 BCE and set down in writing by Hesiod a century later, speaks of "the blameless physician" (Homer), "a great joy to men, a soother of cruel pangs" (Hesiod) who ministered to the common people, criminals and outcasts among them, regardless of the consequences.[2]

Hippocrates, who, for Plato, was simply "the Asklepiad,"[3] carried forward this caring ethic into fifth century BCE Athens, the Age of Pericles. And now, 2,500 years later, what physicians still offer us, we hope, is a sacrosanct kind of caring, a caring validated by the Hippocratic Oath (if only in a modernized version) and codes of professional ethics that formalize and render obligatory what the bioethicist Edmund Pellegrino terms "the good intent inherent in healing."[4] As far back as Scribonius Largus, physician to the Roman emperor Hadrian in the first century CE, physicians have entered their profession by publicly *professing* to care about us.[5] Medical ethics, then and now, obligate *all* physicians to care for us honorably and well; to safeguard our privacy, our rights, our dignity, our worth; to place our interests before all others; and, always, to do good and no harm.

But medical caring is not a Platonic form, a universal template that guides physicians of all times and places in the art and practice of caring. What it means to be a "caring" doctor who cares well and truly for patients changes over time. For those of us born in the mid-twentieth century or earlier, it has changed over the course of our lifetime. Through the nineteenth century and well into the twentieth, the state of medical practice put care and caring in close relationship. Providing care *to* the patient and caring *for* the patient were twin sides of virtuous doctoring; both were integral to a care*giving* informed by the classical virtues of *Humanitas*—the gravity, integrity, modesty, beneficence, and compassion associated with civilized humanity. To be sure, the emergence of medical specialization in the late nineteenth century, with its increasing reliance on diagnostic and laboratory technologies found only in hospitals, strained the linkage between care and caring. But medical specialization, originally a nebulous concept that gave rise to legions of part-time, often opportunistic "specialists," did not strain the linkage unduly. Rather, it was the enormous medical advances of mid-twentieth-century America, which would blossom into the high-tech, hospital-based, cost-containing, and "managed" treatment environment of the 1970s and beyond, that placed the linkage in jeopardy.

The 1950s and '60s, then, are the critical transitional decades. We can discern our contemporary system of health care and many of the failings associated with it in this 20-year span. At the same time, through the 1950s and '60s, most of our medical care remained, quite literally, in the hands of our family doctors.

For almost all of us, things are different now and not entirely for the better. In the second decade of the twenty-first century, what has become of what we have long understood as *traditional* doctoring? And what are the new parameters within which physicians are encouraged and even allowed to care for their patients? These questions pertain to all of medicine, but they are especially salient in the realm of primary care medicine. *Primary care physicians* (PCPs) are our frontline providers—the pediatricians, family physicians, and general internists we seek out when we are unwell, or think we may be unwell, or are anxious at the prospect of becoming unwell. They are the doctors with whom we maintain continuing relationships over time; they are the doctors who counsel us and get to know us and, if we are fortunate, come to care *about* us. This, withal, is what tradition leads us to believe.

In this chapter and the chapters to follow, I am especially concerned with contemporary family physicians (FPs), heirs to the general practitioners (GPs) of a bygone era, the most general of the generalists. In posing questions about what our family doctors (and also our pediatricians and internists) do *to* us and *for* us, about their ability and willingness to doctor us in ways that preserve the tradition of *Humanitas*, I am less concerned with what medical commentators refer to as *scope of practice*—the range of conditions that our frontline doctors are trained to diagnose and treat—than with something more subjective and tenuous: the *quality* of their caring. So we begin with a simple two-part question that captures the two-sidedness of being cared for by a doctor and guides us through this chapter. There is the objective side of the question: *How* do our (family) doctors care for us? And there is the subjective side: How *well* do our (family) doctors care for us?

II.

Among the generation of American general practitioners who trained during and immediately after World War II—not to mention the generations of generalists that preceded them—the quality of caring was anchored in hands-on doctoring: It was instrumental and procedural. The family doctor was a good listener and explainer, but he or she listened and explained preparatory to doing things to the patient, to "doctoring" the patient's body. In *The Last Family Doctor*, my tribute to my father's medicine and the medicine of his cohort of post-World War II American GPs, I underscored this manual aspect of their doctoring.[6] From the 1940s through the 1960s, American GPs not only prescribed, ordered tests, and referred to specialists; they doctored through a laying on of hands, with all that entails. To be sure, there were far fewer procedures than today, and even specialty procedures were far less enmeshed in exotic technologies. For this very reason, a highly motivated family doctor could acquire broad procedural competence across a range of medical specialties simply by reading the journal literature, taking postgraduate courses, and receiving hands-on instruction by surgical specialists on various office-based interventions. This was an era when generalist values could sustain a truly general practice, despite the ongoing growth of specialist values and specialty care.[7] This is not as paradoxical as it sounds, for reasons that will become clear over the course of these chapters.

Consider office surgery. When I ask my family physician and others I have met whether or not they do office surgery, they typically evince mild chagrin and reply to this effect: "Only if I have to. It really messes up office hours." My father's medicine was different. He learned surgery as a surgical tech on the battlefields of France and Germany; during his internship at a small community hospital in southeastern Pennsylvania; through a post-internship mentorship with a local surgeon; and then during a year-long course on minor surgery at Philadelphia's Einstein Medical Center in the late 1950s. He did all kinds of office surgery—and he enjoyed doing it. Like countless GPs of the time, especially those in smaller communities, he tended surgically to all manner of farm- and factory-related injuries. He cleaned, irrigated, and sutured deep and jagged wounds arising from agricultural machinery. He reattached the first joint of countless fingers and toes. He was skilled at performing nerve blocks. He did successful skin grafts in the office. He practiced office dermatology and performed basic urological procedures of the time, such as passing a set of urethral sounds (elongated metal probes) to enlarge the urethral opening of patients with urinary constriction or recurrent bladder infections.

This was rural general practice in the 1950s and '60s. The caring of a family doctor who actually doctors—who treats you and, where possible, *fixes* you—is different from the caring of a family doctor who examines, prescribes, orders studies, manages risk factors, and coordinates multispecialty care. In my father's day, patients felt well cared for; today, more often than not, they feel well managed.

I am not suggesting for an instant that contemporary family physicians, along with the general pediatricians and internists who fill out the primary care ranks, do not care about their patients. Of course they do. But the caring has been attenuated in important ways. Fewer and fewer procedural tributaries flow into the caring. Increasingly primary care training and the caring it sustains are cordoned off from the laying on of hands in medically salient ways. So we end up with PCPs who are touted as gatekeepers to the health care system; as "case managers" or "central coordinators of care";[8] and, more grandiloquently still, as "an essential hub in the network formed by patients, health care organizations, and communities."[9]

Empirical research suggests that the majority of patients (90% by one account) continue to have trusting relationships with their doctors, and that trust is the "basic driver" of patient satisfaction.[10] Patients who trust their doctors tend to have less treatment anxiety and greater pain tolerance;[11] they are more likely over time to be satisfied with the care they receive. But there are different kinds of trust. Can the trust associated with managing, coordinating, and being an "essential hub" approximate the trust that grew out of, and was sustained by, a range of doctoring activities—suturing, delivering babies, doing basic dermatology, gynecology, ENT, allergy testing and allergy treatment?

Trust that has bodily moorings tends to be deeper and more sustaining than the disembodied trust of care coordinators, just like the most vital and enduring of the metaphors that enter into our everyday speech—the "metaphors we live by," the title of the classic book by the linguists George Lakoff and Mark Johnson—tend to be rooted in phenomena and relationships in the physical environment.[12] When it came to forging trusting bonds with their patients, my father's medicine—which lives on among American and Canadian family physicians trained to care for rural and/or underserved populations—had a leg up (indeed, an entire torso up) on contemporary primary care providers. They doctored from infancy onward and from the body outward, so their patients were left not only with the *knowledge* of being well managed but with the *feeling* of being well cared for.

Contemporary providers cannot care in the manner of my father's generation, for their caring is legally, procedurally, and educationally constrained in ways that were alien to GPs of the mid-twentieth century. Like all physicians, PCPs are subject to clinical practice guidelines, treatment eligibility criteria, and reimbursement schedules. Now insurance carriers, relying on credentialing organizations, effectively determine the range of procedures and interventions a given doctor may employ. So in most American and Canadian locales, contemporary PCPs differ from family doctors of my father's generation because third parties largely determine the kind of medicine they may even *aspire* to practice.

I am hardly the first to point out the relationships among physicianly caring, patient trust, and the performance of medical procedures. But the insight has been long in coming among the modern-day proponents of family medicine. The "family practice" specialty, heir to the nonspecialty of general practice medicine, came into being in the late 1960s. Yet, it was only in 2007 that the Group on Hospital Medicine and Procedural Training of the Society for Teachers of Family Medicine (STFM) issued a Group Consensus Statement announcing that "Procedure skills are essential to the definition of a family physician." Indeed, they continued, "Provision of procedural care in a local setting by a family physician can add value in continuity of care, accessibility, convenience, and cost-effectiveness without sacrificing quality."[13] These normative claims strike me as reasonable, even commonsensical. But how do they square with the reality of general medicine since the first "family practice" certifying specialty exam was administered in 1969?

The fact is that primary care physicians of today, with rare exceptions, cannot be proceduralists in the manner of my father's postwar generation, much less the generations that preceded it. Residency training has to date failed to provide them with a set of common procedural skills. As of 2006, the College of Family Physicians of Canada did not even evaluate procedural skills on the Certification Examination in Family Medicine.[14] Unsurprisingly, many family physicians, in Canada and elsewhere, do not find themselves competent "in the skills that they themselves see as being essential for family practice training."[15]

Even older family physicians comfortable with older-style procedural medicine have been pulled away from office-based procedures in the effort to maximize productivity, satisfy insurers, and accommodate the sensibilities of patients. The narrowing scope of primary care medicine is a recurrent theme in the interviews conducted by the health policy analyst Timothy Hoff and collected in the volume *Practice Under Pressure: Primary Care Physicians and Their Medicine in the Twenty-First Century* (2010). Let these remarks by a family physician in his late fifties stand for a number of similar musings. Everyday family medicine, as he practiced it, had all but eliminated hands-on care:

> Anything that calls for procedural type activity, meaning a laceration, an injury, stepping on a nail, whatever, folks have gone from using their primary care physician to using their nearest specialist or urgent care center. That did not used to be the way it was. Our scope of work keeps decreasing. The amount and type of procedures we do has changed, and become a lot less. If we're looking at laceration repairs, for example, I still do them but we're doing a lot fewer. Splits and casts for straight up fractures, for an ankle, a level 1, 2, or 3 sprain, avulsion fractures, fractures of the metatarsal, things we normally would've taken care of—almost without fail the patient now goes off to the orthopedist for the splint and care during and after. . . . Normally, in family practice we would do uncomplicated cyst aspiration. Now, we'll send them to a general surgeon whether they're complicated or uncomplicated. Most family docs today wouldn't even think of doing a cyst aspiration. . . . Also what we call 'lumps and bumps,' excision of suspicious lesions, we don't do a lot of that anymore, either. Invariably, we'll go to plastics or a general surgeon to get it done for the patient. So, we pare down into fairly straight medicine, fairly straight peds [pediatrics].[16]

There is no easy way of remedying the procedural lacunae in contemporary primary care medicine. Efforts to infuse family medicine residency programs with procedural training run up against the reality, ceded by educators, that "Many privileging committees currently use specialty certification and/or a minimum number of procedures performed . . . to award privileges to perform procedures independently."[17] In one recent study, Canadian family medicine residents who took "procedural skills workshops" during their residencies were found no more likely than other residents to employ these skills when they entered private practice. More than a decade earlier, a procedurally gifted family physician in rural south Georgia reported on a series of 751 colonoscopies out of a total of 1,048 performed over a nine-year period. The practitioner, who acquired all his endoscopic training (including 80 supervised procedures) and experience while in solo practice, had results that were fully equal to those of experienced gastroenterologists; indeed, his results were exemplary. Still, he experienced difficulty obtaining colonoscopy privileges at a small community hospital in his own town.[18] My own family physician performed sigmoidoscopy on me in the early '90s. A decade later I asked her if she was still doing the procedure. "No," she replied, because she was no longer covered for it by insurers. "And it's too bad," she added, "because I liked doing them." I recently inspected a simple skin tag on the neck of one of my sons. "Why don't you have your family doctor whisk it off?" I asked. "Actually," he replied, "she referred me to a plastic surgeon."

It is the same story almost everywhere. The "almost" refers to rural training programs which, especially in Canada, produce family physicians with significantly greater procedural competence than their urban colleagues. This tends to be true in the U.S. as well, especially in those rural areas where access to specialists is still limited. But even rural family physicians here have been found to vary greatly in procedural know-how, with a discernible trend away from the use of diagnostic instruments. In the mid-'90s, a random sample of 403 rural FPs in eight Midwestern and Western states found that 57% performed sigmoidoscopy, but only 20% performed colposcopy (examination of vaginal and cervical tissue with a colposcope), and fewer than 5% performed nasopharyngoscopy (examination of the nasal passages and pharynx with a laryngoscope).[19] In his illuminating Afterword to *The Last Family Doctor*, the internist-geriatrician David Stepansky recounts the trend away from procedural competence during his internal medicine residency of the late '70s:

> I recall the increasingly clear demarcation of skills practiced by residents in different areas of medical training. For example, internal medicine residents had traditionally received routine training in certain invasive procedures such as spinal taps, thoracenteses (to remove fluid from the chest cavity) and paracenteses (to remove fluid from the abdomen), and insertion of central intravenous catheters. Although I was trained in these procedures and had some opportunity to perform them, my experience was limited, compared to the training of internal medicine residents who preceded me by only a few years. There arose the general understanding that such technical procedures were best left to those who performed them frequently and well—a concept that is now broadly applied throughout healthcare.[20]

Efforts to upgrade the procedural competence of PCPs have an air of remediation about them. After all, in the United States the residency-based "family practice" specialty came into being in 1969, but the development of a core list of procedures that all family medicine residents should be able to perform awaited the efforts of the STFM's Group on Hospital Medicine and Procedural Training in 2007. And this effort, in turn, followed a spate of research over the past decade from the United States, Canada, Australia, New Zealand, and The Netherlands suggesting that "the procedural skill set expected of new family or general practice physicians is not being adequately taught in residency or registrar programs."[21]

Shoring up the procedural skill set of PCPs runs up against the simple reality that the majority of overworked PCPs are content to refer their patients to specialists for procedures. Indeed, if the PCPs in Hoff's sample are representative, then contemporary medical students and residents increasingly choose primary care medicine because it is a "lifestyle-friendly" specialty in which the predictability of a bounded workday and reduced scope of practice compensate for the routine, lower-paying, procedure-free nature of the work.[22]

Finally, we have reached a point in which a majority of patients *expect* to have procedures performed by specialists. Implicitly if not explicitly, they have come to embrace the difference between procedural training (and the experience that comes from applying a procedure occasionally in a generalist setting) and the mastery associated with routine use of a procedure in a specialty or hospital setting. Exceptions to the rule, like the eminently competent FP colonoscopist mentioned above or the skilled FP proceduralists profiled in Howard Rabinowitz's *Caring for the Country: Family Doctors in Small Rural Towns* (2004)[23] or the dwindling number of FPs who simply make it their business to perform procedures, serve to underscore the rule. And the rule, for doctors and patients alike, is part of the problem.

"The history of medicine," declaimed the internist W. R. Houston in 1937, "is a history of the dynamic power of the relationship between doctor and patient." Houston's address to the American College of Physicians, which, in published form, is the classic article "The Doctor Himself as a Therapeutic Agent," left no doubt about the kind of interactions that powered the doctor's agency. "What the patient most imperatively demands from the doctor," he wrote, "is, as it always was, action." And action, in Houston's sense of the term, always referred back to "the line of procedure," to the act of doing things to and for the patient.[24] The performance of a medical procedure, as Houston well knew, made the doctor the representative of modern scientific medicine. It was the doctor's calming scientific authority channeled through his or her sensory endowment, especially sight and touch. We now know more: that the laying on of hands, even if mediated by medical instruments, activates contact touch, an inborn biological pleasure that, through symbolic elaboration, may come to represent affection and strength.[25] Psychoanalysts would say that a basic physiological pleasure is amplified by an idealizing transference.

Houston, of course, delivered his address before World War II and the growth of specialization that accompanied it and followed it. In America of the 1930s, patients might still expect their personal physicians to know and to implement the "line of procedure," whatever the ailment. But what are we to make of his dictum in our own time? Absent the kind of procedural glue that bonded GPs and patients of the past, how can today's primary care physicians come to know their patients and provide physicianly caring that approximates the procedurally grounded caring of their forebears? Contemporary doctors not only manage their patients; they also care for them. But, given the paucity of procedural interventions, of actually *doing* things to their patients' bodies, what more can they do to make these patients *feel* well cared for? Medical educators have come up with various strategies for reinvigorating doctor-patient relationships, most of which cluster around a recent concept that stands in for a physicianly attitude that is not only old but positively antique. It is the quintessential pouring of old wine in new bottles and goes by the name of "patient-centered medicine."

III.

Beginning in the 1980s, primary care educators became concerned that newly trained family physicians, freighted with technology and adrift in protocols, lacked basic people skills. So they resuscitated an expression coined by the British psychoanalyst Enid Balint in 1969. They began promoting "patient-centered medicine," which, according to Balint's stunningly pedestrian insight, called on the physician to understand the patient "as a unique human being."[26] More recently, patient-centered medicine has evolved into "relationship-centered care," which also goes by the more comprehensive tag "patient-and-relationship-centered care" (PRCC). The latter not only delineates the relational matrix in which care is provided, but also extols the "moral value" of cultivating doctor-patient relationships that transcend the realm of the biomedical. In language that could just as well come from a primer of relational psychotherapy, these educators enjoin clinicians to embrace the clinician-patient relationship as "the unique product of its participants and its context," to "remain aware of their own emotions, reactions, and biases," to move from detached concern to emotional engagement and empathy, and to embrace the reciprocal nature of doctor-patient interactions. Such reciprocity means that the clinical goal of restoring and maintaining health must still "allow[ing] a patient to have an impact on the clinician" in order "to honor that patient and his or her experience."[27]

Recent literature on relationship-centered care evinces an unsettling didacticism about the human dimension of effective doctoring. It is as if medical students and residents not only fail to receive training in communication skills but fail equally to comprehend that medical practice will actually oblige them to comfort anxious and confused human beings. Residency training, in particular, hardly socializes freshly minted physicians into a patient-centered medical world. Two recent time-motion studies of internal medicine interns, one conducted at two academic medical centers in Baltimore and another at a VA hospital in Milwaukee, found that medical interns—20% of whom will go on to practice general adult medicine—spent only 12% of their time in direct patient care and averaged only 7.7 minutes with each patient on their service per day. During these 7.7 minutes, interns introduced themselves to patients only 40% of the time and sat down with them (which included sitting on, or crouching next to, the patient's bed) less than 10% of the time.[28] The interns may be learning many clinically relevant things during their first year of postgraduate training, but they are not learning them from patients. What then are they doing? They are consulting with other providers but otherwise writing admissions and progress notes and reviewing charts, all of which place them in front of a computer screen for 40% of their duty time.

The upshot of these and other time-motion studies is that budding internists learn to practice a kind of medicine that consigns human interaction to the margins of hospital care and leaves no time at all for caring. Physician-writers like Pauline Chen have called attention to this state of affairs and what it portends for these doctors, both interpersonally and diagnostically, when they complete training and begin independent practice.[29] What do medical educators have to offer? They compensate for the dearth of doctor-patient interaction by devising "models" and "frameworks" that will teach residents and fully trained clinicians how to communicate effectively. Painfully commonsensical "core skills" for delivering quality health care are enumerated over and over. The creation and maintenance of an "effective" doctor-patient relationship becomes a "task" associated with a discrete skill set (e.g., listening skills, effective nonverbal communication, respect, empathy). A piece from 2011 on "advanced" communication strategies for relationship-centered care in pediatrics reminds pediatricians that "Most patients prefer information and discussion, and some prefer mutual or joint decisions," and this proviso leads to the formulation of a typical "advanced-level" injunction: "Share diagnostic and treatment information with kindness, and use words that are easy for the child and family to understand."[30]

Other writers shift the relational burden away from caring entirely and move to terrain with which residents and practitioners are bound to be more comfortable. Thus, we read of how electronic health records (EHRs) can be integrated into a relational style of practice and of how "interprofessional collaboration" between physicians and alternative/complementary providers can profit from "constructs" borrowed from the "model" of relationship-centered care. More dauntingly still, we learn of how relational theory may be applied to the successful operation of primary care practices, where the latter are seen as "complex adaptive systems" in need of strategies for organizational learning borrowed from complexity theory.[31]

There is the sense that true doctoring skills—really just the human aptitude and desire to doctor—are so ancillary to contemporary practice that their cultivation must be justified in statistical terms. Journal readers continue to be reminded of studies from the 1990s that suggest an association between physicianly caring and the effectiveness and appropriateness of care, the latter measured by efficiency, diagnostic accuracy, patient adherence, patient satisfaction, and the like.[32] And, *mirabile dictu*, researchers have found that physicians who permit patients to complete a "statement of concerns" report their patients' problems more accurately than those who do not; indeed, failure to solicit the patient's agenda correlates with a 24% reduction in physician understanding.[33]

The problem, as I observed in *The Last Family Doctor*, is that contemporary medical students are rarely drawn to general medicine as a calling and, even if they are, the highly regulated, multispecialty structure of American (and to a somewhat lesser extent, Canadian) medicine militates against their ability to live out the calling. So they lack the aptitude and desire to be primary caregivers—which is not the same as being primary care physicians—that was an a priori among GPs of the post-WWII generation and their predecessors. Contemporary primary care educators compensate by endeavoring to codify the art of humane caregiving that has traditionally been associated with the generalist calling—whether or not students and residents actually feel called. My father, who trained in the late 1940s and early '50s, would probably have appreciated the need for a teachable model of relationship-centered care, but he would also have viewed it as a sadly remedial attempt to transform individuals with medical training into physicians. Gifted generalists of his generation did not require instruction on the role of the doctor-patient relationship in medical care-giving. "Patient-and-relationship-centered care" was intrinsic to their doctoring; it did not fall back on a skill set to be acquired over time.

The PRCC model, however useful in jump-starting an arrested doctoring sensibility, pales alongside the writings of the great physician-educators of the early twentieth century who lived out values that contemporary educators try to parse into teachable precepts. For medical students and primary care residents, I say, put aside the PRCC literature and introduce them *ab initio* to writings that lay bare what Sherwin Nuland terms "the soul of medicine." I find nothing of practical significance in the PRCC literature that was not said many decades ago—and far more tellingly and eloquently—by Francis W. Peabody in "The Care of the Patient" (1927), George Draper in "The Education of a Physician" (1932), Lawrence J. Henderson in "Physician and Patient as a Social System" (1935), W. R. Houston in "The Doctor Himself as a Therapeutic Agent" (1939), and especially William Osler in the addresses gathered together in the volume *Aequanimitas* (1904).[34] Supplement these classic readings with a healthy dose of Oliver Sacks and Richard Selzer and top them off with patient narratives that underscore the terrible cost of physicians' failing to communicate with patients as people (such as Sacks's own *A Leg to Stand On* [1984] and David Newman's powerful and troubling *Talking with Doctors* [2011]),[35] and you will have done more to instill the principles of patient- and relationship-centered care than all the models, frameworks, algorithms, communicational strategies, and measures of patient satisfaction under the sun. And further, you will have made a good start at introducing them to the psychodynamic dimension of giving and receiving medical care.

This latter dimension of doctoring was long described as the role of psychiatry in general medical care, typically abbreviated to "psychiatry in medicine." Of late, family physicians and general pediatricians, who see a large number of children and adolescents with behavioral disorders and learning difficulties, have taken to referring to it as "behavioral medicine." This pathway to patient-centered care has a historical trajectory of its own, beginning with the holistic psychobiological approach to patient care of Adolf Meyer in the early twentieth century, picking up steam with the infusion of Freudian thinking into medicine during the 1920s and '30s, and coming to fruition in the two decades following World War II. Now, sadly, it has slowed to a trickle in the world of contemporary primary care.

IV.

If it is little known in medical circles that World War II "made" American psychiatry, it is even less well known that the war made psychiatry an integral part of general medicine in the postwar decades. Under the leadership of the psychoanalyst (and as of the war, Brigadier General) William Menninger, Director of Neuropsychiatry in the Office of the Surgeon General, psychoanalytic psychiatry guided the armed forces in tending to soldiers who succumbed to combat fatigue, aka war neuroses, and getting some 60% of them back to their units in record time. But it did so less because of the relatively small number of trained psychiatrists available to the armed forces than through the efforts of the general medical officers (GMOs), the psychiatric foot soldiers of the war. These GPs, with at most three months of psychiatric training under military auspices, made up 1,600 of the army's 2,400-member neuropsychiatry service.[36]

The GPs carried the psychiatric load, and by all accounts they did a remarkable job. Of course, it was the psychoanalytic brass—William and Karl Menninger, Roy Grinker, John Appel, Henry Brosin, Franklin Ebaugh, and others—who wrote the papers and books celebrating psychiatry's service to the nation at war. But they all knew the GPs were the real heroes. John Milne Murray, the army air force's chief neuropsychiatrist, lauded them as the "junior psychiatrists" whose training had been entirely "on the job" and whose ranks were destined to swell under the VA program of postwar psychiatric care.[37]

The splendid work of the GMOs encouraged expectations that they would help shoulder the nation's psychiatric burden after the war. The psychiatrist-psychoanalyst Roy Grinker, coauthor with John Spiegel of the war's enduring contribution to military psychiatry, *Men Under*

Stress (1945), was under no illusion about the ability of trained psychiatrists to cope with the influx of returning GIs, a great many "angry, regressed, anxiety-ridden, dependent men" among them. "We shall never have enough psychiatrists to treat all the psychosomatic problems," he remarked in 1946, when the American Psychiatric Association boasted all of 4,000 members. And he continued: "Until sufficient psychiatrists are produced and more internists and practitioners make time available for the treatment of psychosomatic syndromes, we must use heroic shortcuts in therapy which can be applied by all medical men with little special training."[38]

Grinker was seconded by none other than William Menninger, who remarked after the war that "the majority of minor psychiatry will be practiced by the general physician and the specialists in other fields." As to the ability of stateside GPs to manage the "neurotic" veterans, Lauren Smith, psychiatrist-in-chief at the Institute of Pennsylvania Hospital prior to assuming his wartime duties, offered a vote of confidence two years earlier. The majority of returning veterans would present with psychoneuroses rather than major psychiatric illness, and most of them "can be treated successfully by the physician in general practice if he is practical in being sympathetic and understanding, especially if his knowledge of psychiatric concepts is improved and formalized by even a minimum of reading in today's psychiatric literature."[39]

These appraisals, enlarged by the Freudian sensibility that saturated popular American culture in the postwar years, led to the psychiatrization of American general practice in the 1950s and '60s. They bore witness to what Charles Burlingame, psychiatrist-in-chief at the Hartford Institute of Living, termed the "decided development" of postwar psychiatry "along the line of simple, practical psychotherapy aiming at positive results in less time and at lower costs."[40] Just as the GMOs had been the foot soldiers in the campaign to manage combat stress, so GPs of the postwar years were expected to lead the charge against the ever-growing number of "functional illnesses" presented by their patients.[41] Surely these patients were not all destined for the analyst's couch, and in truth they were usually better off in the hands of their GPs. "I contend that every general practitioner's office should be a mental health center," intoned Milton Casebolt in his Chairman's

Address to the AMA's Section on General Practice in 1950. Four years later, Robert Needles echoed Casebolt's injunction in his own address to the Section on General Practice. When it came to functional and nervous illnesses, Needles lectured, "The careful physician, using time, tact, and technical aids, and teaching the patient the signs and meanings of his symptoms, probably does the most satisfactory job."[42]

V.

Many generalists of the postwar era, my father, William Stepansky, among them, practiced psychiatry. Indeed they viewed psychiatry, which in the late '40s, '50s, and '60s typically meant psychoanalytically informed psychotherapy, as intrinsic to their work. My father did office psychotherapy from the time he set out his shingle in 1953. Well-read in the psychiatric literature of his time and additionally interested in psychopharmacology, he supplemented medical school and internship with basic and advanced-level graduate courses on psychodynamics in medical practice. His own cardiac neurosis, a legacy of the death of both his parents from heart disease, his father when he was only 15, led him to seek short-term psychiatric assistance in the mid-'50s. This in turn reinforced his commitment to psychiatry as a critical dimension of general medicine.

Appointed staff research clinician at McNeal Laboratories in 1959, he conducted and published clinical research on McNeal's valmethamide, an early antianxiety agent.[43] Beginning in the 1960s, he attended case conferences at Norristown State Hospital (in exchange for which he gave his services, gratis, as a medical consultant). And he participated in clinical drug trials as a member of the Psychopharmacology Research Unit of the University of Pennsylvania's Department of Psychiatry, sharing authorship of several publications that came out of the unit. In *The Last Family Doctor*, my tribute to him and his cohort of postwar GPs, I wrote:

> The constraints of my father's practice make it impossible for him to provide more than supportive care, but it is expert support framed by deep psychodynamic understanding and no less valuable to his patients owing to the relative brevity of 30-minute 'double' sessions. Saturday

mornings and early afternoons, when his patients are not at work, are especially reserved for psychotherapy. Often, as well, the last appointment on weekday evenings is given to a patient who needs to talk to him. He counsels many married couples having difficulties. Sometimes he sees the husband and wife individually; sometimes he seems them together in couples therapy. He counsels the occasional alcoholic who comes to him. He is there for whoever seeks his counsel, and a considerable amount of his counseling, I learn from [his nurse] Connie Fretz, is provided gratis.[44]

To be sure, this was family medicine of a different era. Today primary care physicians lack the motivation, not to mention the time, to become frontline psychotherapists. Nor would their credentialing organizations (or their accountants) look kindly on scheduling double sessions for office psychotherapy and then billing the patient for a simple office visit. The time constraints under which PCPs typically operate, the pressing need to maintain practice "flow" in a climate of regulation, third-party mediation, and bureaucratic excrescences of all sorts—these things make it more and more difficult for physicians to summon the patience to take in, much less to co-construct and/or psychotherapeutically reconfigure, their patients' illness narratives.

But this is largely beside the point. Contemporary primary care medicine, in lockstep with psychiatry, has veered away from psychodynamically informed history taking and office psychotherapy altogether. For generalists and nonanalytic psychiatrists alike—and certainly there are exceptions—the postwar generation's mandate to practice "minor psychiatry," which included an array of supportive, psychoeducative, and psychodynamic interventions, has effectively shrunk to the simple act of prescribing psychotropic medication.

At most, PCPs may aspire to become, in the words of Howard Brody, "narrative physicians" able to empathize with their patients and embrace a "compassionate vulnerability" toward their suffering. But even this has become a difficult feat. Brody, a family physician and bioethicist, remarks that respectful attentiveness to the patient's own story or "illness narrative" represents a sincere attempt "to develop *over time* into a certain sort of person—a healing sort of person—for whom the primary focus of attention is outward, toward the experience and suffering of the patient, and not inward, toward the physician's own preconceived agenda."[45] The attempt is no less praiseworthy than the goal. But where, pray tell, does the *time* come from? The problem, or better, the *problematic*, has to do with the driven structure of contemporary primary care, which makes it harder and harder for physicians to enter into a world of open-ended storytelling that *over time* provides entry to the patient's psychological and psychosocial worlds.

Whether or not most primary care physicians even *want* to know their patients in psychosocially, much less psychodynamically, salient ways is an open question. Back in the early 1990s, primary care educators recommended special training in "psychosocial skills" in an effort to remedy the disinclination of primary care residents to address the psychosocial aspects of medical care. Survey research of the time showed that most residents not only devalued psychosocial care, but also doubted their competence to provide it.[46]

Perhaps things have improved a bit since then with the infusion of courses in the medical humanities into some medical school curricula and focal training in "patient and relationship-centered medicine" in certain residency programs. But if narrative listening and relationship-centered practice are to be more than academic exercises, they must be undergirded by a clinical identity in which relational knowing is constitutive, not superadded in the manner of an elective. Psychodynamic psychiatry was such a constituent in the general medicine that emerged after World War II. If it has become largely irrelevant to contemporary primary care, what can take its place? Are there other pathways through which our primary doctors, even within the structural constraints of contemporary practice, may get to know us and enter into our stories and provide the human connection we need when we are ill and fearful? Medical educators have developed an answer: Let's teach them the art of human empathy, let's devise curricular innovations that will make them empathic, caring doctors. Let's teach them how to care.

As we will see, the effort to make a didactic project out of our need for patient-and-relationship-centered doctoring is both helpful and an admission of failure. To understand the paradox, it is necessary to step back and consider first how doctors became empathic caregivers in the nineteenth century, long before there was any formal appreciation of the role of psychiatry in medicine and longer still before patient-centered doctoring became a psychosocial skill set to be taught in the manner of diagnosis and treatment.

CHAPTER 3

The Hunt for Caring Doctors

'Introspective' and 'loving' are not adjectives that earn ready acceptance to most medical schools.
　　　　　—Howard Spiro, "Empathy: An Introduction" (1993)

I n the nineteenth century, no one was devising courses, workshops, or coding schemes to foster psychosocial skills and patient-centered care. In both Europe and America, students were expected to learn medicine's existential lessons in the manner they long had: through mastery of Latin and immersion in ancient writings. This fact should not surprise us: knowledge of Latin was the great nineteenth-century signpost of general knowledge. It was less an index of education achieved than testimony to educability per se. As such, it was an aspect of cultural endowment essential to anyone aspiring to a learned profession.

I have written elsewhere about the relationship of training in the classics to medical literacy throughout the century.[1] Here I want to focus on the "felt" aspect of this cultural endowment: the relationship of classical training to the kind of *Humanitas* that was foundational to patient-centered care.

The conventional argument has it that the role of Latin in medicine progressively diminished throughout the second half of the nineteenth century, as experimental medicine and laboratory science took hold, first in Germany and Austria, then in France, and finally in Britain and the United States, and transformed the nature of medical training. During this time, physicians who valued classical learning, so the argument goes, were the older men who clung to what Christopher Lawrence terms "an epistemology of individual experience." In Britain, aficionados of the classics were the older, hospital-based people who sought to circumscribe the role of science in clinical practice. Like their younger colleagues, they used the rhetoric of science to bolster their authority but, unlike the younger men, they "resisted the wholesale conversion of bedside practice into a science—any science." For these men, clinical medicine might well be based on science, but its actual practice was "an art which necessitated that its practitioners be the most cultured of men and the most experienced reflectors on the human condition."[2]

For Lawrence, classical learning signified the gentleman-physician's association of bedside practice with the breadth of wisdom associated with general medicine; as such, it left them "immune from sins begotten by the narrowness of specialization." In America, I believe, the situation was different. Here the classics did not (or did not only) sustain an older generation intent on dissociating scientific advance from clinical practice. Rather, in the final decades of the century, the classics sustained the most progressive of our medical educators in their efforts to resist the dehumanization of sick people inherent, they believed, in specialization. Medical educators embraced experimental medicine and laboratory science, to be sure, but they were also intent on molding physicians whose sense of professional self transcended the scientific rendering of the clinical art. Seen thusly, the classics were more than a pathway to the literacy associated with professional understanding and communication; they were also a humanizing strategy for revivifying the Hippocratic Oath in the face of malfunctioning physiological systems and diseased organs.

Consider the case of Johns Hopkins Medical College, which imported the continental, experimental model to the United States and thereby became the country's first modern medical school in 1892. In the medical value assigned to the classics, three of Hopkins's four founding fathers were second to none. William Welch, the pathologist who headed the founding group of professors (subsequently known as "The Big Four"), only reluctantly began medical training in 1872, since it meant abandoning his first ambition: to become a Greek tutor and ultimately a professor of classics at his alma mater, Yale University. Welch's love of the classics, especially Greek literature and history, spanned his lifetime. "Everything that moves in the modern world has its roots in Greece," he opined in 1907.

William Osler, the eminent professor of medicine who hailed from the Canadian woodlands north of Toronto, began his education as a rambunctious student at the Barrie Grammar School, where he and two friends earned the appellation "Barrie's Bad Boys." On occasion, the little band would give way to "a zeal for study" that led them after lights-out to "jump out of our dormitory window some six feet above the ground and study our Xenophon, Virgil or Caesar by the light of the full moon." Osler moved on to the Trinity College School where, in a curriculum overripe with Latin and the classics, he finished first in his class and received the Chancellor's Prize of 1866. Two years later, he capped his premedical education at Trinity College with examination papers on Euclid, Greek (Medea and Hippolytus), Latin prose, Roman history, pass Latin (Terence), and classics (honors).[3] Ever mindful of his classical training, Osler not only urged his Hopkins students "to read widely outside of medicine," but admonished them to "Start at once a bed-side library and spend the last half hour of the day in communion with the saints of humanity," among whom he listed Plutarch, Marcus Aurelius, Plato, and Epictetus.[4]

When Howard Kelly, the first Hopkins professor of gynecology and arguably the foremost abdominal surgeon of his time, began college in 1873, he was awarded the University of Pennsylvania's matriculate Latin prize for his thesis, "The Elements of Latin Prose Composition." Kelly, like Welch and Osler, was a lifetime lover of the classics, and he relished summer vacations, when he could "catch up on his Virgil and other classics."[5]

Of the fourth Hopkins founding father, the reclusive, morphine-addicted surgeon William Stewart Halsted, there is no evidence of a life-long passion for the ancients, though his grounding in Latin and Greek at Phillips Academy, which he attended from 1863 to 1869, was typically rigorous. Far more impressive bona fides belong to one of Halsted's early trainees, Harvey Cushing, who came to Hopkins in 1897 and became the hospital's resident surgeon in 1898. Cushing, the founder of modern neurosurgery, entered Yale in 1887, where he began his college career "walking familiarly in the classics" with courses that included "geometry, Livy, Homer, Cicero, German, Algebra, and Greek prose." In February 1888 he wrote his father that Yale was giving him and his friends "our fill of Cicero. We have read the Senectute and Amicitia and are reading his letters to Atticus, which are about the hardest Latin prose, and now we have to start in on the orations."[6]

In the early twentieth century, Latin, no less than high culture in general, fell by the wayside in the effort to create modern "scientific" doctors. By the 1920s, medical schools had assumed their modern "corporate" form, providing an education that was standardized and mechanized in the manner of factory production. "The result of specialization," Kenneth Ludmerer has observed, "was a crowded, highly structured curriculum in which subjects were taught as a series of isolated disciplines rather than as integrated branches of medicine."[7] Absent such integration, the very possibility of a holistic grasp of sick people, enriched by study of the classics, was gradually relinquished.

The elimination of Latin from the premed curriculum made eminently good sense to early twentieth-century medical educators. But it was not only the language that went by the wayside. Gone as well was familiarity with the broader body of myth, literature, and history to which the language opened up. Gone, that is, was the kind of training that sustained holistic, perhaps even empathic, doctoring.

When in the fall of 1890—a year after the opening of Johns Hopkins Hospital—Osler and Welch founded the Johns Hopkins Hospital Historical Club, it was with the explicit understanding that medical history, beginning with the Hippocratic and Galenic writings, was a humanizing building block in the formation of a medical identity. The first year of monthly meetings was devoted exclusively to Greek medicine, with over half of 15 presentations dealing with Hippocrates. Osler's two talks dealt, respectively, with "The Aphorisms of Hippocrates" and "Physic and Physicians as Depicted in Plato." Over the next three years, the club's focus broadened to biography, with Osler himself presenting essays on seven different American physicians, John Morgan, Thomas Bond, Nathan Smith, and William Beaumont among them. His colleagues introduced the club to other medical notables, European and American, and explored topics in the history of the specialties, including the history of trephining (boring into the skull with a small circular saw to remove bone), the history of lithotomy (surgery to remove bladder stones through the perineum) in women, and the ancient history of rhinoscopy.[8]

Osler, be it noted, supplemented the meetings of the Historical Club with informal Friday evening gatherings at his home with his clinical clerks. There, as one attendee recounts, he "laid in the student's [sic] minds foundations of an interest in medical history." "So skillfully did Dr. Osler weave into his discussions the importance of medical history," he continued, "and so entertaining and interesting did he make it, that many of the students continued an active interest in the subject through life, and numerous of them made notable contributions to it."[9] Of course, this is the same Osler for whom medical societies were founts of medical history, where meetings might begin by reviewing original accounts of rare diseases. His example is Hezekiah Beardsley's description of hypertrophic stenosis of the pylorus (a narrowing of the opening between the stomach and small intestine in infants), as reported in the Transactions of the New Haven County Medical Society of 1788.[10]

The collective delving into history of medicine that took place within the Hopkins Medical History Club and, for a select few, around Osler's dining room table, not only broadened the horizons of the participants, residents among them. It also promoted a comfortable fellowship conducive to—dare we say it?—patient-centered medicine. The Hopkins professors and their occasional guests were not only leading lights in their respective specialties, but Compleat Physicians deeply immersed in the humanities. Residents and students who attended the meetings of the club saw their teachers as engaged scholars; they beheld professors who, during the first several years of meetings, introduced them, inter alia, to "The Royal Touch for Scrofula in England," "The Medicine of Shakespeare," "The Plagues and Pestilences of the Old Testament," and "An Old English Medical Poem by Abraham Cowley." Professors familiar with doctor-patient relationships throughout history were the very type of positive role models that contemporary medical educators search for in their efforts to counter what they term the "hidden curriculum" of medical school—the culture of academic hierarchies, cynical mixed messages, and commercialism that, taken together, pulls students away from patient-centered values.[11]

Medical history clubs were not uncommon in the early decades of the twentieth century, nor were they limited to the eastern seaboard. The St. Louis Medical History Club met regularly, and its transactions were published in the *Medical Library and Historical Journal*, the official organ of the Association of Medical Librarians.[12] In 1909, John S. Milne, a GP from Hartlepool, England, wrote a paper expressly for the club that was something of an event. The paper in question, "The Apparatus Used by the Greeks and Romans in the Setting of Fractures and the Reduction of Dislocations," was "profusely illustrated," inducing the club to move from its regular location in the medical library to the amphitheater at Washington University Medical College, where the epidiascope (an optical projector) could be used to share Milne's 54 plates with the audience.[13]

The Hopkins Club, along with the New York–based Charaka Club founded in 1899, had staying power. The Charaka Club published its proceedings every several years, and the fifth volume, published in 1920, rated review in the *British Medical Journal*, which singled out papers by C. L. Dana, S. Weir Mitchell, and Osler among the "familiar favorites" of previous volumes. In 1939, the third meeting of the Hopkins Club, which presented a play adapted by Hopkins's medical librarian Sanford Larkey from William Bullein's "A Dialogue Against the Fever Pestilence" (1564), drew a crowd of 460. The following year, when the Hopkins Club celebrated its fiftieth anniversary, Baltimore alone boasted two other medical history clubs: the Osler Society of the Medical and Chirurgical Faculty of the State of Maryland and the Cordell Society of the University of Maryland.[14]

Although medical history clubs are a thing of the past, we see faint echoes of their milieu in contemporary medical student and resident support groups, some modeled on the Balint groups developed by Michael and Enid Balint at London's Tavistock Clinic in the 1950s.[15] All such groups seek to provide a safe space for shared reflection and self-examination in relation to physician-patient relationships. In the late-nineteenth and early-twentieth centuries, history clubs filled this space with topics in medical history. Their meetings broadened the caregiving sensibility of young physicians by exposing them to pain and suffering, to plagues and pestilences, far beyond the misery of everyday rounds. Medical history and the broadened "medical self" it evokes and nurtures—now there's a pathway to patient-centered medicine.

II.

Yes, but the Oslerian world where medical history was understood as a humanizing dimension of medical education is long gone. So what can we do to cultivate a caring sensibility among medical students in an era of evidence-based treatment, informatics, defensive medicine, and patient rights? Maybe the key is to alter medical school admission criteria in order to find medical students whose predisposition to holistic, patient-centered doctoring is strong enough to withstand the dehumanizing rigors of med school and residency. Where do we start?

Perhaps we should start with the Medical College Admission Test (MCAT), which has been around in one form or another since 1928. The test was developed by Fred A. Moss, a psychologist at George Washington University who felt his work on personality assessment and psychological measurement would be strengthened by medical training, which he undertook at GW, receiving his M.D. in 1927.[16] Shortly after graduating, Moss, back in psychologist mode, turned to a problem that arose at his own med school and at med schools throughout the country: Only one-quarter of applicants gained admission to one or another U.S. medical school, yet over 20% of admittees failed to complete medical training.

With this problem in mind, Moss began to study the background and performance of GW's entering medical classes of 1927 and 1928. Then, with these data at hand, and aided by colleagues in the GW psychology department, he attempted to devise a test that would, in his words, "indicate ability to successfully pursue a medical course, and which might be used as one of the determining factors in selecting students for admission to the medical school."[17] A preliminary trial at GW was followed by a larger trial the following year, this time with the support of the American Council on Education, which printed and distributed the tests free of charge to 14 participating med schools.

Each school administered the test to its new freshman class and sent the results to Moss and his team. The first-year grades of each student who had taken the test arrived the following summer, giving Moss a basis for correlating test results with med school performance. In 1930, the test, now dubbed the "Scholastic Aptitude Test for Medical Students," was adopted by the Association of American Medical Colleges as a standard entrance requirement. As such, it would be administered prior to medical school admission, in time for the results to be sent to med school admission officers as an aid in selecting members of their incoming class.[18]

Renamed, successively, the "Professional School Aptitude Test" and in 1948 the "Medical College Admission Test," the exam always had questions drawn from biology, chemistry, and physics as its core, supplemented by one or more units of softer content that changed over time. From the beginning, MCAT science questions relied on what Robert Powers, who retook the exam 10 years out of medical school to strengthen his work as an admissions officer, terms "regurgitant performance"—memory retrieval exercises involving any number of formulas, equations, valences, and the like.[19]

The version of the MCAT in effect from 1992 through 2013 had units on verbal reasoning and a writing sample in addition to the units on the biological and physical sciences. Gone from the 1992 version were units on "Understanding Modern Society" and "General Information" that had been included in the versions in use from 1946 to 1962 and from 1962 to 1977, respectively. William McGaghie, who traced the evolution of the MCAT over its first 75 years, calls attention to the shifting nature of the "peripheral material" that has been added to its core scientific content:

> Peripheral material that has moved in and out of favor includes verbal ability; numeracy or quantitative ability; general information from the liberal arts, social sciences, and humanities; reading ability; and writing skills. Each of these presumptive features of medical aptitude has had one or more vogues depending on the tastes and interests of the successive MCAT design committees. Thus except for a set of core, consensual principles from the biological and physical sciences, the historical definition of aptitude for medical education has not been a fixed entity but has been constructed socially.[20]

This exercise in social construction continues apace. The MCAT has been overhauled yet again, with the latest version approved by the American Association of Medical Colleges (AAMC) in February 2013 and taking effect in 2015. The latest revision of the MCAT devotes almost half its questions to the social sciences and critical reasoning, and the latter includes reading passages that address cross-cultural issues and medical ethics. According to Darrell G. Kirch, president of the AAMC, the new version of the test will aid medical schools in finding students "who you and I would want as our doctors. Being good doctors isn't just about understanding science, it's about understanding people."[21]

To which I reply: Will wonders never cease? We're going to help medical schools create humanistic doctors with better people skills by making sure premed students are exposed to humanistic medicine as it filters through introductory psychology and sociology courses? Really? Had MCAT test designers perused a sampling of introductory psychology and sociology syllabi, they might have paused before deciding to cultivate this new skill set through introductory social science courses, which, in this day and age, devote little time to theories of personality, family structure and dynamics, psychosocial development, and psychodynamics—the very topics that engaged me when I studied introductory psychology at Princeton in the fall of 1969. Still less do today's introductory social science courses permit psychosocial and ethical consideration of health-related issues; for the latter, one must seek out upper-class courses in medical sociology, medical anthropology, and medical ethics, which are often not available at the undergraduate level.

If it's a matter of choosing general nonscience courses that frame some of the ethical and cross-cultural (and racial and gender-related) issues tomorrow's physicians will face, introductory philosophy courses in moral philosophy and/or ethics would be far more to the point. But I am a historian and my own bias is clear: At the top of horizon-broadening and humanizing courses would be surveys of nineteenth- and twentieth-century medicine in its cultural, political, and institutional aspects. I offered two such seminars to upper-class history majors at my university under the titles "Medicine and Society: From Antebellum America to the Present" and "Women, Their

Bodies, Their Health, and Their Doctors: America, 1850 to the Present." Both seminars addressed doctor-patient relationships over the past two centuries, a topic at the heart of the social history of medicine.

But let's face it. Requiring premed students to take a few additional courses is a gesture—something more than an empty gesture but a gesture nonetheless. There is every reason to believe that students who spend their undergraduate years stuffing their brains with biology, organic chemistry, and physics will approach the social science component of premed studies in the same task-oriented way. The nonscience courses will simply be another hurdle to overcome. Premed students will take introductory psychology and sociology to learn what they need to know to do credibly well on the MCATs. And, for most of them, that will be that. Premed education will continue to be an intellectual variant of survivor TV: making the grade(s), surviving the cut, and moving on to the next round of competition. Nor is there any evidence that social science courses give survivors a leg up once the next round has begun: There are no studies suggesting that college preparation in the behavioral and social sciences helps students learn the medically salient aspects of these subjects any better in med school.[22]

The overhaul of the MCAT is premised on the same fallacy that persuades medical educators they can "teach" empathy to medical students through dramatizations, workshops, and the like. The fallacy is that physicianly caring, especially caring heightened by empathy, is a cognitive skill that can be instilled through one-time events or curricular innovations. But empathy cannot be taught, not really. It is an inborn sensibility associated with personality and temperament. It is not an emotion (like rage, anger, joy) but an *emotional aptitude* that derives from the commensurability of one's own feeling states with the feeling states of others. The aptitude is twofold: It signifies (1) that one has lived a sufficiently rich emotional life to have a range of emotions available for identificatory purposes; and (2) that one is sufficiently disinhibited to access one's own emotions, duly modulated, to feel what the patient or client is feeling in the here and now of the clinical encounter. Empathy does not occur in a vacuum; it always falls back on the range, intensity, and retrievability of one's own emotional experiences. For this reason, Heinz Kohut, who believed empathy was foundational to the psychoanalytic method, characterized it as "vicarious introspection," the extension of one's own introspection (and associated feelings) to encompass the introspection (and associated feelings) of another.

Everyone possesses this ability to one degree or another; extreme situations elicit empathy even in those who otherwise live self-absorbed, relationally parched lives. This is why psychologists who present medical students with skits or film clips of the elderly in distressing situations find the students score higher on empathy scales administered immediately after viewing such dramatizations. But the "improvement" is short-lived.[23] An ongoing (read: characterological) predisposition to engage others in caring and comprehending ways cannot result from what one team of researchers breezily terms "empathy interventions."[24]

If one seeks to mobilize a preexisting aptitude for empathic, patient-centered caregiving, there are much better ways of doing it than adding introductory psychology and sociology courses to the premed curriculum. Why not give premed students sustained contact with patients and their families in settings conducive to an emotional connection? Let's introduce them to messy and distressing "illness narratives" in a way that is more than didactic. Let's place them in situations in which these narratives intersect with their own lived experience. To wit, let's have all premed students spend the summer following their junior year as premed volunteers in one or another empathy-eliciting setting: pediatric cancer wards; recovery and rehab units in VA hospitals; public geriatric facilities, especially the Alzheimer's units of such facilities, and the like.

I recommend six weeks of full-time work before the beginning of senior year. Routine volunteer duties would be supplemented by time set aside for communication—with doctors, nurses, and aides, but especially with patients and their families. Students would be required to keep journals with daily entries that recorded their experience, especially how it affected (or didn't affect) them personally and changed (or didn't change) their vision of medicine and medical practice. These journals, in turn, would be included with their senior-year applications to medical school. Alternatively, the journals would be the basis for an essay on doctor-patient relationships informed by their summer fieldwork.

I mean, if medical educators want to jump-start the humane sensibility of young doctors-to-be—if the goal of the MCAT is to locate
students "who you and I would want as our doctors"—why not go the
full nine yards and expose these scientifically minded young people to
aspects of the human condition that will stretch them emotionally?
Emotional stretching will not make them empathic; indeed, it may
engender the same defenses that medical students, especially in the
third year, develop to ward off emotional flooding when they encounter seriously ill patients.[25] But apart from the emotions spurred or
warded off by daily exposure to children with cancer, veterans without
limbs, and elderly people with dementias, the experience will have a
psychoeducational yield: It will provide incoming med students with
a broadened range of feeling states that will be available to them in
the years ahead. As such, their summer in the trenches will lay a foundation for clinical people skills far more durable than what they can
glean from introductory psychology and sociology texts.

Those premed students of caring temperament will perhaps be
pulled in a patient-centered direction; they will have an enlarged reservoir of life experience to draw on when they try to connect with
their patients during medical school and beyond. In slightly different terms, they will emerge from their summer in the trenches with
a broadened range of imagined possibilities to link up with future
patients' real-life predicaments.[26] Those budding scientists who are
drawn to medicine in its research or data-centric "managerial" dimension[27] will at least have broadened awareness of the suffering humanity that others must tend to. Rather than reaching for the grand prize
(viz., a generation of empathic caregivers), the AAMC might lower its
sights and help medical schools create physicians who, even in technologically driven specialties and subspecialties, evince a *little* more
sensitivity. In their case, this might simply mean understanding that
many patients need doctors who are not like them. A small victory is
better than a Pyrrhic victory.

III.

My late father, William Stepansky, was the most empathic caregiver
I have ever known. Until recently, however, I never thought of him
that way. Indeed, I never had the sense that he "practiced" medicine

one way or another, simply that he lived out his medical calling. I thought nothing of having a father who taped the Hippocratic Oath to his dresser and read it every morning.

My father's empathy did not grow out of medical training; it was the stuff of life experience. His family's emigration from Russia followed the Hitler-like savagery of the Ukrainian pogroms that followed World War I. Anti-Semite thugs murdered his grandfather on his own doorstep several years before his father, Pincus, mother, Vittie (then pregnant with him), and older sister, Enta, began their uncertain journey to America in 1921. Pincus, a highly decorated Russian war veteran, a member of the 118th (Shuiskii) Infantry Regiment of the 30th Infantry Division, was the recipient of what my father characterized as the Russian equivalent of our own Congressional Medal of Honor. "He was a sergeant," he would tell me, "but a colonel had to salute him first." On the battlefield he was wounded three times in the chest and once left for dead. Stripped of his decorations by the bandits who raided his native village of Stavishche in 1918, occupied his family's home, and, on leaving, murdered his father, Pincus arrived in the new world penurious and crippled with chest pain.

My father, who was born in Kishinev, Rumania, during the first leg of his family's 1,900-mile journey across continental Europe, was six months old when they arrived in Boston Harbor. A year later, they left Boston and made their home in the densely Jewish enclave in South Philadelphia. Throughout my life, my father shared two memories of his own father; they attest, respectively, to the positive and negative poles of the wounded soldier-tailor's dedication to high culture. The first is of Pincus gamely limping across long city blocks with his young son in tow; he was taking Willie, my father, to his weekly violin lesson with his first teacher, the local postman. Pincus never left the music room, and when the lesson was over, he took his son's violin and lovingly wiped it down with a special cloth brought solely for that purpose.

The second memory is of Pincus imperiously ordering his son to bring his violin and perform whenever neighbors, friends, or relations gathered in the family's small apartment. A shy, retiring child, my father urgently wanted not to play. But his father's directives were issued from on high with military-like peremptoriness that brooked neither contradiction nor delay. And so my father got his violin and he played, perhaps through tears, perhaps through rage.

My father, at age 15, watched *his* father die of heart disease. In February 1943, having completed his third year of pharmacy training, he was called up by the army and served as a surgical technician in a medical battalion attached to the 80th Infantry Division of Patton's Third Army. In France, Belgium, and Germany, he worked alongside battlefield surgeons who fought to keep wounded GIs alive in a surgical clearing company only a short remove from the front line. I learned a bit about the visceral reality of wound management in the European Theatre during his final years, when I interviewed him and several of his surviving comrades for *The Last Family Doctor*. The prosaic summary of his duties in his army discharge of January 1946—"Removed uncomplicated cases of shrapnel wounds, administered oxygen and plasma, sterilized instruments, bandages, clothing, etc. Gave hypodermic injections and performed general first aid duties"—only hints at this reality.

My father, so I learned, held down wounded GIs for anesthesia-less suturing, assisted with frontline battlefield surgery, much of which involved amputation, and then, after the day's work, went outside to bury severed arms and legs. He experienced close fighting in the woods of Bastogne during the freezing winter of 1945, when the techs worked 20-hour shifts to keep up with the inflow of casualties. The brutally cold nights—it was simply impossible to get warm—were punctuated by the visits of Midnight Charlie, as the GIs termed the Germans' nightly flyovers of the woods. One can only wonder at the impact of such things on the constitution of a gentle and soft-spoken 22-year-old pharmacy student whose passion, before and after the war, was the violin, and who carried Tolstoy's *War and Peace* in his backpack throughout his European tour.

A different man might have emerged from my father's childhood and wartime experience emotionally constricted, withdrawn, intimidated by authority figures or, obversely (or concurrently) enraged by them. In my father's case, a lifelong performance anxiety—the legacy of a militaristic father repeatedly *ordering* him to play violin before visitors—was vastly counterbalanced by an enlarged empathic sensibility that enabled him to understand and contain his patients' anxieties about their health, their relationships, their ability to love and to work. Wrestling as he did with his own anxieties and memories of the war, which included the liberation of Dachau and Buchenwald, he became a physician who accepted utterly his patients' prerogative to share their anxieties with him, even to project their anxieties onto him. He was, after all, their doctor.

My father was not only an astute diagnostician but also a gifted psychotherapist, and the amalgam of these twin talents was an ability to titrate his disclosures, to tell patients what they needed to know, certainly, but in a manner he thought they could bear. His psychologically attuned approach to patient care is now associated with the paternalism of a different era. But it was also an aspect of his ability, rare among physicians, to diagnose suffering and to discern the limits of this or that patient's ability to cope with it.[28] This style of practice was wonderfully appreciated by his patients, some of whom, after leaving the area, traveled a distance for yearly appointments with him. No doubt they wanted to experience the "holding environment" of his person.

Premed students who grind away at biology and physics have no idea what my father and his cohort of war-tested physicians, many first- and second-generation immigrants, overcame for the privilege of studying medicine. I would not wish his life story—of which I relate only a few particulars here—on any of them. And yet, we might ponder the desirability of subjecting premed students to some muted version of his experience in order to nurture whatever elements of empathic temperament they possess. My proposal that budding premed students, after completing their junior year, spend six weeks helping care for a sick, traumatized, and/or disadvantaged population, with written reflections on the experience being a component of the med school application, is made in this spirit. It is a matter of ensuring that premeds are not subverted by medicine's "hidden curriculum"—its institutional pull away from patient-centered values and practices toward technology and commerce—while they are still in college, especially when they complete their med school applications and present for their interviews. Medical educators, for their part, should work harder to find clinical teachers who do not endorse shame, humiliation, and intimidation as credible educational strategies for acculturating med students and young doctors into the profession.[29]

If we wish to steer contemporary medical students toward compassionate, or at least adequately sensitive, caregiving—and here I echo what others have said[30]—then we need to provide them with clinical teachers who are dissatisfied with a passive conception of role modeling and actually *model* discrete and specifiable behaviors in their interactions with patients.[31] They need to find more teachers like the infectious disease specialist Philip Lerner, whose deeply caring, hands-on "whole patient" approach to specialty medicine during the 1970s and '80s is beautifully captured in his son's recent memoir.[32] Sadly, the literature continues to provide examples of clinical training during medical school and residency that are denigrating, demoralizing, and ultimately desensitizing. We end up with clinical teachers (not all, by any means, but no doubt a good many) who long ago capitulated to the hidden curriculum and devote themselves to readying the next generation of trainees for a like-minded (or better, a survival-minded) capitulation. With this intergenerational dynamic in place, we are at the point of Marshall Marinker's devastating "Myth, Paradox and the Hidden Curriculum" (1997), which begins: "The ultimate indignity teachers inflict upon students is that, in time, *they* become *us*."[33]

My father and his cohort of med students who trained during and shortly after WWII were resistant to shaming and intimidation. They had experienced too much to be diverted from a calling to practice medicine. But then their teachers too had experienced a great deal, many working alongside their future students—the pharmacists, medics, techs, and GIs—in casualty clearing stations, field hospitals, VA hospitals, and rehab facilities in Europe and America. Teachers emerging from the war years encountered a generation of mature students whose wartime experience primed them to embrace medicine as patient care. And the students, for their part, encountered teachers whose own wartime experience and nascent cold war anxieties militated against Napoleonic complexes. High-tech medicine, bioethics, and patient rights all lay in the future. Generalists like my father were trained to provide care that was caring; their ministrations were largely, as I have written, "medicinal, manual, and mentalistic, which is to say, psychological."[34] In the kind of training they received, the notion of castigating as "unprofessional" med students whose patient-centered concerns and queries slowed down the breakneck pace of team rounds—a documented reality these days[35]—would literally have been nonsensical.

But that was then and this is now. Today medical culture has in key respects become subversive of the ideals that drew my father and his cohort to medicine. And this culture, which revolves around the sacrosanctity of an academic hierarchy that, inter alia, insists on perfection, denigrates uncertainty, privileges outcome over process, and, in the clinical years, engages students adversarially, is far too entrenched to be dislodged with manifestos, position papers, and curricular reforms, much less a new and improved MCAT. What educators *can* do is seek out medical students whose empowerment derives less from high grades and artfully constructed admissions essays and more from life experience in the trenches—in *any* trenches. We don't need to send premeds off to war to make them resistant to the hidden curriculum, but we should encourage premed experience robust enough to deflect its pull and let those of caring temperament develop into caring physicians.

Perhaps we need students who are drawn less to biochemistry than to the vagaries of human chemistry, students who have already undertaken experiential journeys that bring into focus the humanistic skyline of their medical horizons. What Coulehan[36] terms "socially relevant service-oriented learning" should not be confined to residency training. We need more students who come to medicine after doing volunteer work in developing nations; fighting for medical civil rights; staffing rural and urban health clinics; and serving public health internships.[37] And if this suggestion is quixotic, let's at least, as I suggest, have premed students spend the summer before senior year in a trench of one type or another. Such strategies will not create empathic caregivers de novo, but they will nurture the empathic temperament of those so endowed and, one hopes, fortify them a little better against the careerist blandishments of the hidden curriculum. It would be nice if, several generations hence, other sons (and daughters) could write about *their* fathers' (and mothers') special kind of therapeutic empathy.

CHAPTER 4

Is Your Doctor Empathic?

I feel your pain.
> —President Bill Clinton, responding to AIDS activist
> Bob Rafsky at the Laura Belle nightclub, Manhattan,
> March 27, 1992

What passes for psychoanalysis in America these days is a far cry from the psychoanalysis Freud devised in the early years of the last century. A sea change began in the 1970s, when Heinz Kohut, a Vienna-born and Chicago-based psychoanalyst, developed what he termed "psychoanalytic self psychology." At the core of Kohut's theorizing was the replacement of one kind of psychoanalytic method with another. Freud's method—which Freud himself employed imperfectly at best—revolved around the coolly self-possessed analyst, who, with surgeon-like detachment, processed the patient's unfiltered thoughts—his free associations—with "evenly hovering attention" and offered back pearls of interpretive wisdom. The analyst's neutrality signified his unwillingness to become a "real" person who related to the patient in conventionally sympathetic and supportive ways. It rendered him a "blank screen" that elicited the same feelings of love and desire—and also of fear, envy, resentment, and hatred—as the mother and father of the patient's early life. These feelings clustered into what Freud termed the positive and negative transferences.[1]

Kohut, however, found this traditional psychoanalytic method fraught with peril for patients burdened less with Freudian-type neurotic conflicts than with psychological deficits of what analysts term a "preoedipal" nature. Such deficits, that is, were understood as arising very early in development, before the desires, rivalries, and conflicts between older children and their parents coalesced in Freud's Oedipus complex. They gained expression in more primitive types of psychopathology, especially in what Kohut famously termed "narcissistic personality disorder." For these patients—and eventually, in Kohut's mind, for *all* patients—the detached, emotionally unresponsive analyst simply compounded the feelings of rejection and lack of self-worth that brought the patient to treatment. He proffered in its place a kinder, gentler psychoanalytic method in which the analyst was content to listen to the patient for extended periods of time, to affirm and mirror back what the patient was saying and feeling, and over time to forge an empathic bond with him or her from which interpretations would arise. The goal of psychoanalytically informed treatment was to help the patient create a healthy sense of self sustained by a healthy kind of self-esteem. For Kohut, it was a matter of helping the patient forge a firm "psychic structure"—a firm and reliable sense of self in relation to others that included a realistic understanding of one's own strengths and weaknesses alongside the strengths and weaknesses of those important others with whom one's life intersected (parents, siblings, close friends, teachers, and the like).

Following Kohut, empathy has been widely construed as an aspect, or at least a precondition, of talking therapy. For self psychologists and others who draw on Kohut's insights, the ability to sympathize with the patient has given way to a higher-order ability to feel what the patient is feeling, to "feel with" the patient from the inside out. And this process of *empathic immersion,* in turn, permits the therapist to "observe," so to speak, the patient's psychological interior and to comprehend the patient's "complex mental states." For Kohut, the core of psychoanalysis, indeed of depth-psychology in general, was employment of this "empathic mode of observation," an evocative but semantically questionable turn of phrase, given the visual referent of "observe," from the Latin *observare* (to take note of, to watch over). More counterintuitively still, he sought to cloak the empathic listening posture of the therapist in scientific objectivism. His writings refer over and over to the "data" that analysts acquired through their deployment of "scientific" empathy, i.e., through their empathic listening instrument.

I was Heinz Kohut's personal editor from 1978 until his death in the fall of 1981. Shortly after his death, I was given a dictated transcript from which I prepared his final book, *How Does Analysis Cure?*, for posthumous publication.[2] Throughout the 1980s and into the '90s, I served as editor to many of Kohut's colleagues, helping them frame their arguments about empathy and psychoanalytic method and write their papers and books. I grasped then, as I do now, the heuristic value of a stress on therapeutic empathy as a counterpoise to traditional notions of analytic neutrality, which gained expression, especially in the decades following World War II, in popular stereotypes of the tranquilly "analytic" analyst whose caring instincts were no match for his or her devotion to Freud's rigidly "blank screen" method.

The comparative perspective tempers bemusement at what would otherwise be a colossal conceit: that psychoanalytic psychotherapists alone, by virtue of their training and work, acquire the ability to empathize with their patients. I have yet to read an article or book that persuaded me that empathy can be taught, or that the yield of *therapeutic* empathy is the apprehension of "complex psychological states" that are analogous to the "data" gathered and analyzed by bench scientists (Kohut's own analogy).

I *do* believe that empathy can be cultivated, but, as I noted in chapter 3, only in those who are adequately empathic to begin with. In medical, psychiatric, and psychotherapy training, one can present students with instances of patients clinically misunderstood and then suggest how one might have understood them better, i.e., more empathically. Being exhorted by teachers to bracket one's personal biases and predispositions in order to "hear" the patient with less adulterated ears is no doubt a good thing. But it assumes trainees can develop a psychological sensibility through force of injunction, which runs something like: "Stop listening through the filter of your personal biases and theoretical preconceptions! Listen to what the patient *herself* is saying in *her* voice! Utilize what you understand of yourself, the hard-won fruits of your own psychotherapy and self-reflection and clinical training, to put yourself in *her* place! Make trial identifications so that *her* story and *her* predicament resonate with aspects of *your* story and *your* predicament; this will help you feel your way into *her* inner world."

At a less hortatory level, one can provide trainees with teachers and supervisors who are sensitive, receptive listeners themselves and thus "skilled" at what Kohutian self psychologists like to refer to as "empathic attunement." When students, residents, and psychotherapy trainees listen to such instructors and perhaps observe them working with patients, they may learn to appreciate the importance of empathic listening and then, in their own work, reflect more ongoingly on what their patients are saying and on how they are hearing them say it. They may acquire the ability for "reflection-in-action," which Donald Schön, in two underappreciated books of the 1980s, made central to the work of "reflective professionals" in a number of fields, psychotherapy among them.[3] To a certain extent, systematic reflection *in the service* of empathy may help therapists and physicians *become* more empathic with patients in general.

But then the same may be said of any person who undergoes a transformative life experience (even, say, a successful therapy) in which he learns to understand differently—and less tendentiously—parents, siblings, spouses, children, friends, colleagues, and the like. Life-changing events—fighting in wars, losing loved ones, being victimized by natural disasters, living in third-world countries, providing aid to trauma victims—cause some people to recalibrate values and priorities and adopt new goals. Such decentering can mobilize an empathic sensibility, so that individuals return to their everyday worlds with less self-centered ways of perceiving and being with others.

There is nothing privileged about psychotherapy training in acquiring an empathic sensibility. I once asked a senior psychoanalyst what exactly differentiated psychoanalytic empathy from empathy in its everyday sense. He thought for a moment and replied that in psychoanalysis, one deploys "sustained" empathy. What, pray tell, does this mean, beyond the fact that psychoanalysts, whether or not empathic, listen to patients for a living, and that the units of such listening are typically 45-minute sessions? Maybe he simply meant that, in the nature of things, analysts must *try* to listen empathically for longer periods of time, and prolongation conduces to empathic competence.

Well, anything is possible, I suppose. But the fact remains that some people are born empathizers and others not. Over the course of a 27-year career in psychoanalytic and psychiatric publishing, I worked with a great many analysts, psychiatrists, and psychotherapists who struck me as unempathic, sometimes strikingly so. And those who struck me as empathic were not aligned with any particular school of thought, certainly not one that, like Kohutian self psychology, privileges empathy.

Nor is it self-evident that the empathy-promoting circumstances of psychotherapy are greater than the circumstances faced day-in and day-out by any number of physicians. Consider adult and pediatric oncologists, transplant surgeons, and internists and gerontologists who specialize in palliative care. These physicians deal with patients (and their parents and children) *in extremis*; surely their work should elicit "sustained empathy," assuming they begin with an empathic endowment strong enough to cordon off the miasma of uncertainty, dread, and imminent loss that envelops them on daily rounds. Consider at the other end of the medical spectrum postwar generalists such as my father, William Stepansky, and those remaining family doctors who, often in rural settings, provide intergenerational, multispecialty care and continue to treat patients in their homes. The nature of their work makes it difficult for them *not* to observe and comprehend their patients' complex biopsychosocial states; there are extraordinary empathizers among them.

When it comes to techniques for heightening empathy, physicians have certain advantages over psychotherapists, since their patients present with bodily symptoms and receive bodily (sometimes procedural) interventions, both of which have a mimetic potential beyond "listening" one's way into another's inner world. There is more to say about the grounds of *medical* empathy, but let me conclude this section with a concrete illustration of such empathy in the making.

William Stevenson Baer graduated from Johns Hopkins Medical College in 1898 and stayed on at Hopkins as an intern and then assistant resident in William Halsted's dauntingly rigorous surgical training program. In June 1900, at the suggestion of Baer's immediate supervisor, one Harvey Cushing, Halsted asked Baer to establish an orthopedic outpatient clinic at Hopkins the following fall. With no grounding in the specialty, Baer readied himself for his new task by spending the ensuing summer at the orthopedic services of Massachusetts General Hospital and the Boston Children's Hospital. At both institutions, many children in the orthopedic ward had to wear plaster casts throughout the hot summer months. On arrival, Baer's first order of business was to alter his life circumstances in order to promote empathy with, and win the trust of, these young patients. To wit, he had himself fitted for a body cast that he wore the entire summer. His sole object, according to his Hopkins colleague Samuel Crowe, was "to gain the children's confidence by showing them that he too was enduring the same discomfort."[4]

Psychotherapists are generally satisfied that empathy can be acquired in the manner of a thought experiment.[5] "Bracket your biases and assumptions," they admonish, "empty yourself of 'content,' and then, through a process of imaginative identification, you will be able to hear what your patient is saying and feel what she is feeling." Baer's example reminds us that illness and treatment are first and foremost bodily experiences, and that "feeling into another"—the literal meaning of the German *Einfühlung*, which we translate as "empathy"— does not begin and end with complementary (or what psychoanalysts term "concordant") memories amplified by psychological imagination.[6] In medicine, there is an irremediably visceral dimension to empathy. Physicians, drawing on their own reservoir of hurt, must learn to empathize with patients who are not only anxious and confused but actually in pain and sometimes fearful of dying.

How do they do so? There are simply born caregivers, like my father, whose empathic endowment is mobilized by trying life circumstances and coalesces into an abiding sense of medicine as a calling. This was the generalist medicine, at once procedural and humanistic, that typified the early twentieth century and, despite the inroads of specialization that deepened after World War II, came to fruition in the 1950s. It was an empathy that was not taught in medical school but, rather, was fortified by several aspects of medical practice not yet eclipsed by hospital-based specialty care. One such aspect was a legacy of the nineteenth century: the house call.

II.

It is now four decades since George Engel, an internist at the University of Rochester Medical School, formulated his biopsychosocial model of medicine.[7] Concerned with the reductionism and fragmentation inherent in scientifically guided specialist care, Engel called on his colleagues to locate biomedical interventions on a larger biopsychosocial canvas. Drawing on the version of general systems theory popular in the 1970s, Engel argued that clinical assessment properly embraced a hierarchy of discrete levels—the biological, the personal, and the transpersonal—any combination of which might enter into the meaning of illness, whether acute or chronic. Even in ostensibly biomedical conditions such as diabetes, cancer, and heart disease, Engel held, it was not simply deranged cells and dysfunctional organs that accounted for the pathophysiology.

Engel's model made a strong epistemic (knowledge-related) claim: That hierarchically ordered layers of intra- and interpersonal stressors were all *causal* factors in disease as it expressed itself in this or that person. It followed that personality structure; adaptive resources and "ego strength"; psychodynamic conflicts; two-person conflicts; family-related conflicts; conflicts in the workplace—that all these factors, in various combinations, entered into the *scientific* understanding of disease.

In devising the biopsychosocial model, Engel was influenced by the psychoanalysis of his day. It is for this reason that biopsychosocial medicine is typically, and I believe erroneously, identified with the kind of "psychosomatic medicine" that analysis gave birth to in the quarter century following World War II.[8] More generally still, it is conflated with psychosocial *skills*, especially as they enter into doctor-patient communication. Because Engel's model is not an algorithm for determining which levels of the patient "system" are implicated in this or that individualized instance of illness, it has been criticized over the years for failing to guide clinical action, including the ordering of therapeutic goals. Self-evidently, the model has proven very difficult to teach and equally difficult to integrate into the conventional medical school curriculum.[9]

These findings are hardly surprising. It is difficult to teach doctors-in-training how to apply a biopsychosocial model when real-world doctoring rarely places them in regular contact with the transmedical "systems" invoked by the model. This was not always the case. Consider the house call, that site of biopsychosocial consciousness-raising throughout the nineteenth and well into the twentieth century. It was in the home of the patient, after all, that the physician could actually experience the psychosocial "systems" that entered into the patient's illness: The patient's personality, but also the patient as spouse, parent, sibling, son or daughter, all apprehended within the dynamics of a living family system. And of course there was the home environment itself, a psychosocial container of medically salient information. Wise clinicians of the early twentieth century did not need the assistance of a biopsychosocial model to understand the role of the house call in cultivating the physician's biopsychosocial sensibility. Here is Harvard's Francis Peabody in "The Care of the Patient" (1927):

> When the general practitioner goes into the home of a patient, he may know the whole background of the family life from past experience; but even when he comes as a stranger he has every opportunity to find out what manner of man his patient is, and what kind of circumstances make his life. He gets a hint of financial anxiety or of domestic incompatibility; he may find himself confronted by a querulous, exacting, self-centered patient, or by a gentle invalid overawed by a dominating family; and as he appreciates how these circumstances are reacting on the patient he dispenses sympathy, encouragement or discipline. What is spoken of as a 'clinical picture' is not just a photograph of a man sick in bed; it is an impressionistic painting of the patient surrounded by his home, his work, his relations, his friends, his joys, sorrows, hopes and fears.[10]

Three decades after Peabody's lecture, I began riding shotgun when my father, William Stepansky, made his daily round of house calls in rural southeastern Pennsylvania. Sometimes, especially with the older patients he visited regularly, I came into the house with him, where I was warmly welcomed, often with a glass of milk and home-baked treats. Patients came to know me as the doctor's traveling companion, and, in those instances where I waited in the car, they occasionally sent him out with gifts for me. J. Hansell French (of the pharmaceutical "Smith, Kline, & French" Frenches), whom my father visited several days a week, was a passionate stamp collector, and he sent my father back to the car with packets of stamps, always with the same instructions: I was to go through them, take what I needed for my own collection, and send the rest back with my father at his next visit. A. W. Jury, into whose home in Evansburg I had entry and whose wife always welcomed me with home-baked cakes and cookies, gave me a handcrafted 111-piece jigsaw puzzle that he made on his jigsaw, so the box tells me, on January 29, 1929. It remains in my closet to this day. One patient invited us to his farm to fish in his pond. Sixteen-millimeter film shows my younger brother David and me standing side by side, and then has me reeling in a modestly sized catfish, the first catch of my life. A wealthy patient who bred racehorses invited us over whenever we wished to inspect his prize thoroughbreds and swim in his pool. We did so many times.

Other patients were not so fortunate and the offering was entirely from my father. Many older couples were initially able to drive to the office, but as age and infirmity made the husband's drive increasingly difficult, my father added them to the list of regular house calls. Sometimes the families he saw at home were related, and there were tensions among them. In such cases, he graciously accepted the role of mediator, conciliator, and relational problem-solver; his house calls straddled the boundaries of medicine, psychiatry, and casework.

When the physician and essayist Lewis Thomas accompanied his physician father on house calls early in the last century, the elder Dr. Thomas enjoined his young son to understand that most illnesses simply ran their course and the patient either recovered or died, whatever the doctor might do. His fatalistic admission ran in the face of his patients' insistence that Dr. Thomas, *their* doctor, was a wondrous healer whose care led to miraculous recoveries, often from incurable conditions. "My father's early instructions to me, sitting in the front of his car on his rounds," recalled his son, "were that I should be careful not to believe this of myself if I became a doctor." "It was important to my father," continued Thomas, "that I understand this; it was a central feature of the profession, and a doctor should not only be prepared for it but be even more prepared to be honest with himself about it."[11]

Of course, Thomas began accompanying his father on house calls in 1918, the year the influenza pandemic gripped the nation, and there were ample grounds for therapeutic pessimism all around. My own experience in the postwar 1950s and early '60s—the era of childhood vaccination and antibiotic therapy—was much less cautionary and much more upbeat. During the drives to patients' homes, we would pick an organ of the body, and my father would proceed to tell me all about it—its anatomy and physiology, its functioning, and its pathology—always, be it noted, in an eminently age-appropriate and loving manner. Then when he emerged from the house call that followed and we set out for the next one, he would quiz me on the organ we had covered during the last drive. Then I (or he or we) would pick another part of the body and the process would begin anew. It was great fun, and it led me to believe that, even as a young child, I was not merely accompanying my father on his calls but learning from him and with him the whole time we were making our rounds. I'm sure it also contributed to my budding sense that my father did not merely "practice" medicine but rather lived it out, day by day, as a calling.

In rural communities in the 1950s, house calls established durable bonds that eased patients through the tribulations of illnesses that could not be managed within their homes. For many, even in the postwar period, hospital care remained a frightening prospect, and the family physician's support was indispensable: he formed a human bridge over which patients and their families crossed to a strange new land of tests and technologies. Here is a letter to my father of December 21, 1954, in which a patient's aunt must find the words to express what her reticent niece, quite overwhelmed by a recent stay in the hospital, could not:

> Dear Dr. Stepansky,
>   What better time than at Christmas to write a little note of gratitude. For some time I've been wanting to tell you how much we appreciated your kindness to my niece, Betty Jo Hanson. You went out of your way to arrange for the stay at the Pottstown hospital and that was especially nice of you, then in addition, your personal kindness. I do want to tell you that Betty Jo thinks you're just wonderful. She was very afraid about the whole thing, physically, I mean, in addition to the emotional complications, and she told me that she felt all right as soon as you got there that night at the hospital. To put it conservatively, Betty Jo isn't much of a talker, as you of course noticed, and most probably she didn't tell you or even give you the impression that she appreciated all you did for her. I know she did, though, and I want to say thanks again for all of us.[12]

From my time on the road, I learned and occasionally saw how my father's clinical gaze met and absorbed the anxious gazes of family members. It was Betty Jo Hanson and her aunt (or her parents or her siblings or her children) over and over again. It became clear to me that his medical obligation was not only to the patient, but to the patient-as-member-of-a-family and to the family-as-medically-relevant-part-of-the-patient. In a lecture to the junior class of his alma mater, Jefferson Medical College, in 1965, he made this very point in differentiating the scope of the family physician's clinical gaze from that of the pediatrician and internist. Unlike the latter, he observed, the family physician's interventions occurred "within the special domain of the family," and his treatment of the patient had to be continuously attentive to the "needs of family as an entity." It was for this reason, he added, that "family medicine must teach more than the *arithmetic sum* of the contents of specialties."[13]

My father's lecture of 1965 anticipated by eight years Ransom and Vandervoort's influential call for a new kind of "family medicine" that, in contradistinction to "family practice" and "primary care," as conceptualized at the time, would actually teach students and residents to view illness through the lens of the family and its vicissitudes.[14] Here in the mid-'60s, my father anticipates their call for a systems approach to health and illness by positing a medical-interventional substratum to what would emerge a decade or so later, in the realm of psychotherapy, as family systems theory and "structural family therapy." And then, 12 years before Engel came on the scene, he offered his conception of "a solid intellectual approach to medicine":

> To me this means relating the effects of the body systems one upon the other in health and disease through knowledge of the basic sciences—i.e., biochemistry and physiology—through some understanding of the social and environmental stresses on the patient, and finally through insight into the psychological influences of personality structure as it affects health and disease.[15]

Of course, physicians long before my father and long before Francis Peabody understood that medical treatment of the individual might entail interventions with transpersonal systems. Witness the Victorian physicians of well-off American families of the 1870s and 1880s described by the historian Nancy Theriot.[16] Making home visits to overwrought postpartum women in the throes of what was then termed "puerperal insanity"—we have only the far less evocative "postpartum depression"—these knowing family physicians dissuaded their patients from the drastic surgical interventions, such as ovariotomy, available to them. They recommended instead a change in the family "system" to accommodate the parturient's urgent need for "time out" from the burdens of household management, childrearing, and husband pleasing, to which care of a newborn was now superadded. Is it any wonder that the matrons of these well-run Victorian households became "insane," and that their insanity took the form, inter alia, of vile language, refusal to dress appropriately, refusal to resume housework, indifference to their children's daily needs, and even—*horribile dictu*—refusal to hold their newborns? And yet these same women, flouting Victorian conventions with postpartum abandon, often returned to bourgeois sanity after the family physician, with the weight of medical authority, simply prescribed a daily period of solitude when the new mother, perhaps sitting alone in the family garden, was not to be disturbed—not by *anyone*. Biopsychosocial intervention aimed at the family system was never so elegantly simple.

Interventions of this sort are hardly unknown among contemporary providers, some small percentage of whom continue to visit their patients in their homes. Further, as one of my readers reminded me, all family medicine residencies employ full-time behaviorists, usually psychologists, who help trainees develop a biopsychosocial model of care. But outside of these programs the biopsychosocial model remains where it has always been—on the fringe of a medical world of fragmented and technology-driven specialist care. In this sense, it is no different than the house call, which lives on among some 4,000 physicians in the U.S. (1,300 of whom belong to the American Academy of Home Care Medicine) and through a small number of university hospital-based "home visit programs" that target the frail elderly.[17] But let there be no mistake: these physicians and these programs remain at the far margins of primary care. The house call is all but dead, and periodic testimonials to its value among physicians, patients, and their families barely mask this fact.[18] A random sample of 5% of 1993 Medicare Part B claims data found that only 0.88% of 1,357,262 elderly Medicare patients, mainly those with terminal conditions, received house calls.[19] In 1997, writing in the

New England Journal of Medicine, the internist Edward Campion pronounced the house call a "rarity" that was "in danger of becoming extinct."[20] When the American Academy of Family Physicians polled its active members in 2008 on the settings in which they saw patients, respondents from urban and rural regions alike reported an average of *0.6* house calls a week. (My father, in the '50s and '60s, probably averaged three or four a day.) If this figure represents the rate at which house-call–making doctors make house calls, then it is fair to say that the house call has long since ceased to be an intrinsic—and intrinsically humanizing—dimension of primary care medicine. This is why I pay tribute to the Great American House Call. It is a relic of an era when biopsychosocial medicine suffused general practice without the aid of a biopsychosocial model.

Addendum: In 1998, in a belated effort to revitalize the house call, Medicare provided a new code and increased reimbursement for comprehensive home visits. But the intent was not primarily to provide patients with what Campion calls "the low-technology luxury of having a physician come to see them at home."[21] Rather, it was to cut down on hospital-based acute care costs among select populations of debilitated older patients. Most physicians never learned about the changes in Medicare payment, which did not factor in travel time to and from the patient's home, and so the miniscule number of physician house calls remained unchanged.[22] Unbeknown to many, the Patient Protection and Affordable Care Act passed by Congress in March 2010 contains an "Independence at Home Act" that provides physicians with financial incentives to treat their oldest and sickest patients in their homes. To wit, house-call–making doctors will share in cost saving if they can "prove" their in-home care reduced hospital use and left their patients satisfied. So much for the scientific bona fides of biopsychosocial medicine. It's about the money, stupid.

CHAPTER 5

Can We Teach Doctors to Care?

These properties of care and of compassion, although sometimes dismissed as merely 'bedside manner,' are the fundamental and most important tools of any clinician. With them, he can often give healing or comfort where science fails or does not exist. Without them, his science is unsatisfactory, no matter how excellent.

—Alvan Feinstein, *Clinical Judgment* (1967)

M edical students of today no longer have the life experience of the World War II generation to counter the pull of fragmented high-tech specialty care and elicit a more holistic patient-centered approach to caregiving. What newly minted physicians have by the time they graduate from medical school is, for the most part, enormous debt, burgeoning family obligations, and the prospect of three to five years of specialty training, followed by at least two years of fellowship training in a medical or surgical subspecialty. And yet medical educators do not give up. If the nature of medical training and the structure of medical practice militate against patient-centered care, against an appreciation of the patient as a suffering human being embedded in his own illness narrative, then we must approach the problem from the standpoint of the medical curriculum. We must *teach* students and physicians in residency training to be caring providers. We must remedy the absence of humanism in contemporary medicine by teaching students and residents to care. We must, so they tell us, "teach" them to be empathic. The project is much needed and highly problematic.

Dipping into the vast[1] literature on clinical empathy, one quickly discerns the dominant storyline. Everyone agrees that empathy, while hard to define, hovers around a kind of physicianly caring that incorporates emotional connection with patients. The connection conveys sensitivity to the patient's life circumstances and personal psychology, and gains expression in the physician's ability to encourage the patient to express emotion, especially as it pertains to his medical condition. Then the physician draws on her own experience of similar emotions to communicate an "accurate" empathic understanding of how the patient feels and why he should feel that way. In its most simplistic rendering, this activity is reduced to an "interview skill" that follows from a few didactic rules and the willingness to "take a few minutes" to empathize with a patient or his caregiver.[2]

Almost all commentators agree that empathy, whatever it is, is a good thing indeed. They cite empirical research linking it to more efficient and effective care, to patients who are more trusting of their doctors, more compliant in following instructions, and more satisfied with the outcome of treatment. Patients want doctors who give them not only an appointment time but the time of day, and when they feel better understood, they simply feel better. Furthermore, doctors who are empathic doctor better. They learn more about their patients and, as a result, are better able to fulfill core medical tasks such as history taking, diagnosis, and treatment. Given this medley of benefits, commentators can't help but lament the well-documented decline of empathy—the devaluation of humanistic, patient-centered caregiving among medical students and residents—and to proffer new strategies for reviving it. So they present readers with a host of training exercises, coding schemes, and curricular innovations to help medical students retain the empathy with which they began their medical studies, and also to help overworked, often jaded, residents refind the ability to empathize that has succumbed to medical school and the dehumanizing rigors of specialty training.[3]

It is at this point that empathy-promoting narratives fork off in different directions. Empathy researchers typically opt for a cognitive-behavioral approach to teaching empathy, arguing that if medical educators cannot teach students and residents to feel *with* their patients, they can at least train them to discern what their *patients* feel, to encourage the expression of these feelings, and then to respond in ways that affirm and legitimize the feelings. This interactional approach leads to the creation of various models, step-wise approaches, rating scales, and coding systems, all aimed at cultivating a cognitive skill set that, from the patient's perspective, gives the impression of a caring and emotionally attuned provider. Duly trained in the art of eliciting and affirming emotions, the physician becomes capable of what one theorist terms "skilled interpersonal performances" with patients. Seen thusly, empathic connection becomes a "clinical procedure" that takes the patient's improved psychobiological functioning as its outcome.[4]

The cognitive-behavioral approach is an exercise in what researchers term "communication skills training." It typically parses doctor-patient communication into micro-interactions that can be identified and coded as "empathic opportunities." Teaching students and residents the art of "accurate empathy" amounts to alerting them to these opportunities and showing how their responses (or nonresponses) either exploit or miss them. One research team, in a fit of linguistic inventiveness, tagged the physician's failure to invite the patient to elaborate an emotional state (often followed by a physician-initiated change of subject), an "empathic opportunity terminator." Learning to pick up on subtle, often nonverbal, clues of underlying feeling states and gently prodding patients to own up to emotions are integral to the process. Thus, when patients don't actually express emotion but instead provide a clue that may point to an emotion, the physician's failure to travel down the yellow brick road of masked emotion becomes, more creatively still, a "potential empathic opportunity terminator." Whether protocol-driven questioning about feeling states leads patients to feel truly understood or simply the object of artificial, even artifactual, behaviors has yet to be systematically addressed. Medical researchers ignore the fact that empathy, however "accurate," is not effective unless it is perceived as such by patients.[5]

Medical educators of a humanistic bent take a different fork in the road to empathic caregiving. Shying away from protocols, models, scales, and coding schemes, they embrace a more holistic vision of empathy as growing out of medical training leavened by character-broadening exposure to the humanities. The foremost early proponent of this viewpoint was Howard Spiro, whose article of 1992, "What Is Empathy and Can It Be Taught?" set the tone and tenor for an emerging literature on the role of the humanities in medical training. William Zinn echoed his message a year later: "The humanities deserve to be a part of medical education because they not only provide ethical guidance and improve cognitive skills, but also enrich life experiences in the otherwise cloistered environment of medical school." The epitome of this viewpoint, also published in 1993, was the volume edited by Spiro and his colleagues, *Empathy and the Practice of Medicine*. Over the past 20 years, writers in this tradition have added to the list of nonmedical activities conducive to clinical empathy. According to Halpern, they include "meditation, sharing stories with colleagues, writing about doctoring, reading books, and watching films conveying emotional complexity." Johanna Shapiro, Rita Charon, and their colleagues single out courses in medicine and literature, attendance at theatrical performances, and assignments in "reflective writing" as specific empathy enhancers.[6]

Spiro practiced and taught gastroenterology in New Haven, home of Yale University School of Medicine and the prestigious Western New England Psychoanalytic Institute. One quickly discerns the psychoanalytic influence on his approach. The humanistic grounding he sought for students and residents partakes of this influence, whether in the kind of literature he wanted students to read (i.e., "the new genus of pathography") or in his approach to history taking ("The clues that make the physician aware at the first meeting that a patient is depressed require free-floating attention, as psychoanalysts call it.").

A variant of the "humanist" approach accepts the cognitivist assumption that empathy is a teachable skill but veers away from communications theory and cognitive psychology to delineate it. Instead, it looks to the world of psychotherapy, especially the psychoanalytic self psychology of Heinz Kohut, with which we began chapter 4. Articles about medical empathy that take up Kohut, most of which were published in the 1990s, are replete with psychoanalytic conceptualizations and phraseology; they occasionally reference Kohut himself but more frequently cite work by psychoanalytic self psychologists Michael Basch and Dan Buie, the psychiatrist Leston Havens, and the psychiatrist-anthropologist Arthur Kleinman.

Authors following a psychoanalytic path to empathy assign specific tasks to students, residents, and practicing clinicians, but the tasks are more typically associated with the opening phase of long-term psychotherapy. Clinicians are enjoined to begin in a patiently receptive mode, avoiding the "pitfalls of premature empathy" and realizing that patients "seldom verbalize their emotions directly and spontaneously," instead offering up clues that must be probed and unraveled. Empathic receptiveness helps render more understandable and tolerable "the motivation behind patient behavior that would otherwise seem alien or inappropriate." For Charon, it all begins with what she understands as "narrative competence," the physician's ability to grasp and process the patient's story, which will emerge as a "complicated narrative of illness told in words, gestures, physical findings, and silences and burdened not only with the objective information about the illness but also with the fears, hopes, and implications associated with it."[7]

The physician's ability to follow the patient's "narrative thread," to be moved by it and "in some way" to enter into it—this, for Charon and others allied with humanist psychoanalysis, is tantamount to "empathic engagement." Through "self-monitoring and self-analyzing," the empathic clinician learns to rule out endogenous causes for heightened emotional states and can "begin to understand its source in the patient." In difficult confrontations with angry or upset patients, physicians, no less than psychoanalysts, must cultivate "an ongoing practice of engaged curiosity" that includes systematic self-reflection. Like psychoanalysts, that is, they must learn to analyze their subjective and sometimes inappropriate reactions to patients—their countertransference—for clues about their patients' feelings.[8]

There is a mildly overwrought quality to the medical appropriation of psychoanalysis, as if an analytic sensibility per se—absent lengthy analytic training—can be superadded to the mindset of task-oriented, often harried, residents and clinicians and thereupon imbue them with heightened "empathic accuracy." Enshrining and objectifying "narrative competence" as the sine qua non of empathic doctoring simply begs the question: It ignores the constructed nature of patient stories, which are subject to any number of conventions, such as the patient's desire to tell a "good" story that will please the physician or to graft his or her experience onto a "stock" storyline that is idealized in our culture.[9] Narrative competence cannot be severed from an empathic (or, more plausibly, a sympathetic) willingness to wrestle with the vagaries of patient stories in the first place. Absent a story-listening disposition—which falls back on a measure of inborn or acquired empathy (or again, just sympathy)—a physician is hard-pressed to make therapeutic use of a patient's "story."

Given the tensions among the gently analytic vision of empathic care, the claims of patient autonomy, and the managerial, data-oriented, and evidence-based structure of contemporary practice, one welcomes as a breath of fresh air the recent demurral of Anna Smajdor and her colleagues, who remind us that the development of objectivity, not clinical empathy, "helps doctors to do extraordinary things—not least, cutting into living flesh." Patients, they suggest, really don't want empathic doctors who enter their worlds and feel their pain, only doctors who communicate clearly and treat them with courtesy and a modicum of respect. Indeed, many patients take comfort in knowing that the doctors who see and act on their bodies do not feel with them in the "usual" human way. Subjectivity and empathy may yet have a role in treatment, they allow, but only in specific areas, such as "general practice," in which longer-term relationships may develop.[10]

The problem here is that their claim easily segues into a reductio ad absurdum in which medical care is a zero-sum game in which one must choose between care that is clinically objective and care that is empathic. Withal, Smajdor and her colleagues provide a helpful corrective to the empathy literature, a reminder that, in the words of the bioethicist Edmund Pellegrino, competence and not compassion is the physician's "prime humane precept and the one most peculiar to the physician's function in society." It is difficult to imagine a more passionate champion of compassionate caregiving than Pellegrino, yet it is Pellegrino who cautions that contemporary demands for greater compassion from our doctors "must not obfuscate the centrality of competence in the physicians' existence."[11]

And so the empathy narratives move on. Over the past decade, neuroscientists have invoked empathy as an example of what they term "interpersonal neurobiology," i.e., a neurobiological response to social interaction that activates specific neural networks, probably those networks involving the mirror neuronal system. It may be that empathy derives from an "embodied simulation mechanism" that is neurally grounded and operates outside of consciousness.[12] In all, this growing body of research may alter the framework within which empathy training exercises are understood.

Of course, long before the term "empathy" was used, much less operationalized for educational purposes, and long before "narrative skills" were posited as requisite to meaningful engagement of patients, there were deeply caring, patient-centered physicians who knew how to listen to patients' stories. Medical educators know we cannot go back to their world. No one is calling for a return to Latin and the classics—the world of ancient history and mythology that fostered medical humanism and patient-centeredness throughout the nineteenth century, and was especially important to those pivotal figures who introduced "modern medicine" to America at the turn of the last century.[13] Nor is there any real likelihood that the house call, in all its socializing, humanizing, and even empathy-promoting glory, is going to make a comeback anytime soon, the incentives in the Patient Protection and Affordable Care Act of 2010 notwithstanding.

So contemporary researchers will continue to devise new, often discordant, approaches to empathy training, absent any real evidence that such exercises have durable results and actually make physicians more caring and patient-centered than they would otherwise be. Placing empathy training, literary reading groups, and "reflective" writing workshops to the side, are there more general strategies of humanistic renewal that medical educators can direct us to? Are there implementable precepts that can help medical students and residents doctor more effectively and more humanely? Perhaps so.

II.

Medical educators certainly have their differences, but one still discerns an emerging consensus about the kind of changes that will improve health care delivery and simultaneously re-humanize physician-patient encounters. Here we summarize several of the most progressive trends in medical education in order to underscore all that can be done to create caring physicians without the strained, if not despairing, effort to "teach" them to be empathic.

Contemporary medical training stresses the importance of teamwork and militates against the traditional narcissistic investment in solo expertise. Teamwork, which relies on the contributions of nonphysician mid-level providers such as physician assistants and nurse practitioners, works against the legacy of socialization that, for many generations, rendered physicians "unfit" for teamwork. The trend now is to re-vision training so that the physician becomes fit for a new kind of collaborative endeavor. It is teamwork, when all is said and done, that "transfers the bulk of our work from the realm of guesswork and conjecture to one in which certainty and exactitude may be at least approached."

Must group practice militate against personalized care? Perhaps not. Recently, medical groups large and small have been enjoined to remember that "a considerable proportion of the physician's work is not the practice of medicine at all. It consists of counseling, orienting, extricating, encouraging, solacing, sympathizing, understanding."

Contemporary medical training understands that the patient him- or herself has become, and by rights ought to be, a member of the health care team. Medical educators ceded long ago that patients, in their own best interests, "should know something about the human body." Now we have more concrete expressions of this requirement, to wit, that if more adequate teaching of anatomy and physiology were provided in secondary schools, "physicians will profit and patients will prosper." "Just because a man is ill," notes one educator, "is no reason why he should stop using his mind, especially as he [i.e., the patient] is the important factor in the solution of his problem, not the doctor."

For many contemporary educators the knowledgeable patient is not only a member of the "team," but the physician's bona fide collaborator. They assume, that is, that physician and patient "will be able to work together intelligently." Working together intelligently suggests a "frank cooperation" in which physician and patient alike have "free access to all outside sources of help and expert knowledge." Of course the Internet, for better and worse, is the great equalizer when it comes to free access to such knowledge. Working together also means recognizing, without prejudice or personal affront, that the patient's "inalienable right is to consult as many physicians as he chooses." Even today, one educator observes, "doctors have too much property interest in their patients," despite the fact that patients find their pronouncements something less than, shall we say, "oracular." Contemporary training inherits the mantle of the patient rights revolution of the 1970s and '80s. Educators today recognize that "It is the patient who must decide the validity of opinion from consideration of its source and probability." Another speaks for many in reiterating that

> If the doctor's opinion does not seem reasonable, or if the bias of it, due to temperament or personal and professional experience is obvious, then it is well for the patient to get another opinion, and the doctor has no right to be incensed or humiliated by such action.

Contemporary medical training stresses the importance of primary care values that are lineal descendants of old-style general practice. This trend grows out of the realization that a physician "can take care of a patient without caring for him," that the man or woman publicly considered a "good doctor" is invariably the doctor who will "find something in a sick person that aroused his sympathy, excited his admiration, or moved his compassion." If empathy exercises can help physicians locate this "something" and use it to mobilize their sympathy for the patient, then I am all for them.

Optimally—and here we find a more original suggestion— multispecialty and subspecialty groups might retain their own patient-centered generalists—call them, perhaps, "therapeutists"—to provide integrative patient care beyond diagnostic problem-solving and even beyond the conventional treatment modalities of the group. Such doctors would be analogous to contemporary hospitalists, internists who work entirely in hospitals, where they assume monitoring, evaluative, and coordinating roles. The group-based therapeutist, while trained in the root specialty of his colleagues, would also have specialized knowledge of alternative treatments outside the specialty. He would, for example, supplement familiarity with mainstream drug therapies with a whole-patient, one might say a "wholesome," distrust of drugs.

Contemporary training recognizes the importance of first-hand experience of illness in inculcating the values that make for "good doctoring." Indeed, innovative curricula now land medical students in the emergency rooms and clinics with (feigned) symptoms and histories that invite discomfiting and sometimes lengthy interventions. Why has it taken educators so long to enlarge the curriculum in this humanizing manner? If, as one educator notes, "It is too much to ask of a physician that he himself should have had an enigmatic illness," it should still be a guiding heuristic that "any illness makes him a better doctor." Another adds: "It is said that an ill doctor is a pathetic sight; but one who has been ill and has recovered has had an affective experience which he can utilize to the advantage of his patients."

The affective side of a personal illness experience may entail first-hand experience of medicine's dehumanizing "hidden curriculum." Fortunate the patient whose physician has undergone his or her own medical odyssey, so that life experience vivifies the commonplace reported by one seriously ill provider: "I felt I had not been treated like a human being." A physician-writer who experienced obscure, long-term infectious illness early in his career and was shunted from consultant to consultant understands far better than healthy colleagues that physicians "are so prone to occupy themselves with the theoretical requirements of a case that they lose sight entirely of the human being and his life story." Here is the painful reminiscence of another ill physician of more literary bent:

> There had been no inquiry of plans or prospects, no solicitude for ambitions or desires, no interest in the spirit of the man whose engine was signaling for gas and oil. That day I determined never to sentence a person on sight, for life or to death.

Contemporary medical training increasingly recognizes that all medicine is, to one degree or another, psychological medicine. Clinical opinions, educators remind us, can be truthful but still contoured to the personality, especially the psychological needs, of the patient. Sad to say, the best clinical educators are those who know colleagues, whatever their specialty, who either "do not appreciate that constituent of personality which psychologists call the affects . . . and the importance of the role which these affects or emotions play in conditioning [the patient's] destiny, well or ill, or they refuse to be taught by observation and experience."

This realization segues into the role of psychiatric training in medical education, certainly for physicians engaged in primary care, but really for all physicians. Among other things, such training "would teach him [or her] that disease cannot be standardized, that the individual must be considered first, then the disease." Even among patients with typical illnesses, psychiatric training can help physicians understand idiosyncratic reactions to standard treatment protocols. It aids comprehension of the individual "who happens to have a very common disease in his own very personal manner." The fact that contemporary primary care physicians no longer have the time or inclination to practice office psychotherapy does not mean they cannot be sensitized during residency to the psychodynamic dimension of primary care, including the act of prescribing psychotropic drugs. They might learn, for example, about the various psychodynamic meanings of drug use and their relationship to patient compliance.[14]

III.

These trends encapsulate the reflections and recommendations of progressive medical educators who are responsive to the public demand for more patient-centered caregiving but envision pathways to this goal outside of formal empathy training. The trends are also responsive to the mounting burnout of physicians—especially primary care physicians—who, in the cost-conscious, productivity-driven, and regulatory climate of our time, find it harder than ever to practice patient-centered medicine. But are these trends really so contemporary? I confess to a deception. The foregoing paraphrases, quotations, and recommendations are not from contemporary educators at all. They are culled from the popular essays of a single physician, the pioneer neurologist Joseph Collins, all of which were published in *Harper's Monthly* between 1924 and 1929.[15]

Collins is a fascinating figure. An 1888 graduate of New York University Medical College, he attended medical school and began his practice burdened with serious, sometimes debilitating, pulmonary and abdominal symptoms that had him run the gauntlet of consultant diagnoses—pneumonia, pulmonary tuberculosis, "tuberculosis of the kidney," chronic appendicitis, even brain tumor. None of these authoritative pronouncements was on the mark, but taken together they left Collins highly critical of his own profession and pushed him in the direction of holistic, collaborative, patient-centered medicine. After an extended period of general practice, he segued into the emerging specialty of neurology (then termed neuropsychiatry) and, with his colleagues Joseph Fraenkel and Pearce Bailey, founded in 1909 the first specialty hospital for disorders of the nervous system, the New York Neurological Institute.[16] Collins was chief of the First Division of the hospital and executive officer of the institute, but his career as a neurologist never dislodged his commitment to generalist patient-centered care. Indeed, the neurologist, as he understood the specialty in 1911, was the generalist best suited to treat chronic disease of any sort.[17]

Collins's colorful, multifaceted career as a popular medical writer and literary critic is beyond the scope of this chapter.[18] I invoke him here to circle back to a cardinal point: "Patient-centered/relationship-centered care," humanistic medicine, narrative medicine, empathic caregiving, physician acceptance of patients' rights—these additives to the medical school curriculum are as old as they are new. What is new is the relatively recent effort to cultivate such sensibilities through curricular innovations. Taken together, public health, preventive medicine, childhood vaccination, and modern antibiotic therapy have (mercifully) cut short the kind of experiential journey that for Collins secured the humanistic moorings of the biomedical imperative. Now, as we have observed, medical educators rely, inter alia, on communication skills training, empathy-promoting protocols, core-skills workshops, and seminars on "The Healer's Art" to close the circle, rescue medical students from evidence-based and protocol-driven overkill, and bring them back in line with Collins's hard-won precepts.

It is not quite right to observe that these precepts apply equally to Collins's time and our own. They give expression to the caregiving impulse, to the ancient injunction to cure through caring, that in all its ebb and flow, whether as figure or ground, weaves through the fabric of medical history writ large. Listen to Collins one final time as he expounds his philosophy of practice in 1926:

> It would be a wise thing to devote a part of medical education to the mind of the physician himself, especially as it concerns his patients. For the glories of medical history are the humanized physicians. Science will always fall short; but compassion covereth all.[19]

CHAPTER 6

Medical Tools and Medical Touch

The plethora of tests available to the young clinician has significantly eroded the skills necessary to obtain adequate histories and careful physical examinations. Day in and day out, I encounter egregious examples of misdiagnosis engendered by inadequacies in these skills.

—William Silen, M.D., "The Case for Paying Closer Attention to Our Patients" (1996)

"Treat the Patient, Not the CT Scan," adjures Abraham Verghese in a *New York Times* op-ed piece of February 26, 2011. Verghese targets American medicine's overreliance on imaging tests, but, like others before him, he is really addressing the mindset that fosters such overreliance. Preclinical medical students, he reminds us, all learn physical examination and diagnosis, but their introduction to the art dissipates under the weight of diagnostic tests and specialist procedures during their clinical years. "Then," he writes, "they discover that the currency on the ward seems to be 'throughput'—getting tests ordered and getting results, having procedures like colonoscopies done expeditiously, calling in specialists, arranging discharge." In the early 1990s, William Silen, Harvard's Johnson and Johnson Distinguished Professor of Surgery, Emeritus,[1] made the same point with greater verve. In one of his wonderful unpublished pieces, "Lumps and Bumps," he remarked that "the modern medical student, and most physicians, have been so far removed from physical diagnosis, that they simply do not accept that a mass is a mass is a mass unless the CT scan or ultrasound tells them it is there."

Verghese and Silen get no argument from me on the clinical limitations and human failings associated with technology-driven medicine. But these concerns are hardly unique to an era of CT scans and MRIs. There is a long history of concern about overreliance on new technologies; Silen has a delightfully pithy, unpublished piece on the topic that is simply titled "New Toys."

One limitation of such critiques is the failure to recognize that all "toys" are not created equal. Some new toys become old toys, at which point they cease being toys altogether and simply become part of the armamentarium that the physician brings to the task of physical examination and diagnosis. For example, we have long since stopped thinking of x-ray units, EKG machines, blood pressure meters (i.e., sphygmomanometers), and stethoscopes as "new toys" that militate against the acquisition of hands-on clinical skill.

But it was not always so. When x-rays became available in 1896, clinical surgeons were aghast. What kind of images were *these*? Surely not photographic images in the reliably objectivistic late-nineteenth-century sense of the term. The images were wavy, blurry, and imprecise, vulnerable to changes in the relative location of the camera, the x-ray tube, and the object under investigation. There was nothing objective about them; what exactly they represented was clear neither to physicians nor jurists. That such monstrously opaque images might count as illustrative evidence in courts of law, that they might actually be turned against the surgeon and his "expert opinion"—what was the world coming to?[2] Military surgeons quickly saw the usefulness of x-rays for locating bullets and shrapnel, but their civilian colleagues remained suspicious of the new technology for a decade or more after its invention. No fools, they resorted to x-rays only when threatened by malpractice suits.

Well before the unsettling advent of x-ray photography, post-Civil War physician-educators were greatly concerned about the use of mechanical pulse-reading instruments. These ingenious devices, so they held, would discourage young physicians from learning to appreciate the subtle diagnostic indicators embedded in the pulse. And absent such appreciation, which came only from prolonged training of their fingertips, they could never acquire the diagnostic acumen of their seniors, much less of the great pulse readers of the day. Thus they cautioned students and young colleagues to avoid the instruments. It was only through "the habit of discriminating pulses instinctively" that the physician acquired "valuable truths . . . which he can apply to practice." So inveighed the pioneering British physiologist John Burdon-Sanderson in 1867. His judgment was shared by a generation of senior British and American clinicians for whom the trained finger remained a more reliable measure of radial pulse than the sphygmograph's arcane tracings. In *The Pulse*, his manual of 1890, William Broadbent cautioned his readers to avoid the sphygmograph entirely, since interpretation of its tracings could "twist facts in the desired direction." Physicians should "eschew instrumental aids and educate the finger," echoed Graham Steell in *The Use of the Sphygmograph in Medicine* at the century's close.[3]

Lower still on the totem pole of medical technology, indeed about as low down as one can get—is the stethoscope, "invented" by René Laennec in 1816 and first employed by him in the wards of Paris's Hôpital Necker. In 1898, James Mackenzie, the founder of modern cardiology, relied on the stethoscope, used in conjunction with his own refinement of the Dudgeon sphygmograph of 1881 (i.e., the Mackenzie polygraph of 1892), to identify the fast, irregular beating of the heart's two upper chambers, what we now term atrial fibrillation. In the years to follow, Mackenzie, a master of instrumentation, became the principal exponent of what historians refer to as the "new cardiology." His "New Methods of Studying Affections of the Heart," a series of articles published in the *British Medical Journal* in 1905, signaled a revolution in understanding cardiac function.[4] "No man," remarked his first biographer, R. McNair Wilson, in 1926, "ever used a stethoscope with a higher degree of expertness." And yet this same Mackenzie lambasted the stethoscope as the instrument that had "not only for one hundred years hampered the progress of knowledge of heart affections, but had done more harm than good, in that many people had had the tenor of their lives altered, had been forbidden to undertake duties for which they were perfectly competent, and had been subject to unnecessary treatment because of its findings."[5]

Why did Mackenzie come to feel this way? The problem with the stethoscope was that the auscultatory sounds it made audible, while diagnostically illuminating, could cloud clinical judgment and lead to unnecessary treatments, including draconian restrictions of lifestyle. Similarly, for Mackenzie sphygmomanometers were essentially educational aids that would corroborate what medical students were learning to discern through their senses, in this case through their trained fingertips. And, of course, he allowed for the importance of such gadgetry in research. His final refinement of pulse-reading instrumentation, the Mackenzie ink jet polygraph of 1902, was just such a tool. But it was never intended for generalists, whose education of the senses was expected to be adequate to the meaning of heart sounds. Nor was Mackenzie a fan of the EKG, when it found its way into hospitals after 1905. He perceived it as yet another new toy that provided no more diagnostic information than the stethoscope and ink jet polygraph. And for at least the first 15 years of the machine's use, he was right.

Lest we dismiss such instrumental skepticism as a relic of the nineteenth century, it bears remembering that as late as 1949, the eminent cardiologist Samuel Levine belittled the EKG by remarking that "The greater the time spent in taking three electrocardiographic leads and later nine and now twelve leads, the less time is left to elicit an adequate history of the case or to auscultate the heart properly."[6] And nearly two decades later, Alvan Feinstein, in his opus, *Clinical Judgment*, took issue with the usefulness of the phonocardiograph, a massive machine that, in conjunction with highly sensitive crystal microphones placed on the patient's chest, could "hear" and graphically record via a writing stylus faint heart sounds inaudible to the stethoscope and too subtle to appear on an EKG readout.

Despite the advances made through phonocardiography since the mid-1930s—the sequencing of heart sounds, the understanding of the "splitting of sounds" during what clinicians term the second heart sound (S_2), and the interpretation of a number of previously inaudible heart murmurs[7]—Feinstein questioned the accuracy of a device that converted sound to sight. Yes, he acknowledged, the phonocardiograph was a boon to the timing of noises, but its graphic tracings omitted the high-frequency sounds of heart murmurs, so that its graphic tracings might "falsify the actual intensity, duration, and timing of the murmur." Further, he held, the tracings were subject to electric cancellations that produced the "visual illusion" of no heart sounds in the face of what clinicians clearly heard through their stethoscopes. "For the sensory perceptions of quality and of certain other critical properties of noises," he concluded, "a clinician is thus often better than inanimate devices. Moreover, he and his stethoscope are always portable, and constantly available."[8] It is John Burdon-Sanderson, William Broadbent, and James Mackenzie all over again.

In point of fact, Feinstein's concerns typified a mechanical era in which interpretations of subtle physiological processes were limited by the recording technologies then available. The limitations of phonocardiographic tracings were occasionally remarked on in literature of the 1940s and 1950s, but, by the 1960s, primitive "oscilloscopic" phonocardiography that recorded the intensity of heart sounds had given way to "spectral" phonocardiography that displayed the frequency scale of these sounds, so Feinstein's concerns were of little moment by the time of his writing.[9] Now, in the era of twenty-first-century digital technology, his defense of the naked ear has an antique ring. Engineers are currently at work on a way for doctors to place their mobile phones on a patient's chest and record a high-fidelity display of heart sounds. If they succeed, "it will revolutionize the physical exam and perhaps make auscultation obsolete."[10] Even as matters stand, visual images of heart sounds have taken the lead: They guide medical students and physicians back to the bedside to see if they can hear and appreciate what they have already seen.

Now, of course, the stethoscope, the sphygmomanometer, and, for adults of a certain age, the EKG machine are integral to the devalued art of physical examination. Digitized phonocardiographic phone apps may soon render the stethoscope itself a minor adjunct to physical examination, no longer shoved into white jackets and draped around the necks of students, residents, and nurses.[11]

Critics who bemoan the overuse of CT scans and MRIs, of echocardiography and angiography, would be happy indeed if medical students and residents spent more time examining patients and learning all that can be learned from stethoscopes, blood pressure monitoring,

baseline EKGs, and phonocardiographs. But at the time of their introduction these instrumental prerequisites of physical examination and
diagnosis were themselves new toys, and educators were wary of what
medical students would lose by relying on them at the expense of educating their senses. Now educators worry about what students lose by
not relying on them, though, with the venerable stethoscope, we may
be at the point of closing the circle. "I value my stethoscope highly,"
wrote the Baylor University cardiologist Robert Rosenthal in 2013,
"but if the phonocardiogram had been invented before the stethoscope, I believe the stethoscope, when it came along, would have been
regarded as no more than a curiosity—a cardiac party toy—no longer
carried in our jacket pockets."[12] Indeed.

Toys aside, I too hope those elements of physical diagnosis that fall
back on one tool of exquisite sensitivity—the human hand—will not
be lost among reams of lab results and diagnostic studies. As unhappy
as one might be at the eclipsing of the trained clinical ear, one shud-
ders at the thought of a clinical medicine utterly bereft of the laying
on of hands, which is not only an instrument of diagnosis but an
amplifier of therapy. The great pulse readers of the late nineteenth
century are long gone and of interest only to a handful of medical historians. Will the same be true, a century hence, of the great palpators
of the late twentieth?

II.

We are back to the laying on of hands, to all that we feel when
our doctors and nurses touch us. Etymologically, the word "touch"
(from the old French *touchier*) is a semantic cornucopia. In English,
of course, common usage embraces dual meanings. We make tactile
contact and we receive emotional contact. The latter meaning is usually passively rendered, in the manner of receiving a gift: We are the
beneficiary of someone else's emotional offering; we are "touched"
by a person's words, gestures, or deeds. Sometimes a single expression embraces the duality: We can be "out of touch" with another in
either communicative or psychological ways. The former typically has
a spatial or temporal component; the latter a strong, here-and-now
emotional valence.

The duality extends to the realm of health care: As patients, we are touched physically by our physicians (or other providers) but, if we are fortunate, we are also touched emotionally by their kindness, concern, empathy, even love. Here the two kinds of touching are complementary. We are examined and often experience a measure of contact comfort through the touch. Then, hopefully, we are comforted by the physician's sympathetic words; we are touched by the human contact that grows out of physical touch. The sympathy is informed by authority; we are especially looking for the reassurance that derives from authoritative touch.

For nurses, caregiving as touching and being touched has been central to professional identity. The foundations of nursing as a modern profession were laid down on the battlefields of Crimea and the American South during the mid-nineteenth century. Crimean and Civil War nurses could not "treat" their patients, but they "touched" them literally and figuratively and, in so doing, individualized their suffering. Their nursing touch was amplified by the caring impulse of mothers: They listened to soldiers' stories, sought to keep them warm and especially to nourish them, struggling to pry their food parcels away from corrupt medical officers. In the process, they formulated a professional ethos that, in privileging patient care over hospital protocol, was anathema to the kind of professionalism associated with male medical authority.[13]

This alternative, comfort-based vision of professional care is one reason that nursing literature is more nuanced than medical literature in exploring the phenomenology and dynamic meanings of touch.[14] It has fallen to nursing researchers to isolate and appraise the tactile components of touch (such as duration, location, intensity, and sensation) and also to differentiate between comforting touch (also referred to as caring touch and expressive touch) and the touch associated with performing procedures, i.e., procedural or instrumental touch.[15] We must look to this literature for studies that survey patient reactions to comforting touch of different parts of the body and examine the various patient, nurse, and contextual (e.g., work environment, work stress level, nurse-patient relationship) variables that influence patients' experience of touch.[16]

Buttressing the phenomenological viewpoint of Husserl and Merleau-Ponty with recent neurophysiologic research, Catherine Green has recently argued that nurse-patient interaction, with its "heavily tactile component," promotes an experiential oneness: It "plunges the nurse into the patient's situation in a direct and immediate way." To touch, she reminds us, is simultaneously to be touched, so that the nurse's soothing touch not only promotes deep empathy of the patient's plight but actually "constitutes" the nurse herself (or himself) in her (or his) very personhood.[17] Other nurse researchers have questioned the inter-subjective convergence of touching and being touched presumed by Green. A survey of hospitalized patients, for example, documents that some patients are ambivalent toward the nurse's touch, since for them it signifies not only care but also control. More generally, according to the anthropologist Susan Christine Edwards, hospitalized patients' expectation of being touched may be attributed to the depersonaliza-tion and subordination associated with hospitalization. So the com-forting intention of nursing touch, usually welcome and appreciated, may not always correspond with touch as experienced by the patient. It follows that hospital nurses must be aware of cultural differences in attitudes toward touch and learn to pick up clues, both verbal and nonverbal, that an individual patient is receptive or aversive to inti-mate nursing touch.[18]

After World War II, the rise of sophisticated monitoring equipment in hospitals pulled American nursing away from the hands-on, one-on-one bedside nursing that revolved around touch. By the 1960s, hospital nurses, no less than physicians, were "proceduralists" who relied on cardiac and vital function monitors, electronic fetal moni-tors, and the like for "data" on the patients they "nursed." They moni-tored the monitors and, for educators critical of this turn of events, especially psychiatric nurses, they had become little more than moni-tors themselves.

As the historian Margarete Sandelowski has elaborated, this trans-formation of hospital nursing had both an upside and a downside. It elevated the status of nurses by aligning them with postwar scientific medicine in its blossoming technological power. Nurses, the skilled human monitors of the machines, were key players on whom hospital-ized patients and their physicians increasingly relied. In the hospital setting, they became "middle managers,"[19] with command author-ity of their wards. They had an administrative power and a claim to respect far removed from the directive to touch and power to comfort of their premonitoring forbears.

Those nurses with specialized skills—especially those who worked in the newly established intensive care units (ICUs)—were at the top of the nursing pecking order. They were the most medical of the nurses, trained to diagnose and treat life-threatening conditions as they arose. As such, they achieved a new collegial status with physicians, the limits of which were all too clear. Yes, physicians relied on nurses (and often learned from them) in the use of the new machines, but they simultaneously demeaned the "practical knowledge" that nurses acquired in the service of advanced technology—as if educating and reassuring patients about the purpose of the machines; maintaining them (and recommending improvements to manufacturers); and utilizing them without medical supervision was something any minimally intelligent person could do.

A special predicament of nursing concerns the impact of monitoring and proceduralism on a profession whose historical raison d'être was hands-on caring, first on the battlefields and then at the bedside. Self-evidently, nurses with advanced procedural skills had to relinquish that most traditional of nursing functions: the laying on of hands. Consider hospital-based nurses who worked full time as x-ray technicians and microscopists in the early 1900s; who, beginning in the 1930s, monitored polio patients in their iron lungs; who, in the decades following World War II, performed venipuncture as full-time IV therapists; and who, beginning in the 1960s, diagnosed and treated life-threatening conditions in the machine-driven ICUs. Consider as well obstetrical nurses who, beginning in the late 1960s, relied on electronic fetal monitors to gauge the progress of labor and who, on detecting "nonreassuring" fetal heart rate patterns, initiated oxygen therapy or terminated oxytocin infusions without physician oversight. These "modern" OB nurses were worlds removed from their pre-1940s forebears, who monitored labor with their hands and eyes in the patient's own home. Nursing educators grew concerned that, with the growing reliance on electronic monitoring, OB nurses were "literally and figuratively 'losing touch' with laboring women."[20]

Nor did the dilemma for nurses end with the pull of machine-age monitoring away from what nursing educators have long construed

as "true nursing." It pertained equally to the compensatory efforts to
restore the personal touch to nursing in the 1970s and '80s. This is
because "true nursing," as understood by Florence Nightingale and
successive generations of twentieth-century nursing educators, fell
back on gendered touching; to nurse truly and well was to deploy the
feminine touch of caring women. This was the touch of the mother-
ing nurses of the Crimean and American Civil Wars, and this was the
touch celebrated and embellished in the first nurse training schools of
the 1870s.

If "losing touch" through technology was the price paid for elevated status in the hospital, then restoring touch brought with it the
re-gendering (and hence devaluing) of the nurse's charge: She was,
when all was said and done, the womanly helpmate of physicians,
those masculine (or masculinized) gatekeepers of scientific medicine
in all its curative glory.[21] And yet, in the matter of touching and being
touched, gender takes us only so far. What then of male nurses, who,
despite persistent stereotypes that sexualize male touch, insist on the
synergy of masculinity, caring, and touch?[22] Is their touch ipso facto
deficient in some essential ingredient of true nursing?

As soon as we enter the realm of soothing touch, with its attendant
psychological meanings, we encounter a number of binaries. Each pole
of a binary is a construct, an example of what the sociologist Max Weber
termed an "ideal type." The question-promoting, if not questionable,
nature of these constructs only increases their heuristic value. They give
us something to think about. So we have "feminine" and "masculine"
touch, as noted above. But we also have the nurse's touch and, at the
other pole, the physician's touch. In the gendered world of many feminist writers, this binary replicates the gender divide, despite the historical and contemporary reality of women physicians and male nurses.

But the binary extends to women physicians themselves. In their
efforts to gain entry to the world of male American medicine, female
medical pioneers adopted two radically different strategies. At one
pole, we have the touch-comfort-sympathy approach of Elizabeth
Blackwell, which assigned women their own feminized domain of
practice (child care, nonsurgical obstetrics and gynecology, womanly
counseling on matters of sanitation, hygiene, and prevention). At the
opposite pole we have the research-oriented, scientific approach of

Mary Putnam Jacobi and Marie Zakrezewska, which held that women physicians must be physicians in any and all respects. Only with state-of-the-art training in the medical science (e.g., bacteriology) and treatments (e.g., ovariotomy) of the day, they held, would women docs achieve what they deserved: full parity with medical men. The binary of female physicians as extenders of women's "natural sphere" versus female physicians as physicians pure and simple runs through the second half of the nineteenth century.[23]

Within medicine, we can perhaps speak of the generalist touch (analogous to the generalist gaze[24]) that can be juxtaposed with the specialist touch. Medical technology, especially tools that amplify the physician's senses, invites another binary. There is the pole of direct touch and the pole of touch mediated by instrumentation. This binary spans the divide between "direct auscultation," with the physician's ear on the patient's chest, and "mediate auscultation," with the stethoscope linking, and for some nineteenth-century patients coming between, the physician's ear and the patient's chest.

Broader than any of the foregoing is the binary that pushes beyond the framework of comfort care per se. Consider it a meta-binary. At one pole is *therapeutic touch* (TT), whose premise of a preternatural human energy field subject to disturbance and hands-on (or hands-near) remediation is nothing if not a recrudescence of Anton Mesmer's "vital magnetism" of the late eighteenth century, with the TT therapist, usually a nurse, taking the role of Mesmer's *magnétiseur*.[25] At the opposite pole is *transgressive touch*. This is the pole of *boundary violations*, typically, though not invariably, associated with touch-free specialties such as psychiatry and psychoanalysis.[26] Transgressive touch signifies inappropriately intimate, usually sexualized, touch that violates the boundaries of professional caring and results in the patient's dis-comfort and dis-ease, sometimes to the point of leaving the patient traumatized, i.e., "touched in the head." It also signifies the psychological impairment of the therapist who, in another etymologically just sense of the term, may be "touched," given his or her gross inability to maintain a professional treatment relationship.

These binaries invite further scrutiny, less on account of the extremes than of the shades of grayness that span each continuum. Exploration of touch is a messy business, a hands-on business, a psycho-physical business. It may yield important insights but perhaps only fitfully, in the manner of—to invoke a meaning that arose in the early nineteenth century—touch and go.

III.

But, in the matter of caring, what about medical tools? Is there a binary within the realm of medical technology that embraces the experiential dimension of tool use by doctors and nurses? Is there a feeling-tone associated with the touch of an instrument? Can we perceive the instruments as caring for us?

The critique of contemporary medical treatment as impersonal, uncaring, and disease-focused suggests there is no binary at all, since dehumanization, or at least the threat of it, seems to inhere in what we think of as "high" technology. The problem is that high technology, historically speaking, is a moving target. In the England of the 1730s, obstetrical forceps were the high technology of the day; William Smellie, London's leading obstetrical physician, opposed their use for more than a decade, despite compelling evidence that the technology revolutionized childbirth by permitting obstructed births—fetuses who became wedged into the birth canal during labor—to become live births.[27]

For much of the nineteenth century, as we have observed, stethoscopes and sphygmomanometers (blood pressure meters) were considered technological contrivances that distanced the doctor from the patient. For any number of Victorian patients (and doctors too), the kindly ear against the chest and the trained finger on the wrist helped make the physical examination an essentially human encounter. Interpose instruments between the physician and the patient and, ipso facto, you distance the one from the other. In late-nineteenth-century Britain, "experimental" or "laboratory" medicine was itself a revolutionary technology, and it elicited bitter denunciation from antivivisectionists (among whom were physicians) that foreshadows contemporary indictments of the "hypertrophied scientism" of modern medicine.[28] Late nineteenth-century defenders of new instruments, like the Philadelphia neurologist S. Weir Mitchell, lauded the increase in precise measurement and diagnostic accuracy they made possible.[29] But critics thought the cost of such accuracy might be too high. We might well end up with a generation of physicians whose atrophied senses left them unable to connect with patients as people, to touch them in both senses of the term.

The concerns of nineteenth-century clinicians about high technology blossomed in the early twentieth century, when diagnostic technologies (urinalysis, blood studies, x-rays, EKGs) multiplied and their use switched to hospital settings. Older pediatricians opposed the use of the newfangled incubators for premature newborns. They not only had faulty ventilation that deprived infants of fresh air but were a wasteful expenditure, given that preemies of the working classes were never brought to the hospital immediately after birth, when the incubator might have done some good.[30] Cautionary words were always at hand for the younger generation given to the latest gadgetry. At the dedication of Yale's Sterling Hall of Medicine, the neurosurgeon Harvey Cushing extolled family physicians as exemplars of his gospel of observation and deduction and urged Yale students to engage in actual "house-to-house practice" without the benefit of "all of the paraphernalia and instruments of precision supposed to be necessary for a diagnosis." This was in 1925.[31]

Concerns about the impact of technology on doctor-patient relationships blossomed again in the 1960s and '70s and played a role in the rebirth of primary care medicine in the guise of the "family practice movement." Reading the papers of the recently deceased G. Gayle Stephens, written at the time and collected in his volume *The Intellectual Basis of Family Practice* (1982), is a strong reminder of the risks attendant to loading high technology with relational meaning. Stephens, an architect of the new structure of primary care training in America, saw the "generalist role in medicine" as an aspect of 1970s counterculture that questioned an "unconditional faith in science" that extended to medical training, practice, and values. And so he aligned the family practice movement with other social movements of the '70s that sought to put the brakes on scientism run rampant: agrarianism, utopianism, humanism, consumerism, and feminism. With its clinical focus on the whole person and liberal borrowings from psychiatry and the behavioral sciences, family practice set out to liberate medicine from its "captivity" to a flawed view of reality that was mechanistic, protoplasmic, and molecular.[32]

Technology was deeply implicated in Stephens's critique, even though he failed to stipulate which technologies he had in mind. His was a global indictment: Medicine's obsession with its "technological legerdemain" blinded the physician to the rich phenomenology of "dis-ease" and, as such, was anti-Hippocratic. He meant that reliance on technology pulled physicians away from a Hippocratic sensibility, a commitment to a healing art characterized by close observation, cautiously administered therapeutics, high ethics, humility, and comportment "in a godly manner"—in all the elements of the oath devised by the Greek physician Hippocrates (or perhaps one of his students) more than four centuries before the birth of Christ. To this very day a modernized version of the oath is taken by newly minted physicians as part of their medical school graduation ceremony.

For Stephens, the "mechanical appurtenances of healing" had to be differentiated from the "essential ingredient" of the healing process that pulled together Hippocrates's interlacing precepts, namely, "a physician who really cares about the patient." "We have reached a point of diminishing returns in the effectiveness of technology to improve the total health of our nation." So he opined in 1973, only two years after the first crude CT scanner was demonstrated in London and long before the development of MRIs and PET scans, of angioplasty with stents, and of the broad array of laser- and computer-assisted operations available to contemporary surgeons.[33] Entire domains of technologically guided intervention—consider technologies of blood and marrow transplantation and medical genetics—barely existed in the early '70s. Robotics was the stuff of science fiction.

It is easy to sympathize with both Stephens's critique and his mounting skepticism about the family practice movement's ability to realize its goals.[34] He placed the movement on an ideological battleground in which the combatants were of unequal strength and numbers. There was the family practice counterculture, with the guiding belief that "something genuine and vital occurs in the meeting of doctor and patient" and the pedagogical correlate that "A preoccupation with a disease instead of a person is detrimental to good medicine." And then there were the forces of organized medicine, of medical schools, of turf-protecting internists and surgeons, of hospitals with their "business-industrial models" of health care delivery, of specialization and of technology—all bound together by a cultural commitment to science and its "reductionist hypothesis about the nature of reality."[35] In 1981 he looked back at the struggles of the preceding decade with bitter disappointment. Commenting specifically on the American College of Surgeons' efforts to keep FPs out of hospital operating rooms, he wrote of "issues of political hegemony masquerading as quality of patient care, medicolegal issues disguised as professional qualifications, and economic wolves in the sheepskins of guardians of the public safety."[36]

Perceptive and humane as Stephens's critique was, it fell back on the very sort of reductionism he imputed to the opponents of family practice. Again and again, he juxtaposed "high technology," in all its allure (and allegedly diminishing returns), with the humanistic goals of patient care. So did the Canadian family medicine educator Ian McWhinney, for whom the "objective knowledge" produced by medical technology cultivated an obsession with "unnecessary precision" that militated against understanding the patient as a person.[37] But are technology and humane patient care really so antipodal? Technology in and of itself has no ontological status within medicine. It promotes neither a mechanistic worldview that precludes holistic understanding of patients as people nor a humanizing of the doctor-patient encounter. In fact, technology is utterly neutral with respect to the values that inform medical practice and shape individual doctor-patient relationships. Technology does not make (or unmake) the doctor. It no doubt affects the physician's choice of specialty, pulling those who lack doctoring instincts or people skills in problem-solving directions (think diagnostic radiology or pathology). But this is hardly a bad thing.

For Stephens, who struggled to formulate an "intellectual" defense of family practice as a new medical discipline,[38] technology was an easy target. Infusing the nascent behavioral medicine of his day with a liberal dose of sociology and psychoanalysis, he envisioned the family practice movement as a vehicle for recapturing "diseases of the self" through dialogue.[39] To the extent that technology—whose very existence all but guaranteed its overuse—supplanted the sensibility and associated communicational skills that enabled such dialogue, it was ipso facto part of the problem. McWhinney went even further. Reliance on technology, he held, marginalized the subjective knowledge at the very heart of clinical understanding. Teetering at the brink of the Galenic doctoring of antebellum America, when doctors often supplemented their bleedings, purgatives, and emetics with regimens tailored to the lifestyle of the individual patient, he held that "The physician's response to cues and his formulation of hypotheses are highly subjective processes which defy rational explanation. So individual are patients' problems and so personal are clinical styles that, although they may follow general rules, no two clinicians will solve a problem in exactly the same way."[40]

Now there is no question that overreliance on technology, teamed with epistemic assurance that technology invariably determines what is best, can make a mess of things, interpersonally speaking. Late-nineteenth-century physicians who dismissed hypertension (high blood pressure) as a "sphygmomanometric disease," an artifact of instrument-generated numbers that could distort diagnosis, experienced this mess in nascent form.[41] So did early-twentieth-century cardiologists, who "saw" abnormal patterns on their early EKG machines but were hard-pressed to understand which such patterns were clinically significant and justified changes in the patient's lifestyle.

But is the problem with the technology or with the human beings who use it? Technology, however high or low, is an instrument of diagnosis and treatment, not a signpost of treatment well or ill rendered. Physicians who are not patient-centered will assuredly not find themselves pulled toward doctor-patient dialogue through the tools of their specialty. But neither will they become *less* patient-centered on account of these tools. Physicians who *are* patient-centered, who enjoy their patients as people, and who comprehend their physicianly responsibilities in broader Hippocratic terms—these physicians will not be rendered *less* human, *less* caring, *less* dialogic, because of the technology they rely on. On the contrary, their caregiving values, if deeply held, will suffuse the technology and humanize its deployment in patient-centered ways.

When my retinologist examines the back of my eyes with the high-tech tools of his specialty—a retinal camera, a slit lamp, an optical coherence tomography machine—I do not feel that my connection with him is depersonalized or objectified through the instrumentation. Not in the least. On the contrary, I perceive the technology as an extension of his person. I am his patient, I have retinal pathology, and I need his regular reassurance that my condition remains stable and that I can continue with my work. He is responsive to my anxiety and sees me whenever I need to see him. The high technology he deploys in evaluating the back of my eye does not come between us; it is a mechanical extension of his physicianly gaze that fortifies his judgment and amplifies the reassurance he is able to provide. Because he cares for me, his technology cares for me. It is caring technology because he is a caring physician.

Modern retinology is something of a technological tour de force, but it is no different in kind from other specialties that employ colposcopes, cytoscopes, gastroscopes, proctoscopes, rhinoscopes, and the like to investigate symptoms and make diagnoses. If the physician who employs the technology is caring, then all such technological invasions, however unpleasant, are caring interventions. The cardiologist who recommends an invasive procedure like cardiac catheterization is no less caring on that account; such high technology does not distance him from the patient, though it may well enable him to maintain the distance that already exists. It is a matter of personality, not technology. Even technology of the lowest order can be used (and even invented) to preserve distance between physicians of a certain sensibility and their patients.

I extend this claim to advanced imaging studies as well. When the need for an MRI is explained in a caring and comprehensible manner, when the explanation is enveloped in a trusting doctor-patient relationship, then the technology, however discomfiting, becomes the physician's collaborator in caregiving. This is altogether different from the patient who demands an MRI or the physician who, in the throes of defensive medicine, remarks offhandedly, "Well, we better get an MRI" or simply, "I'm going to order an MRI." In such instances the technology is uncaring, because the physician has not seen fit to absorb it into a personalized regimen of care that is also caring. Physicians for whom invasive studies and hospital-based scans are part of everyday work need to remember that patients do not perceive medical technology in an interpersonal vacuum. In the realm of hospital machinery, in particular, they will "trust" the machinery to the extent that they trust the "work system" in which the machinery is embedded. That is, they will trust large-scale technology to the extent they believe their doctors and nurses trust it, are well-trained and experienced in its use, and are confident that it will be helpful, even necessary, to treating *and caring for* the patient. To borrow the language of systems engineering, patients will find large technology trustworthy to the extent they trust the physician, nurse, and technicians who, conjointly, make use of it.[42]

Bringing technology back to the personal level of an individual patient in the hands of an individual physician, medical tools at their best function as the problem-solving equivalent of a prosthetic limb. They are inanimate extenders of the physician's mental grasp of the problem "at hand." To the extent that technology remains tethered to the physician's caring sensibility, to her understanding that *her* diagnostic or treatment-related problem is *our* existential problem—and that we may be fraught with "fear and trembling," even "sickness unto death,"[43] on account of it—then we may welcome the embrace of high technology, just as polio patients of the 1930s and '40s with paralyzed intercostal muscles welcomed the literal embrace of the iron lung, which, however forbidding and confining, enabled them to breathe fully and deeply and without pain.

No doubt, many physicians fail to comprehend their use of technology in this fuzzy, humanistic way—and we are probably the worse for it. Technology does not structure interpersonal relationships; it is simply there for the using or abusing. The problem is not that we have too much of it, but that we impute a kind of relational valence to it, as if otherwise caring doctors are pulled away from patient care because technology gets between them and their patients. For some doctors, this may indeed be the case. But for others, the opposite is true. For James Mackenzie, the founder of cardiology and inventor of the most sophisticated pulse-reading device of the nineteenth century, instruments of precision only underscored the utterly noninstrumental nature of true doctoring. It is not the press of technology per se that reduces physicians to, in a word Stephens disparagingly uses, "technologists." With such doctors, the problem is not in their tools but in themselves.

IV.

It is little known that René Laënnec, the Parisian physician who invented the stethoscope at the Necker Hospital in 1816, found it distasteful to place his ear to the patient's chest to listen to heart sounds.

The distastefulness of "direct auscultation" was compounded by its impracticality in the hospital where, he observed, "it was scarcely to be suggested for most women patients, in some of whom the size of the breasts also posed a physical obstacle."[44] The stethoscope, which permitted "mediate auscultation," not only amplified heart and lung sounds in diagnostically transformative ways; it enabled Laënnec to avoid repugnant ear-to-chest contact.

Many women patients of Laënnec's time and place did not see it that way. Accustomed to the warmly human pressure of ear on chest, they were uncomfortable when an elongated wooden cylinder was interposed between the two. Nor did he escape criticism, sometimes harsh and personal, from his colleagues. In his native France, he and his stethoscope were ridiculed by the influential military surgeon F. J. V. Broussais, whose belief that acute and chronic inflammation of the gastrointestinal tract caused all illness was then in vogue. In London, Henry James Cholmeley, a physician to prestigious Guy's Hospital, expressed his disgust for the newfangled gadget by bringing one to the hospital and, at a succession of ward tables, inserting a flower into its top and loudly exclaiming, "What a capital bouquet holder!"[45] Of course, by the closing decades of the nineteenth century the situation was inverted: The stethoscope, in its modern binaural form, had become so integral to physical examination that patients hardly viewed it as a tool at all. It had become emblematic of hands-on doctoring and, as such, a sensory extender of the doctor. Even now, in an era of echocardiography, angiography, and MRIs, the stethoscope continues to stand in for the doctor, so that a retiring physician will announce that he is, or will be characterized by others as, hanging up his stethoscope.[46] A book review of Kenneth Iserson's *Demon Doctors: Physicians as Serial Killers*, published in 2004, bears the title "When Satan Wears a Stethoscope."[47]

Eighty years after Laënnec introduced the stethoscope to the chagrin of his colleagues, the supremely gifted American throat specialist (laryngologist) Chevalier Jackson perfected the design of a tube-shaped speculum (i.e., an instrument for opening up a bodily orifice) that, depending on its length, enabled him to examine the patient's bronchi (to perform bronchoscopy) or to peer farther down into the esophagus (to perform esophagoscopy). The diameter of the elongated tube

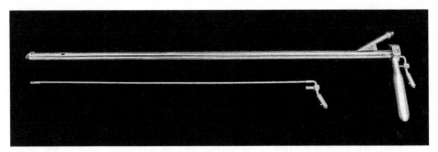

Figure 6.1 Chevalier Jackson's bronchoscope, 15 inches in length, with the light carrier inserted through the instrument shown separately. (Image used with kind permission of The College of Physicians of Philadelphia. Photograph by Evi Numen 2015.)

allowed insertion of tiny hooks and forceps that permitted Jackson to remove foreign objects that blocked air or food passages. The first such objects were a tooth-plate from an adult's esophagus and a coin from a child's; they would go on to include a staggering variety of household and workplace objects, open safety pins, fence staples, and double-pointed tacks among them.[48]

Jackson was not the first to perform what was subsequently termed "rigid bronchoscopy"; in Germany, Gustav Killian, using a more primitive instrument, removed a piece of bone from a patient's bronchus several years earlier, in 1895.[49] But it was Jackson's improved design of the bronchoscope/esophagoscope that revolutionized laryngology and, via attachment of a tiny distal lamp in 1902, extended it into the realm of gastroscopy, i.e., the endoscopic examination of the digestive system and stomach. A collection of 2,374 foreign objects that Jackson removed from patients' throats, esophaguses, and lungs are housed at the Mütter Museum of the College of Physicians in Philadelphia.

Jackson was by all accounts an artist with his instruments, able to perform esophagoscopy in infants without any anesthesia at all and boasting a remarkable 98% success rate in the removal of objects among the patients at his bronchoscopic clinics.[50] In 1908, he was deemed "practically a pioneer in the new field of gastroscopy," and 15 years later, colleagues readily conceded that no one else had attained his skill and judgment, that "humanity and medical science" owed him "a tremendous debt."[51] Yet, Jackson's introduction of the instrument all but derailed his career. In announcing his early results, he failed to alert colleagues to the technical difficulties and potential pitfalls associated with the new instrument. His own near-perfect technique was not tantamount to mastery of the technique by others. As a result, colleagues who initially used it had disastrous results, with attendant mortality. The new instrument "was condemned," Jackson recounted in his memoirs, and he was left heartbroken, demoralized, "filled with remorse, and disconsolate beyond words."[52]

The lesson here is that not all technologies are created equal, which is to say they are not equally accessible to those who employ them. Caring tools are tools competently employed, and, in the early period of a tool's life history, the competence can be hard earned, with tragic consequences along the way. In 1908, the very year one colleague lauded Jackson as a pioneer, another remarked that esophagoscopy was "still in its infancy or, at most, early childhood," with only a "comparatively few" laryngologists having had "any experience in its application."[53] Now, of course, bronchoscopy/esophagoscopy is one of many routine endoscopies that employ either a rigid or flexible endoscope and can be performed safely and quickly either in the outpatient unit of a hospital or in a doctor's office. Being "scoped" is not fun, to be sure, but it is far from a life-threatening ordeal.

It is easy to argue for the "oneness" of the physician and his or her instruments when it's a matter of simple tools that amplify sensory endowment (stethoscopes), provide a hands-on bodily "reading" (of temperature or blood pressure), or elicit a tendon reflex (e.g., the reflex hammer). And the argument can be extended without much difficulty to the more high-tech scopes used by medical specialists to see what is invisible to the naked eye. Instruments become so wedded to one or another medical specialty that it is hard to think of our providers without them. What is an ophthalmologist without her ophthalmoscope? An ENT without his nasal speculum? A gynecologist without her vaginal speculum? An internist without her blood pressure meter? Such hand-held devices are diagnostic enablers, and as such they are, or at least ought to be, our friends. Even more invasive scopes—the sigmoidoscope to examine the rectum and sigmoid colon, the cytoscope to examine the bladder, the colposcope to examine the vagina and cervix, and, yes, the bronchoscope and esophagoscope—retain this enabling status.

But I have suggested that even large-scale technology administered by technicians, and therefore outside the physician's literal grasp, can be linked in meaningful ways to the physician's person. A caring explanation of the need for this or that study, informed by a relational bond, can humanize even the most forbidding high-tech machinery. To be sure, medical machinery, whatever the discomfort and/or bodily bombardment it entails, is still disconcerting, often intimidating. But it is alienating only when we come to it in an alienated state, when it is not an instrument of physicianly engagement but a dehumanized object—a piece of technology.

Critical care nurses, whose work is both technology-laden and technology-driven, have had much to say on the relationship of technology to nursing identity and nursing care. Their literature includes provocative contributions that examine how technology—its availability, its use, its mastery—mediate nurses' standing in a hospital hierarchy that comprises staff physicians, residents, administrators, patients, and patients' families.

For some Coronary Care Unit (CCU) nurses, the use of technology and the acquisition of technological competence segue into issues of power and autonomy that are linked to issues of gender, medical domination, and "ownership" of the technology.[54] A less feminist sensibility informs interview research that yields unsurprising empirical findings, namely, that comfort with technology and the ability to incorporate it into a caring, "touching" disposition hinge on the technological mastery associated with nursing experience. Student and novice nurses, for example, find the machinery of the CCU anxiety-inducing, even overwhelming. They resent the casual manner in which physicians relegate to them complex technological tasks, such as weaning patients from respirators, without appreciating the long list of nursing duties to which such tasks are appended.[55] Withal, beginners approach the use of technology in task-specific ways and have great difficulty "caring with technology."[56] Theirs is not a caring technology but a technology that causes stress and jeopardizes fragile professional identities.

Experienced CCU nurses, on the other hand, evince a technological competence that lets them pull the machinery to them; they use it as a window of opportunity for being with their patients.[57] Following

Christine Little, we can give the transformation from novice to expert a phenomenological gloss and say that as technological inexperience gives way to technological mastery, technological skills become "ready-to-hand" (Heidegger) and "a natural extension of practice."[58]

Well and good. We want critical care nurses comfortable with the machinery of critical care—with cardiac and vital signs monitors, respirators, catheters, and infusion pumps—so that implementing technological interventions and monitoring the monitors do not blot out the nurse's "presence" in the patient's care. But all this is from the perspective of the nurse and her role in the hospital. What, one wonders, does the patient make of all this technology?

Humanizing technology means identifying with it in ways that are not only responsive to the patient's fears but also conducive to a shared appreciation of its role in treatment. It is easier for patients to feel humanly touched by technology, that is, if their doctors and nurses appropriate it and represent it as an extender of care. Perhaps some doctors and nurses do so as a matter of course, but one searches the literature in vain for examples of nurse-patient or doctor-patient interactions that humanize technology through dialogue. And such dialogue, however perfunctory in nature, may greatly matter.

Consider the seriously ill patient whose nurse interacts with him without consideration of the technology-saturated environment in which care is given. Now consider the seriously ill patient whose nurse incorporates the machinery into his or her caregiving identity, as in "This monitor [or this line or this pump] is a terrific thing for you and for me. It gives me information I would not otherwise have and lets me take better care of you." Such reassurance, which can be elaborated in any number of patient-centered ways, is not trivial; it may turn an anxious patient around, psychologically speaking. And it is all the more important when, owing to the gravity of the patient's condition, the nurse must spend more time assessing data and tending to machinery than caring for the patient. Here especially the patient needs to be reminded that the nurse's responsibility for machinery expands his or her role as the patient's guardian.[59]

The touch of the physician's sensory extenders, if literally uncomfortable, may still be comforting. For it is the physician's own ears that hear us through the stethoscope and whose own eyes gaze on us through the ophthalmoscope, the laryngoscope, the esophagoscope, the colposcope. It is easier to appreciate tools as beneficent extenders of care in the safe confines of one's own doctor's office, where instrumental touching is fortified by the relational bond that grows out of continuing care. In the hospital, absent such relational grounding, there is more room for dissonance and hence more need for shared values and empathy. A nurse who lets the cardiac monitor pull her away from patient care will not do well with a frightened patient who needs personal caring. A woman in labor who welcomes the technology of the labor room will connect better with an obstetrical nurse who values the electronic fetal monitor (and the reassuring visualization it provides the soon-to-be mother) than a nurse who is unhappy with its employment in low-risk births and prefers a return to intermittent auscultation.

In the best of circumstances, tools elicit an intersubjective convergence grounded in an expectation of objectively superior care. It helps to keep the "objective care" part in mind, to remember that technology was not devised to frighten us, encumber us, or cause us pain, but to help doctors and nurses evaluate us, keep us stable and comfortable, and enable treatments that will make us better, or at least leave us better off than our technology-free forebears.

V.

My retinologist reclines the examination chair all the way back and begins prepping my left eye for its second intravitreal injection of Eylea, one of the newest drugs used to treat macular disease. I am grateful for all the technology that has brought me to this point: the retinal camera, the slit lamp, the optical coherence tomography machine. I am especially grateful for the development of fluorescein angiography, which allows my doctor to pinpoint with great precision the lesion in need of treatment. And of course I am grateful to my retinologist, who brings all this technology to bear with a human touch, calmly reassuring me through every step of evaluation and treatment.

I experienced almost immediate improvement after the first such injection a month earlier and am eager to proceed with the treatment. So I am *relatively* relaxed as he douses my eye with antiseptic and anesthetic washes in preparation for the needle. Then, at the point of injection, he asks me to look up at the face of his assistant, a young woman with a lovely smile. "My pleasure," I quip, slipping into gendered mode. "I love to look at pretty faces." I am barely aware of the momentary pressure of the needle that punctures my eyeball and releases this wonderfully effective new drug into the back of my eye. It is not the needle that administers treatment but my trusted and caring physician. "Great technique," I remark. "I barely felt it." To which his young assistant, still standing above me, smiles and adds, "I think I had something to do with it." And indeed she had.

CHAPTER 7

The Needle's Touch

... the children's population of this century has been submitted progressively as never before to the merciless routine of the 'cold steel' of the hypodermic needle.

—Karl E. Kassowitz, "Psychodynamic Reactions of Children to the Use of Hypodermic Needles" (1958)

O f course, like so much medical technology, injection by hypodermic needle has a prehistory dating back to the ancient Romans, who used metal syringes with disk plungers for enemas and nasal injections. Seventeenth- and eighteenth-century physicians extended the sites of entry to the vagina and rectum, using syringes of metal, pewter, ivory, and wood. Christopher Wren, the Oxford astronomer and architect, introduced intravenous injection in 1657, when he inserted a quill into a patient's exposed vein and pumped in water, opium, or a purgative (laxative).

But, like so much medical technology, things only get interesting in the nineteenth century. In the first half of the century, the prehistory of needle injection includes the work of G. V. Lafargue, a French physician from the commune of St. Emilion. He treated neuralgic (nerve) pain—his own included—by penetrating the skin with a vaccination lancet dipped in morphine and later by inserting solid morphine pellets under the skin through a large needle hole. In 1844, the Irish physician Francis Rynd undertook injection by making a small incision in the skin and inserting a fine cannula (tube), letting gravity guide the medication to its intended site.[1]

The leap to a prototype of the modern syringe, in which a glass piston pushes medicine through a metal or glass barrel that ends in a hollow-pointed needle, occurred on two national fronts in 1853. In Scotland, Alexander Wood, secretary of Edinburgh's Royal College of Physicians, had been trying to dull his patients' neuralgias, their nerve pain, according to the method of Francois Valleix, the Parisian authority whose *Traité des névralgies* (*Treatise on Neuralgias*) had been published in 1841. First, following Valleix, he created a series of blisters on the skin above the affected nerve. Then, after a period of time, he applied an ointment containing morphine to the raw skin exposed beneath the blister. The morphine, according to Valleix, would seep through the skin and relieve the nerve pain, and Wood experienced a measure of success with his patients.

Well enough. But Wood couldn't leave well enough alone and mused whether a more direct application of morphine by injection would be more effective still. In 1853 he decided to make the experiment, which entailed both a minor innovation and a major one. Wood used sherry wine as his solvent, believing it would prove less irritating to the skin than alcohol and less likely to rust his instrument than water. And then came the breakthrough: He administered the liquid morphine right into the painful pressure points of the nerve through a piston-equipped syringe that ended in a pointed needle. Near the end of the needle, on one side, was an opening through which medicine could be released when an aperture on the outer tube was rotated into alignment with the opening. It was designed and made by the London instrument maker Daniel Ferguson, whose "elegant little syringes," as Wood described them, were intended to inject iron perchloride (a blood-clotting agent, or coagulant) into skin lesions and birthmarks in the hope of making them less unsightly. It never occurred to Ferguson that his medicine-releasing, needle-pointed syringes could be used for subcutaneous injection as well.[2]

Across the channel in the French city of Lyon, the veterinary surgeon Charles Pravaz employed a piston-driven syringe of his own making to inject iron perchloride into the blood vessels of sheep and horses. Pravaz was not interested in unsightly birthmarks; he was

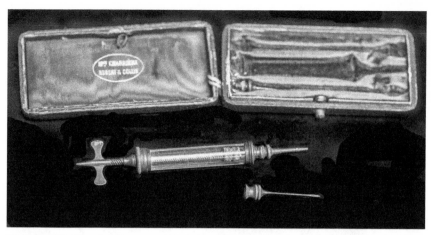

Figure 7.1 Daniel Ferguson's "elegant little syringe," with which Alexander Wood injected liquid morphine in 1853. (Image used with kind permission of The College of Physicians of Philadelphia. Photograph by Evi Numen 2015.)

searching for an effective treatment for aneurysms (enlarged arteries, usually due to weakening of the arterial walls) that he thought could be extended to humans. Wood was the first in print—his "New Method of Treating Neuralgia by the Direct Application of Opiates to the Painful Points" appeared in the *Edinburgh Medical & Surgical Journal* in 1855[3]—and, shortly thereafter, he improved Ferguson's design by devising a hollow needle that could simply be screwed on to the end of the syringe. Unsurprisingly, then, he has received the lion's share of credit for "inventing" the modern hypodermic syringe. Pravaz, after all, was only interested in determining whether iron perchloride would clot blood; he never administered medication through his syringe to animals or people.

Wood and followers like the New York physician Benjamin Fordyce Barker, who brought Wood's technique to Bellevue Hospital in 1856, were convinced that the injected fluid had a local action on inflamed peripheral nerves. Wood allowed for a secondary effect through absorption into the bloodstream but believed the local action accounted for the injection's rapid relief of pain. It fell to the London surgeon Charles Hunter to stress that the system-wide or "systemic" effect of injectable narcotic was primary. It was not necessary, he

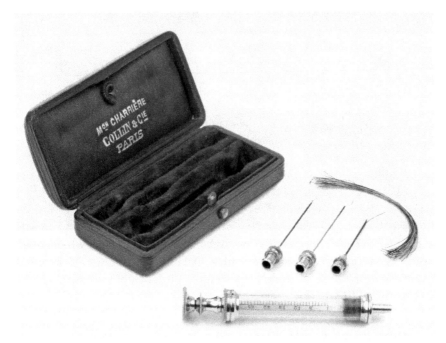

Figure 7.2 Charles Pravaz's hypodermic syringe, seen here with extra needles, needle cleaning wires, and the elegant leather case in which they were packaged and sold. (Photograph by www.phisick.com, used with permission.)

argued in 1858, to inject liquid morphine into the most painful spot; the medicine provided the same relief when injected far from the site of the lesion. It was Hunter, seeking to underscore the originality of his approach to injectable morphine, especially its general therapeutic effect, who introduced the term "hypodermic," from the Greek compound meaning "under the skin."[4]

It took time for the needle to become integral to doctors and doctoring. In America, physicians greeted the hypodermic injection with skepticism and even dread, despite the avowals of patients that injectable morphine provided them with instantaneous, well-nigh miraculous relief from chronic pain.[5] The complicated, time-consuming process of preparing injectable solutions prior to the manufacture of dissolvable tablets in the 1880s didn't help matters. Nor did the trial-and-error process of arriving at something like appropriate doses of

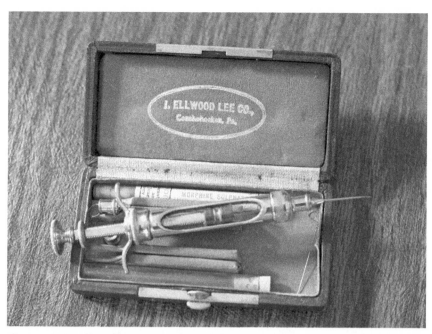

Figure 7.3 Ellwood Lee syringe from the 1890s. Note the protective metal mount around the glass barrel and the obligatory vial of dissolvable morphine sulfate tablets in the carry case. (From the collection of Paul E. Stepansky. Photograph by Phil Leo 2015.)

the solutions. But most importantly, until the early twentieth century, very few drugs were injectable. Through the 1870s, the physician's injectable arsenal consisted of highly poisonous (in pure form) plant alkaloids such as morphine, atropine (belladonna), strychnine, and aconitine, and, by decade's end, the vasodilator heart medicine nitro-glycerine. The development of local and regional anesthesia in the mid-1880s relied on the hypodermic syringe for subcutaneous injections of cocaine solution, but as late as 1905, only 20 of the 1,039 drugs in the U.S. *Pharmacopoeia* were injectable.[6]

The first disposable "syringes" of a sort—collapsible tin tubes (like small toothpaste tubes) with a fixed amount of morphine—were patented in 1912 by James Greeley, an army surgeon who served with the 1st New Hampshire Infantry during the Spanish-American War. Greeley's single-use morphine dispensers were used on the battlefields of World War I and became the prototype of the morphine syrette developed by Squibb Corporation after the war. But it was the availability of injectable insulin in the early 1920s that heralded a new, everyday reliance on hypodermic injections, and over the course of the century, the needle, along with the stethoscope, came to stand in for the physician. Now, of course, as the medical sociologist Atul Kotwal has observed, needles and doctors (and needles and nurses) "seem to go together" with the former signifying "the power to heal through hurting" even as it "condenses the notions of active practitioner and passive patient."[7]

The child's fear of needles, always a part of pediatric practice, has generated a literature of its own. In the mid-twentieth century, in the heyday of Freudianism, children's needle anxiety gave rise to psychodynamic musings. In 1958, Karl Kassowitz of Milwaukee Children's Hospital made the rather obvious observation that younger children were immature and hence more anxious about receiving injections than older children. By the time kids were eight or nine, he found, most had outgrown their fear. Among the less than 30% who hadn't, Kassowitz gravely counseled, continuing resistance to the needle might represent "a clue to an underlying neurosis."[8] Ah, the good old Freudian days.

In the second half of the last century, anxiety about receiving injections was "medicalized" like most everything else, and in the more enveloping guise of BII (blood, injection, injury) phobia, found its way into the fourth edition of the American Psychiatric Association's *Diagnostic and Statistical Manual* in 1994. Needle phobia thereupon became the beneficiary of all that accompanies medicalization—a specific etiology, physical symptoms, associated EKG and stress hormone changes, and strategies of management. The latter are impressively varied and range across medical, educational, psychotherapeutic, behavioral, cognitive-behavioral, relaxation, and desensitizing approaches.[9] Recent literature also highlights the vasovagal reflex associated with needle and blood phobia. Patients confronted with the needle become so anxious that an initial increase in heart rate and blood pressure is followed by a marked drop, as a result of which they become sweaty, dizzy, pallid, nauseous (any or all of the above), and sometimes faint (vasovagal syncope). Another interesting finding is that needle phobia (especially in its BII variant) along with its associated vasovagal reflex probably have a genetic component, as there is a much higher concordance within families for BII phobia than other kinds of phobia. Researchers who study twins put the heritability of BII phobia at around 48%.[10]

Needle phobia is still prevalent among kids, to be sure, but it has long since matured into a fully grown-up condition. Surveys find injection phobia in anywhere from 9 to 21% of the general population and even higher percentages of select populations, such as U.S. college communities.[11] A study by the Dental Fears Research Clinic of the University of Washington in 1995 found that over a quarter of surveyed students and university employees were fearful of dental injections, with 5% admitting they avoided or canceled dental appointments out of fear.[12] Perhaps some of these needlephobes bear the scars of childhood trauma. Pediatricians now urge control of the pain associated with venipuncture and intravenous cannulation (tube insertion) in infants, toddlers, and young children, since there is evidence such procedures can have a lasting impact on pain sensitivity and tolerance of needle picks.[13]

But people are not only afraid of needles; they also overvalue them and seek them out. Needle phobia, whatever its hereditary contribution, is a creation of Western medicine. The surveys cited above come from the U.S., Canada, and England. Once we shift our gaze to developing countries of Asia and Africa we behold a different needle-strewn landscape. Studies attest not only to the high acceptance of the needle but also to its integration into popular understandings of disease. Laypeople in countries such as Indonesia, Tanzania, and Uganda typically want injections; indeed, they often insist on them because injected medicines, which enter the bloodstream directly and (so they believe) remain in the body longer, must be more effective than orally ingested pills or liquids.

The strength, rapid action, and body-wide circulation of injectable medicine—these things make injection the only cure for serious disease.[14] So valued are needles and syringes in developing countries that most laypeople, and even registered medical practitioners in India and Nepal, consider it wasteful to discard disposable needles after only a single use. And then there is the tendency of people in developing countries to rely on lay injectors (the "needle curers" of Uganda; the "injection doctors" of Thailand; the informal providers of India and Turkey) for their shots. This has led to the indiscriminate use of penicillin and other chemotherapeutic agents, often injected without attention to sterile procedure. All of which contributes to the spread of infectious disease and presents a major headache for the World Health Organization.

The pain of the injection? Bring it on. In developing countries, the burning sensation that accompanies many injections signifies curative power. In some cultures, people also welcome the pain as confirmation that real treatment has been given.[15] In pain there is healing power. It is the potent sting of modern science brought to bear on serious, often debilitating disease. All of which suggests the contrasting worldviews and emotional tonalities collapsed into the fearful and hopeful question, "Will it hurt?"

II.

. . . and although the patient had long been a sufferer from dyspnea, chronic bronchitis, and embarrassed heart, we believed that the almost miraculous resurrection which took place would be permanent. He died, however, on the second day.
—Cameron MacDowall, "Intra-Peritoneal Injections in Cholera" (1883)[16]

Among the early British and American proponents of subcutaneous hypodermic injection, especially of liquefied morphine, the seeming miracle of instantaneous pain relief sufficed to bring physician and patient into attitudinal alignment. The convergence of sensibilities is unsurprising. We are, after all, a century removed from the psychoanalytic mindset that encouraged physicians to explore the personal side of hypodermic injection and to develop strategies for overcoming patients' anxieties about needle puncture, their "needle phobia."

There is no need to read between the lines of nineteenth-century clinical reports to discern the convergence of physician delight and patient amazement at the immediate relief provided by hypodermic injection. The lines themselves tell the story, and the story is all about the pain. Patients who received hypodermic injections in the aftermath of Alexander Wood's successful use of Daniel Ferguson's "elegant little syringe" were often in extremis. Here is a woman of 40, who presented with a case of acute pleurisy (inflammation of the membrane around the lungs) in 1867:

> The pain was most intense; great dyspnea [difficulty breathing] existed; sharp, lancinating pains at each rapid inspiration completely prostrated the patient, whose sufferings had been continuous for twelve hours. About one-sixth of a grain of the acetate of morphia was used hypodermically, and with prompt relief, a few minutes only elapsing after its injection before its beneficial results followed. The ordinary treatment being continued, a recovery was effected in a short time.[17]

Consider this "delicate elderly spinster" of 1879, who presented to her physician thusly:

> I found her nearly unconscious, cramped all over body and legs, vomiting violently every minute or two, purging every few minutes, the purging being involuntary and under her. She was showing the whites of the eyes, and the countenance was changed. She was certainly all but gone. Gave at once two-fifths of a grain of sulphate of morphia hypodermically. She did not feel the prick of the needle in the least.[18]

And here is a surgeon from Wales looking in on a 48-year-old gardener in severe abdominal pain at the Crickhowell Dispensary on August 1, 1882:

> On my visiting him at 11:30 on the morning of the above date, I found him in great agony, in which condition his wife informed me he had been during the greater part of the previous night. He implored me to do something for relief, saying he could endure the suffering no longer; and as I happened to have my hypodermic syringe in my pocket, I introduced into his arm four minims of a solution of acetate of morphia. I then left him.[19]

A bit better off, one supposes—if only a bit—were patients who suffered severe chronic pain, whether arthritic, gastrointestinal, circulatory, or cancerous in nature. They too were beneficiaries of the needle. We encounter a patient with "the most intense pain in the knee-joint" owing to a six-year-long attack of gout. Injection of a third of a grain of acetate of morphia was followed by "the most delightful results," with "the patient expressing himself in glowing terms as to the efficacy and promptness of this new remedy." Instantaneous relief, compliments of the needle, enabled him to turn the corner; he "rallied rapidly, having none of the depression and debilitating effects, the resultant of long-continued pain, to recover from, as in former times."[20]

So it was with patients with any number of ailments, however rare or nebulous in nature. A 31-year-old woman was admitted to Massachusetts General Hospital in 1883 with what her physician diagnosed as multiple sarcomas (malignant skin tumors) covering her upper arms, breasts, and abdomen. She was given subcutaneous injections of Fowler's Solution, an eighteenth-century tonic that was 1% arsenic. Discharged from the hospital two weeks later, she self-administered daily injections of Fowler's for another five months, by which time the lesions had cleared completely; a year later she remained "perfectly well to all appearance." In the 1890s, the decade when subcutaneous injections of various glandular extracts gripped the clinical imagination,[21] it is hardly surprising to read that injection of liquefied gray matter of a sheep's brain did remarkable things for patients suffering from nervous exhaustion (neurasthenia). Indeed, its tonic effect comprised "increase of strength, appetite and weight, restoration of spirits and *bien-être*, disappearance of pain, sexual impotence and insomnia." At the other end of the psychophysical spectrum, patients who became manic, even violently delirious, during their bouts with acute illnesses such as pneumonia or rheumatic fever, "recovered in the ordinary way" after one or more injections of morphia, sometimes in conjunction with inhaled chloroform.[22]

Right through century's end, the pain of disease was compounded by the pain of pre-injection treatment methods. What the Boston surgeon Robert White, one of Wood's first American followers, termed the "revolution in the healing art" signaled by the needle, addressed both poles of suffering. Morphia's "wonderful effects" on all kinds of pain—neuralgic pain, joint pain, digestive pain (dyspepsia), the pain of tumors and blockages—were heightened by the *relative* painlessness of injection. Indeed, the revolutionary import of hypodermic injection, according to White, meant that "The painful and decidedly cruel endermic mode of applying medicines [i.e., absorption through the skin] may be entirely superseded, and the pain of a blistered surface completely avoided."[23] When it came to hemorrhoids, carbuncles, and small tumors, not to mention "foul and ill-conditioned ulcers," hypodermic injections of carbolic acid provided "the only absolute and *painless cure* [original emphasis] of these exceedingly painful affections."[24]

And what of the pain of the injection itself? When it rates mention, it is only to put it in perspective, to underscore that "some pain at the moment of injection" gives way to "great relief from the pain of the disease"—a claim which, in this instance, pertained to alcohol solution injected in and around malignant tumors.[25] Very rarely indeed does one find references to the pain of injection as a treatment-related consideration.[26]

Recognition of the addictive potential of repeated morphine injections barely dimmed the enthusiasm of many of the needle's early proponents. In his text of 1880, *The Hypodermic Injection of Morphia*, H. H. Kane, who came to the topic after a decade of studying the opium habit in New York, found that 131 of 328 surveyed physicians reported 184 cases of addiction subsequent to morphine injections. But Kane laid the blame squarely on those colleagues who allowed patients to inject themselves—a recipe for disaster. As long as the physician never let the syringe out of his hands and exercised reasonable care with dosages, there was "but little fear" that the habit would be contracted.[27] Further, then as now, physicians devised rationalizations for preferred treatment methods despite well-documented grounds for concern. They carved out diagnostic niches that, so they claimed, were exempt from mounting evidence of addiction. A Melbourne surgeon who gave morphine injections to hospitalized parturients suffering from "puerperal eclampsia" (convulsions and coma following childbirth) found his patients able "to resist the dangerous effects of the drug; it seems to have no bad consequences in cases, in which, under ordinary circumstances, morphia would be strongly contra-indicated." A physician from Virginia, who had treated puerperal convulsions with injectable morphine for 16

years, seconded this view. "One would be surprised to see the effect
of morphine in these cases," he reported in 1887. It was "as if bringing the dead to life. It does not stupefy the patients, but renders
them brighter."[28] A British surgeon stationed in Burma "cured" a
patient of tetanus with repeated injections of atropine (belladonna),
and held that his case "proved" that tetanus "induced" a special tolerance to an alkaloid known to have serious, even life-threatening,
side effects.[29] Physicians and patients alike stood in awe before a
technology that not only heightened the effectiveness of the pharma-
copeia of the time but also brought it to bear on an extended range
of conditions.

Even failure to relieve suffering or postpone death spoke to the
importance of hypodermic injection. For even then, injections played
a critical role in differential diagnosis: They enabled clinicians to differentiate, for example, "choleric diarrhea," which morphine injections
greatly helped, from, respectively, "malignant" (or Asiatic) cholera and
common dysentery, which they helped not at all.[30]

To acknowledge that not all injections even temporarily relieved
suffering or that not all injections were relatively painless was, in the
context of nineteenth-century therapeutics, little more than a foot-
note. Of course this was the case. But it didn't seem to matter. There
was an understandable wishfulness on the part of nineteenth-century
physicians and patients about the therapeutic benefits of hypodermic
injection per se, and this wishfulness arose from the fact that, prior to
invention of the hypodermic syringe and soluble forms of morphine
and other alkaloids, "almost miraculous resurrection" from intractable pain was not a possibility, or at least not a possibility arising from
a physician's quick procedural intervention.

For those physicians who, beginning in the late 1850s, began
injecting morphine and other opioids to relieve severe pain, there was
something magical about the whole process—and, yes, it calls to mind
the quasi-magical status of injection and injectable medicine in some
developing countries today. The magic proceeded from the dramatic
pain relief afforded by injection, certainly. But it also arose from the
realization, per Charles Hunter, that an injected opioid somehow
found its way to the site of pain regardless of where it was injected. It
was pretty amazing.

The magic, paradoxically, derived from the new scientific under-standing of medicinal therapeutic action in the final three decades of the nineteenth century. The development of hypodermic injection is a small part of the triumph of scientific medicine, of a medicine of specific remedies for specific illnesses, of remedies increasingly devel-oped in laboratories but bringing the fruits of laboratory science to the bedside. We see the search for specific remedies in early trial-and-error efforts to find specific injectables and specific combinations of injectables for specific conditions—carbolic acid for hemorrhoids and carbuncles; morphine and atropia (belladonna) for puerperal convul-sions; whisky and water for epidemic cholera; alcohol for tumors; ether for sciatica; liquefied sheep's brain for nervous exhaustion; and on and on. In Kane's text of 1880, the properties of injectable morphine and atropia, alone and in combination, for a variety of conditions, rated an entire chapter. His survey of 360 colleagues suggested that morphine alone had its "most marked curative effects" with cases of epilepsy, idiopathic tetanus, and neuralgia.[31]

This is a primitive empiricism, to be sure, but a proto-scientific empiricism nonetheless. The very search for injectables specific to one or another condition is worlds removed from the Galenic medicine of the 1830s and '40s, according to which all diseases were really varia-tions of a single disease that had to do with the degree of tension or excitability in the blood vessels.

Despite the paucity of injectable medicines into the early twentieth century, hypodermic injection caught on because, despite the fantas-tical claims (to our ears) that abound in nineteenth-century medical journals, it was aligned with scientific medicine in ascendance. Yes, the penetration of the needle was merely subcutaneous, but skin puncture was a portal to the bloodstream and to organs deep inside the body. In this manner, hypodermic injection partook of the exalted status of "heroic surgery" in the final quarter of the nineteenth century.[32] The penetration of the needle, shallow though it was, stood in for a bold new kind of surgery, a surgery able to penetrate to the very anatomi-cal substrate of human suffering. Beginning in the late 1880s, certain forms of major surgery became recognizably modern, and the lowly needle was along for the ride. The magic was all about the pain, but it was also all about the science.

III.

Fear of the needle is usually acquired in childhood. The psychic trauma to millions of the population produced in this way undoubtedly creates obstacles to good doctor-patient relationships, essential diagnostic procedures, and even life-saving therapy.

—Janet Travell, "Factors Affecting
Pain of Injection" (1955)[33]

It was during the 1950s that the administration of hypodermic injections became a fraught enterprise and a topic of medical discussion. With World War II over and American psychoanalysis suffusing postwar culture, including the cultures of medicine and psychiatry, it is unsurprising that physicians should look with new eyes at needle penetration and the fears it provoked.

In the nineteenth century, it had been all about pain relieved, sometimes miraculously, by injection of opioids. Alongside the pain relieved, the pain of the injection was quite tolerable, even minor, a mere afterthought. But in the mid-twentieth century pain per se took a back seat. It was no longer only about the painful condition that prompted injection. Nor, really, was it about the actual pain of the injection. Psychodynamic thinking trumped both kinds of pain. Increasingly, the issue before physicians, especially pediatricians, was about two things: The anxiety *attendant* to injection pain and the lasting psychological *damage* that was all too often the legacy of needle pain. Elimination of injection pain mattered, certainly, but it became the means to a psychological end. Relieve the pain, they reasoned, and you eliminate the apprehension that exacerbates the pain and potentially leaves deep psychic scars.

And so physicians were put on notice. They were enjoined to experiment with numbing agents, coolant sprays, and various counterirritants to minimize the pain that children and a good many adults dreaded. They were urged to keep their needles sharp and their patients' skin surfaces dry. Coolant sprays and antiseptic solutions that left a wet film, after all, could be carried into the skin as irritants. For the muscular pain attendant to deeper injections, still stronger anesthetics, such as procaine, might be called for. Physicians were also encouraged to reduce injection pain through new technologies, to use, for example, hyposprays and spring-loaded presto injectors. Injection "technique" became a topic of discussion, especially for intramuscular injections of new wonder drugs such as streptomycin. To be sure, new technologies and refined technique often failed to eliminate injection pain, especially when a large volume of solution was injected. But, then again, pain relief was only a secondary goal. The point of the recommendations was primarily psychological, that is, to eliminate "the psychological reaction to piercing the skin."[34] It was *anticipation* of pain and the *fear* it engendered that jeopardized the doctor-patient relationship and threatened lasting psychological damage.

And it might jeopardize even more, such as the willingness of parents to let their children participate in field trials of what promised to be the latest wonder drug—the Salk polio vaccine—in the spring of 1954. In the form letter mailed to parents in 211 participating counties, Basil O'Connor, director of the National Foundation for Infantile Paralysis (NFIP), naturally took pains to reassure parents that Salk's killed-virus solution was totally safe. But he added that the injection itself would be "only slightly painful" and with "no unpleasant effects." Administration of the vaccine (or placebo substitute) would be via a disposable glass syringe/needle combination—the B-D Hypak—mass-produced by the Rutherford, New Jersey, surgical instrument firm Becton, Dickinson in time for the trial and supplied to the NFIP at no profit. Each syringe, touting B-D advertising, was sterile, pyrogen-free, and nontoxic, while its "new, sharp needle point" provided "greater patient comfort."[35] When the first student to receive the vaccine, Randy Kerr of Franklin Sherman Elementary School in McLean, Virginia, was asked how it went, he replied in the truthful manner of a six-year-old for whom an injection could only be about the pain: "I could hardly feel it. It hurt less than a penicillin shot."[36]

Psychoanalysts, far removed from the everyday concerns of pediatricians and general practitioners, had little to say about injection fear and its sequelae. They were content to call attention now and again to needle symbolism—invariably phallic in nature—in dreams and childhood memories. In 1954, the child analyst Selma Fraiberg recalled "The theory of a two-and-a-half-year-old girl who developed a serious neurosis following an observation of coitus. The child maintained that 'the man made the hole,' that the penis was forcibly thrust into the

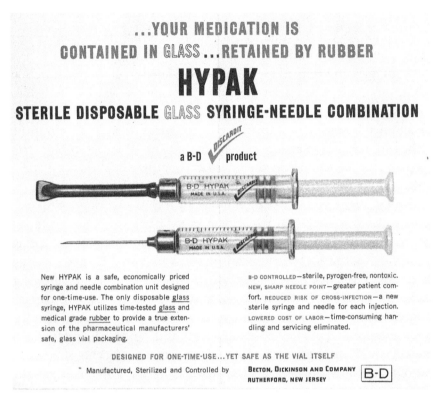

Figure 7.4 Becton, Dickinson 1954 advertisement of the Hypak syringe with its "new, sharp needle point." (Courtesy and © Becton, Dickinson and Company. Reprinted with permission.)

woman's body like the hypodermic needle which had been thrust into her by the doctor when she was ill." Pity the toddler, sorry child of the Freudian '50s.

Inferences about male sadism and castration anxiety were integral to this train of thought. In 1950s-era psychoanalysis, needle injection could symbolize not only "painful penetration" but also the sadistic mutilation of a little girl by a male doctor.[37] One wants to say that such strained psychoanalytic renderings are long dead and buried, but the fact is they still find their way into the literature from time to time, usually in the context of dream interpretations. Here is one from 1994:

Recently Ms. K mentioned a dream in which she was diabetic and had little packets of desiccated insulin which were also like condoms. All she needed now was a hypodermic syringe and a needle. I pointed out the sexual nature of the dream with its theme of penetration; she then remembered that in the dream a woman friend had lifted her skirt and Ms. K had 'whammed the needle right in'.[38]

Psychoanalytic interpretive priorities change over time, whether or not in therapeutically helpful ways being a perennial subject of debate. By the 1990s, however, there was belated recognition that children's needle phobias really didn't call for analytic unraveling; they derived from the simple developmental fact that "children are exposed to hypodermic needles prior to their ability to understand what is going on," and, as such, were more amenable to behavioral intervention than psychoanalytic treatment. In the hospital setting, in particular, children needed simple strategies to reduce fear, not psychoanalytic interpretations.[39]

In 1950s medicine, psychoanalysis was at its best when its influence was subtle and indirect. Samuel Stearns's thoughtful consideration of the "emotional aspects" of treating patients with diabetes, published in the *New England Journal of Medicine* in 1953, is one such example. Stearns worked out of the Abraham Rudy Diabetic Clinic of Boston's Beth Israel Hospital, and he expressed indebtedness to the psychiatrist-psychoanalyst Grete Bibring and other members of her department for "many discussions" on the topic.

For most diabetics, of course, daily injections, self-administered whenever possible, were an absolute necessity. And resistance to the injections, then as now, undercut treatment and resulted in poor glycemic control.[40] How then to cope with the diabetic's resistance to the needle, especially when "the injection of insulin is sometimes associated with a degree of anxiety, revulsion or fear that cannot be explained by the slight amount of pain involved."[41]

Psychoanalysis provided a framework for overcoming the resistance. It was not a matter of "simple reassurance" about insulin injections, Stearns observed, but—and it is Bibring's voice we hear—

Recognition that apparently trivial and unfounded complaints about insulin injections may be based on deeply rooted anxiety for which the patient finds superficial rationalizations enables the physician to be more realistic and tolerant, and more successful in dealing with the problem.

Realism, tolerance, acceptance—this was the psychoanalytic path to overcoming the problem. Physicians had to accept that diabetics' anxiety about injections arose from "individual personalities," and that each diabetic had his or her own adaptively necessary defenses. Exhortation, criticism, and direct confrontation had to be jettisoned on behalf of the kindness and understanding that would lead to a "positive interpersonal relation." This entailed an understanding of the patient's transference to the physician:

> It is particularly apparent that most of the reactions of juvenile diabetic patients to discipline, authoritativeness or criticism by the physician are really identical with their reactions to similar situations involving their parents.

And it included a like-minded willingness to wrestle with the physician's subjective reaction to the patient's resistance, which typically took the form of impatience, frustration, even anger. This was what the analysts termed the physician's "countertransference," and it was an obstacle to treatment:

> Even the occasional display of an untherapeutic attitude by the physician is enough to interfere with the development of a relation that will enable him to obtain maximal cooperation from the patient. If the physician cultivates awareness of his own reactions to a difficult patient, he will be less easily drawn into retaliation or other negative behavior.[42]

The point of the analytic approach was to lay the groundwork for a "positive interpersonal relation" that would enlist the patient's cooperation, and "not through anxiety or fear of the disease or the physician, but rather through the wish to be well and to gain the physician's approval."[43] Sympathetic acceptance of the patient's fears, of the defenses against those fears, of the life circumstances that led to the defenses—this was the ticket to the kind of positive transference relationship that the physician could use to his and the patient's advantage.

IV.

Stearns's paper of 1953 remains helpful to this day. It exemplifies the application of general psychoanalytic concepts to real-world medical problems that, as I suggested in the final chapter of *Psychoanalysis at the Margins* (2009), may yet breathe new life into a beleaguered profession. The reasonableness of Stearns's recommendations stands in contrast to the insular irrelevance of George Moran's "Psychoanalytic Treatment of Diabetic Children," published three decades later. Running with the psychoanalytic ball, as it were, and simultaneously running away from the everyday realities of pediatric practice, Moran proposed that poor glycemic control among children was a "metaphorical expression[s] of psychological disturbance," the latter framed in terms of "entrenched defensive structures" and "drive derivatives." As such, it called for psychoanalytic treatment, sometimes via "prolonged stays" of up to several months in pediatric wards.[44] Moran's draconian recommendation hearkened back to psychoanalytic literature of the 1930s and '40s, when analysts such as George Daniels and William Menninger, agog with Freud's treatment method, linked the onset of clinical diabetes to instinctual conflicts and anxiety neuroses. Menninger postulated a "diabetic personality" characterized by diminished alertness, indifference, hypochondriacal complaints, anxiety, and depression. Moran presented the case of a male diabetic in whom, so he held, diabetes "represented the last stand of the neurosis," the "final resolution" of which would likely "succeed in curing the diabetes."[45]

Stearns, who was content to examine the resistance of diabetic children to insulin injections, was not orbiting earth in a hermetically sealed Freudian spaceship. His cautionary remarks were much more down to earth, much more, as the analysts themselves would say, "reality-tested." And yet, there is something missing from Stearns's temperate suggestions. Like other writers of his time, he was concerned lest needle anxiety become an obstacle to a good doctor-patient relationship. Cultivate the relationship through sympathetic insight into the problem, he reasoned, and the obstacle would diminish, perhaps even disappear. What he ignored—indeed, what all these hospital- and clinic-based writers of the time ignored—is the manner in which a pre-existing "good doctor-patient relationship" can defuse needle anxiety in the first place.

Nineteen fifty-three, the year Stearns's paper was published, was also the year my father, William Stepansky, opened his general practice at 16 East First Avenue, Trappe, Pennsylvania. My father was a Compleat

Physician in whom wide-ranging procedural competence commingled with a psychiatric temperament and deeply caring sensibility. In the world of 1950s general practice, his office was, as the British pediatrician and psychoanalyst Donald Winnicott would say, a holding environment. My father's patients loved him and relied on him to provide care. If injections were part of the care, then ipso facto, they were caring interventions, whatever momentary discomfort they entailed.

The 40 years of my father's practice spanned the first 40 years of my life, and, from the time I was around 13, we engaged in ongoing conversations about his patients and work. Never do I recall his remarking on a case of needle anxiety, which is not to deny that any number of patients, child and adult, became anxious when injection time arrived. My point is that he contained and managed their anxiety so that it never became clinically significant or worthy of mention. At the opposite end of the spectrum, I know of elderly patients who welcomed him into their homes several times a week for injections—sometimes just vitamin B-12 shots—that amplified the human support he provided.

Before administering an injection, my father firmly but gently grasped the underside of the patient's upper arm, and the patient felt held, often in just those ways in which he or she needed holding. When one's personal physician gives an injection, it may become, in some manner and to some extent, a personal injection. And personal injections never hurt as much as injections impersonally given. This simple truth gets lost in contemporary literature that treats needle phobia as a psychiatric condition in need of focal treatment. A primary care physician remarked to me recently that she relieved a patient's severe anxiety about getting an injection simply by putting the injection on hold and sitting down and talking to the patient for five minutes. In effect, she reframed the meaning of the injection by absorbing it into a newly established human connection. Would that all our doctors would sit down with us for five minutes and talk to us as friendly human beings, as fellow sufferers, before getting down to procedural business. Of course, taking even five minutes to defuse a patient's needle anxiety runs in the face of 15-minute office visits and other relationship-straining aspects of contemporary primary care.

I count myself more fortunate than most. For me the very antici-pation of an injection has a positive valence. It conjures up the sights and smells and tactile sensations of my father's treatment room when I was a child. Now in my mid-60s, I still have in my nostrils the bracing scent of the alcohol he used to clean the injection site, and I still feel the firm, paternal grasp of his hand on my arm at the point of injec-tion. I once remarked to a physician that she could never administer an injection that would bother me, because at the moment of needle penetration, her hand became my father's.

Psychoanalysts who adopt the viewpoint of what is termed "object relations theory" speak of "transitional objects," those special inani-mate things—stuffed animals, blankets, and the like—that, especially in early life, stand in for our parents and help calm us in their absence. Such objects become vested with soothing human properties; this is what imparts their "transitional" status. In a paper of 2002, the ana-lyst Julie Miller ventured the improbable view, based on a single case, that the needle of the heroin addict represented a "transitional object" that fostered a maternal connection the addict never experienced in early life.[46] For me, I suppose, the needle is also a transitional object, albeit one that intersects with actual lived experience of a far more benign nature. To wit, when I receive an injection it is always with my father's hand, life-affirming and healing. It is the needle that attests to a paternal connection *realized*, in early life and in life thereafter. It is an injection that stirs loving memories of my father's medicine. So how much can it hurt?

CHAPTER 8

My Doctor, My Friend

It is so obvious to those of us who have been practicing medicine privately that our patients should be our friends that we do not often stop to ask the question, 'Why?'
—Paul Dudley White, "La Médecine du Coeur" (1949)

We want our doctors to care for us competently and professionally. We also want them to care for us in a caring manner. Caring care need not entail empathy, but it does presuppose a decent measure of sympathy and support. Does it follow then that we want our doctors to be our friends? In the nineteenth century, the question would not have computed; it would have been tautological. Medical care, more often than not, was all about caring, and caring gained expression through bonds of friendship. It was the doctor's friendship that affirmed the patient's trust and, in so doing, potentiated the healing potential of care caringly rendered.

One cannot venture far into the sea of nineteenth-century doctor-patient friendships without encountering William Osler, the brilliant lighthouse who illuminates the art of doctoring across a vast expanse. He was not only the preeminent clinician of his day but the embodiment of the doctor who befriended his patients and, in turn, welcomed their own gift of friendship—all in the interest of a healing relationship. In 1854, George Cheyne Shattuck, he of the second of five generations of Boston's most illustrious medical family, left an endowment establishing the lectureship for the Massachusetts Medical

Society that bears his name and continues to this day. Osler delivered the fourth Shattuck Lecture in 1893, and in 1990, on the occasion of the 100th Shattuck Lecture, H. Brownell Wheeler returned to Osler. In his own time, Wheeler held, Osler was not only a hero to the public and to his profession, but "for a hundred years has been regarded as the preeminent role model for a physician." Osler's astonishing competence alone did not provide an explanation, so Wheeler looked in another direction. Osler, he wrote,

> mastered the art of medicine as few have ever done. He knew that patients are unique individuals and that often their illnesses develop from the fabric of their lives. By adroit and good-natured questioning, he could skillfully perceive the person, as well as the disease. He had a genius at establishing friendships with his patients, in part because he had a genuine and deep interest in them. He could comfort and inspire patients and give them confidence in their ability to get well.[1]

From his professorial perch at McGill, then University of Pennsylvania, then Johns Hopkins, and finally Oxford, where he accepted the Regius Professorship of Medicine in 1905, Osler was a friend from on high who withheld his kindness and concern from no one down below. At the time of Osler's death, his colleague at Hopkins, the gynecologist Thomas Cullen, opined that "brotherly love was his finest and most enduring contribution to American medicine."[2]

But Osler was far from alone in this regard. His colleague at Hopkins, the surgeon John M. T. Finney, later to become first president of the American College of Surgeons, began working in the Johns Hopkins Hospital's dispensary at the hospital's opening in 1889. Denied admitting privileges by William Halsted, he started a surgical private practice, operating on patients in their homes or in a private hospital. In his memoir, he writes of a "warm friendship" growing out of an emergency appendectomy. The grateful patient, a German émigré and successful investor, aided his surgeon-friend by coming to the Finney home weekly to review the surgeon's finances with Mrs. Finney.[3]

A world removed from university consultants and surgeons, turn-of-the-century generalists all knew their patients well. They had to. Treatment plans of the time fell back on a detailed knowledge of daily routines far beyond the realm of our own data-driven treatment protocols. In *Doctor and Patient*, his popular work of 1888, the Philadelphia neurologist S. Weir Mitchell—he of the infamous "rest cure" for nervous women—warned patients that any doctor "who gives much medicine and many medicines . . . and who does not insist with care on knowing all about your habits as to diet, mealtimes, sleep, modes of work, and hours of recreation, is, on the whole, one to avoid."[4] A generation later, Richard Cabot, one of Boston's finest, in his lightly drawn *Training and Rewards of the Physician* (1918), urged the family physician to learn all he could about the "Human Menagerie—the types and varieties such as Balzac hoped exhaustively to map out in his 'Comedie Humaine'." And he illustrated the menagerie thusly:

> When a doctor is consulted by a stock broker or a cattleman, a laundress or an actress, he needs to know all that he can about what fills their days and their thoughts—the routine detail of their lives, what they take for granted, what they instinctively like and dislike, fear or admire. The ways and habits of old ladies, young "clubman," candy-eating girls— the laxities and explosions called the artistic temperament, the proportion of thick-headedness usually associated with "hard-headedness" in business men. For these are matters which may form the basis of a correct diagnosis and a successful course of treatment.[5]

The adventures involved in obtaining this kind of "routine detail" about patients and then persuading (or failing to persuade) them to make the lifestyle alterations that followed from it—this is the stuff of any number of physician memoirs from the time. This was the house-call–making era of Arthur Hertzler and William Carlos Williams and countless equally keen observers of patients, families, and households.[6] It is impossible to read accounts of nineteenth- and early-twentieth-century country doctoring without appreciating how the professional gulf between doctor and patient frequently dissolved, leaving as residue frustration, exasperation, despair—but also the special bond of friends. And the curing, more often than not, grew out of the bond, out of the patient's faith in the healing intention of the doctor. Osler appreciated the healing power of the doctor-patient relationship as well as anyone, and he realized that it was not reserved for high-powered consultants who wrote textbooks of medicine. "Faith in the gods or in the saints cures one, faith in little pills another, hypnotic suggestion a third, faith in a plain common doctor a fourth," he quipped in 1901.[7]

The situation in turn-of-the-century urban America was different. Here hospital outpatient departments or "dispensaries" provided low- or no-cost care for the indigent, especially immigrants new to these shores. Much of the care was clinic-like and perfunctory, to be sure. But there were many immigrants among dispensary doctors, especially at hospitals like New York's Jews' Hospital (renamed Mt. Sinai Hospital in 1872) and German Hospital (renamed Lennox Hill Hospital in 1918), whose founding raison d'être was to serve immigrant communities. At such hospitals, common background and ethnicity often overcame circumstances of treatment and led to uncommon connections and abiding friendships between doctors and patients. One cannot read the memoirs of two émigré Hungarians destined for surgical prominence in America—Arpad Gerster, who trained in Vienna in the early 1870s, and Max Thorek, who trained at Chicago's Rush Medical College in the early 1900s—without appreciating this fact.[8] Thorek, a lifelong devotee of the performing arts, both befriended and cared for members of the troupes that made stops in Chicago. In 1911, he founded the 25-bed American Hospital to care for ailing performers like Buffalo Bill ("my patient as well as my friend"), Harry Houdini ("my lifelong friend"), Florence Reed ("one of my most valued friends as well as my patient"), and scores of thespian unknowns. "Much has been added to the richness and variety of my professional life through friendships and associations with these rough-and-tumble knights of the sawdust ring," he reminisced in 1943. "It is the warm human friendship which counts the most. I have a long record of such friendships in my heart."[9]

But that was then and this is now. Now physicians see us during vanishingly brief office visits. They do not visit us in our homes. Nor do they establish dispensaries because they like us and are like us. They diagnose us and treat us according to well-established protocols, often anchored in the research findings of "evidence-based medicine." They relate to us differently, and we expect both more *from* them but less *of* them. So the question must be asked anew: Do our doctors still befriend us? And, more to the point, do we even want them to be our friends?

II.

In an editorial in the *Boston Globe* of August 22, 2011, "Blurred Boundaries Between Doctor and Patient," columnist and primary care internist Suzanne Koven wrote movingly of her patient Emma, whom Koven befriended over the last 15 years of Emma's life. "Emma and I met frequently to gossip, talk about books and politics, and trade stories about our lives," she remarked. "She came to my house for dinner several times, and my husband and kids joined me at her 90th birthday party. When, at 92, Emma moved reluctantly into a nursing home, I brought her the bagels and lox she craved—rich, salty treats her doctor had long discouraged her from eating. Here's the funny part: I was that doctor."

Koven writes perceptively of her initial concern with doctor-patient boundaries (heightened, she admits, by her status as "a young female physician"), her ill-fated efforts to maintain her early ideal of professional detachment, and, as with Emma, her eventual understanding that the roles of physician and friend could be for the most part "mutually reinforcing."

As a historian of medicine interested in the doctor-patient relationship, I reacted to Koven's piece appreciatively but, as I confessed to her, sadly. For her initial concern with "blurred boundaries" and her realization after years of practice that friendship between doctor and patient is compatible with primary medical care suggests that Osler and his generation have fallen by the wayside in the fragmented and depersonalized world of contemporary medicine, primary care included. Now, it appears, the intimacy that once characterized routine doctoring has been replaced with a connection so shallow and partial that we are given to scrutinize doctor-patient "friendship" as a problematic (Is it good? Is it bad? Should there be limits to it?) and to celebrate instances of such friendship as signal achievements. Psychoanalysts, be it noted, have been pondering these questions in their literature for decades, but they at least have the excuse of their method, which centrally implicates the analysis and resolution of "the transference" with patients who tend to become inordinately dependent on them.

In the mid-1980s, a decade after the promulgation of the "Patient Bill of Rights" by the Joint Commission on Accreditation of Hospitals and the American Hospital Association,[10] bioethicists preoccupied with patient autonomy and self-determination shared Koven's early concerns. For writers like Robert Veatch and Patricia Illingworth, the "friendship" model of doctor-patient relationships was for most patients an encumbrance that compromised their autonomy.[11] Rather than highlighting the patient's "wounded humanity" and "petitioner" status in the manner of Edmund Pellegrino, these writers viewed medical patients as autonomous agents who valued "personal" doctoring much less than competent, businesslike medical attention. Such patients might desire friendly rapport with their doctors, to be sure, but they did not seek friendship in the strong sense of Aristotle. They did not, that is, seek "perfect trust" with their doctors, nor did they desire their doctor's good as much as their own.

For these patients, the doctor's proffered friendship, with the reciprocal obligation to befriend the doctor, was burdensome; it mitigated their freedom to choose their own friends according to their own needs and desires. More insidiously still, even patients who sought to befriend their doctors could be acting in bad faith. According to Illingworth, they might be freighted with "psychological oppression," the sense that simple payment to the doctor for services rendered would not secure their best interests, so that the additive of friendship became a safeguard against mediocre medical care.[12] In this glum vision of things, the Hippocratic Oath has succumbed utterly to the cynicism that accompanies patient empowerment.

These ethicist musings, as noted, originated in an era in which patient rights dominated public concern about medicine and doctors. In retrospect, we see that they miss the boat on several counts when it comes to friendship. They render abstract what is never abstract but always personal and particular and contingent on life circumstances. As a consequence, they deny the historical singularity of medicine as a caring profession, for only by severing medical care from medical caring does the friendship between doctor and patient become extraneous, even epiphenomenal.[13]

In making the excision, these ethicists drain the very concept of friendship of its phenomenological and experiential richness. After all, choosing to accept dependency on a physician in the belief that his or her care and caring will aid in the restoration of health and activity—Pellegrino would add in the restoration of freedom and full humanity—can *be* an act of autonomy. And once the patient's expectation of competent treatment is "humanized," i.e., once it incorporates the assumption that medical care from this or that physician will be conjoined with medical caring, then, ipso facto, the patient has accepted a bond that *is* a kind of friendship.

Nor is it any different for the doctor: to accept "into one's care" a person who is ill and anxious, possibly in distress, is to embrace the "caring" dimension of care in all its amplitude. It is to offer oneself as the kind of friend who is entitled to the patient's confidences and bodily intimacies. It is to ask for, and be responsive to, the patient's bestowal of trust as it concerns his or her health and well-being. What is this if not friendship in the *medically appropriate* sense of the term?

My father, William Stepansky, like many of the WWII generation, befriended his patients, but he befriended them *as their doctor*. That is, he understood his medicine to include human provisions of a loving and essentially Hippocratic sort. Friendly two-way extramedical queries about his family, contact at community events, attendance at local weddings and other receptions—these were not boundary-testing land mines but aspects of community-embedded caregiving. And here's the rub: My father befriended his patients as their doctor; his friendship was simply the caring dimension of his caregiving. What, after all, did he have in common with the vast majority of his patients? They were Protestants and Catholics, members of the Rotary and Kiwanis Clubs who attended the local churches and coached little league baseball and Pop Warner football. He was a soft-spoken, bookish East European Jew, a serious lifelong student of the violin whose leisure time was spent practicing, reading medical journals, and tending to his lawn.

And yet to his patients, he was always a special kind of friend, though he himself would admit nothing special about it: his friendship was simply the human expression of his calling. It had nothing to do with religion or ethnicity or cultural background. It was simply the friendship conveyed by warmly caring human contact. It was the warmth of Osler transposed to community medicine of the postwar era. My father did not (to my knowledge) bring anyone bagels and lox or pay visits to chat about books or politics, but he provided treatment (including ongoing supportive psychotherapy) at no charge, accepted payment in kind, and visited patients in their homes when they became too elderly or infirm to come to the office. Other tokens of friendship included charging for a single visit when a mother brought a brood of sick children to the office during the cold season. And when elderly patients became terminal, they did not have to ask—he simply began visiting them regularly in their homes to provide what comfort he could and let them know they were on his mind. Certain patients of modest means he treated for little or nothing at all. He was uncomfortable with financial transactions and never touched money in the office—this too another revenant from the Oslerian world.

When he announced his impending retirement to his patients in the fall of 1990, his farewell letter began "Dear Friend" and then expressed regret at "leaving many patients with whom I have shared significant life experience from which many long-term friendships have evolved." "It has been a privilege to serve as your physician for these many years," he concluded. "Your confidence and friendship have meant much to me." When, in my research for *The Last Family Doctor*,[14] I sifted through the bags of cards and letters that followed this announcement, I was struck by the number of patients who not only reciprocated my father's sentiment but summoned the words to convey deep gratitude for the gift of their doctor's friendship. With many patients the friendship deepened over the years, though never straying beyond the bounds of medical friendship. To some, he became "Dr. Bill." (I wonder: do adult patients these days ever append "Dr." to the first name of a physician who has over time become a physician-friend?) One elderly woman whom he treated for much of his practice refers to him even now, always and only, as "My Friend." Another patient whom my father began treating in the 1950s and stayed in touch with him until his death in 2008, reminded me in 2011 how during office visits, "your Dad and I would wander off the 'medical desert,' and swerve into international affairs." He continued: "I explained to him that when I was young, I'd wish that I was Jewish, in that, the Old Testament intrigued me, due to the historical events of Moses' great personal sacrifice and leadership. To be a joint heir of God's covenant with Abraham, as well as under the recipient of His blessings, was just something to be greatly valued." This is not the kind of thing one ordinarily throws out to one's physician, Jewish or not, but to a longtime friend at a regular office visit? Sure, why not.

There are all kinds of wandering in postwar small-town general practice. I remember well one Alice McFarland, who was bedridden with intractable back pain from spinal stenosis, lived two miles down the road from us, and was adamant that her periodic injections of Demerol were not adequate to her suffering. Alice required and received several house calls a week from her doctor, my father, who administered additional pain medication, often augmented by vitamin B-12 shots. The medical treatments were simply a pretext for giving Alice the human support she desperately needed. Alice became part of our dinnertime and weekend family life. She called the house most days and never identified herself, always beginning, with whichever of the doctor's four sons happened to pick up the phone, "H-o-n-e-y, is D-a-d-d-y there?" Her voice, at once long-suffering and endearing, was unmistakable and sent one or another son scampering down the center hallway, yelling at a run, "Dad! It's Alice!"

III.

In our own era of fragmented multispecialty care, hemmed in by patient rights, defensive medicine, and concerns about boundary violations, it is far more difficult for a physician to "friend" a patient *as a physician*, to be and remain a *physician*-friend. Furthermore, physicians now wrestle with the ethical implications of "friending" in ways that have little to do with the obligations attendant to caring for patients. Many younger physicians choose to forego professional distance at the close of a workday. No less than the rest of us, physicians seek multicolored self states woven of myriad connective threads; no less than the rest of us, they are the Children of Facebook.

A number of recent reports suggest that medical school deans, clinical supervisors, and hospital administrators have their hands full monitoring the online activities of medical students and residents, the most savvy and uninhibited of the medical Children of Facebook. Much has been written of the challenge—some say the impossibility[15]—of keeping separate the professional self and the private self of physicians who, like their patients, are immersed in social networking and often inattentive to the importance of Facebook "privacy settings" or the advisability of withholding full names and medical identities from their Twitter accounts.[16]

This is especially so for students and residents, who frequently evince poor judgment in managing their online identities. The "online disinhibition effect"[17] fostered by social media—the illusory sense of detachment and anonymity associated with online posting—has prevented the budding professionalism of many of these young doctors and doctors-in-training from taking root. Inattentive to the long-term consequences of their digital footprint, many allow patients into their private worlds, oblivious to the short- and long-term impact of their disclosures on their professional selves. Keeping Facebook profiles open to the public in many cases,[18] they post content and photos deemed inappropriate by medical school faculty, fully trained colleagues, and, according to one recent survey, the public at large.[19]

The content in question ranges beyond disclosures of sexual orientation, political ideology, and religious affiliation, though such revelations alone "could cause a patient to withhold information, to form preconceived biases or simply to feel uncomfortable with that individual as their doctor."[20] Some also post images of binge drinking and images that are sexually suggestive or explicit; occasionally they post content in clear violation of the Health Insurance Portability and Accountability Act.[21] In one especially upsetting instance cited by several commentators, physician members of a Puerto Rican humanitarian mission to Haiti posted online photos of naked, unconscious patients in operating suites, along with photos of physicians drinking or posing with grins and "thumbs up" in front of patients or coffins.[22] Whether or not such lapses are better understood through the binary of "public" and "private" online identities or the "appropriateness" of specific postings "in a public space"[23] seems largely beside the point, which has to do with seriously poor judgment that can affect colleagues, hospitals, and especially patients present and future.

The official response to departures from online professionalism has taken the form of guidelines intended to heighten professional consciousness and thereby bring medical students' and physicians' use of social media into alignment with the physician's Hippocratic injunction to "first, do no harm."[24] "First, do no harm" in this context means "taking care to remain professional at all times," even on Twitter; to adopt online "dual citizenship" with separate private and professional online identities; in all to become aware of the "negative professional consequences" attendant to the "current and future practice of sharing information that could be misinterpreted."[25]

Both the Federation of State Medical Boards and the American Medical Association have entered the fray with their own sets of guidelines for medically appropriate use of social media and social networking.[26] Implicit in all such formulations is the assumption that medical professionalism, as traditionally understood, remains in full force in the realm of social media. The Internet simply enlarges the realm in which professional norms operate, and, in so doing, amplifies the consequentiality of the lapses, insensitivities, and indiscretions to which medical students and young doctors are prone. Unsurprisingly, the online behaviors that prompt state medical board investigation and possible reprimand parallel the same behaviors offline, i.e., inappropriate use of alcohol, derogatory speech, violations of patient privacy, conflicts of interest.[27]

Consciousness-raising takes the form of exhortation: medical faculty, senior physicians, state boards, and professional organizations join hands in seeking to impress on medical students and residents that, in the realm of online postings, their generationally shaped sense of what is and what is not appropriate may be out of sync with the norms of both their medical elders and the nonmedical public, not to mention the law. Conversational tweets about medical matters aimed at "virtual colleagues," they are reminded, are available to a limitless number of Twitter users and may be retweeted throughout the network and beyond.[28] "In most cases," they are told, "the risks of interacting with patients on online social forums appear to outweigh any current potential benefits."[29] There are more specific recommendations on how to respond to patients' requests to become online friends, along with the predictable strictures of the older generation (e.g., "Use conservative privacy settings, coupled with sober use of language and professional decorum, to afford oneself sufficient latitude to use the website while avoiding online interactions with patients."[30]) For those students and doctors who feel "compelled" to share access with patients, "closely policing one's privacy status and profile content is imperative."[31] In the knowledge that such admonitions may prove unavailing, residency program directors have been urged to monitor the public sites of residents to identify "gaps in professionalism" that require "correction."[32]

IV.

Guidelines to medical users of social media revolve around the issue of professionalism, which, physicians are advised in no uncertain terms, cannot be parked at the electronic portal. On the contrary, social networking requires heightened vigilance to the requirements of professional behavior. Communications with medical content, physicians are advised over and over, may be interpreted or misinterpreted by patients, prospective patients, medical educators, state review boards, and the public at large.

These discussions are timely and important, but they sequester the status of doctor-patient friendship in the traditional, deeply personal sense of the term. In fact, according to one commentator, Internet "friending" is problematic precisely because "friendships with patients have *not* been a customary part of the patient-doctor relationship."[33] Really? This facile claim leaves Osler dead and buried. It is profoundly inattentive to history, to the crucial role of friendship as a potentiator of treatment and promoter of cure. It is a claim that, at the most primal level, dehumanizes medicine, as it leaves no space at all for the special *kind* of friendship between doctors and patients that has long been intrinsic to general medical practice. And it flies in the face of contemporary research demonstrating that many patients desire physicians who are friends, and "that those who perceived their relationship with their doctor as that of a friend rather than patient had greater levels of confidence in their care,"[34] with all the attendant benefits of a trusting doctor-patient relationship on health care outcomes.[35]

And it is precisely this kind of friendship that is jeopardized by Internet "friending." In a world where everyone can simply *be* a friend, no one can actually *become* a friend. Indeed, the neutered friending permitted by social media discourages the development of kinds of friendship in general. Once we put aside Aristotle, Bacon, and Montaigne, for whom friendship was a sublime meeting of minds, something akin to a psycho-intellectual merger experience, we return to the everyday reality that we have many kinds of friends—work friends, neighbor friends, tennis friends, club friends, sports friends—and the "kinds" are meaningful to us in all their respective limitations and particularities. One downside of social media friending is that it scatters connective energy, and the greater the scattering, the more difficult it becomes for friendships of one or another kind to take root and deepen *over time*. Friendships between doctors and patients are necessarily restrained in certain ways; they are "measured" friendships. But such friendships are no less authentic, no less mutual and binding, on that account.

When, as a society, we construe the friendship of doctors as extra-medical, when we pull it into the arena of deanimated connecting fostered by social media, we risk marginalizing the deeper kind of friendship associated with the medical calling: the physician's nurturing love of the patient. And we lose sight of the fact that, until the final two decades of the nineteenth century, when advances in cellular biology, experimental physiology, bacteriology, and pharmacology ushered in an era of specific remedies for specific ailments, most effective doctoring—excluding treatment for a limited number of conditions along with a limited range of corrective surgeries—amounted to little more than just such friendship, such comfortable and comforting *be*friending of sick and suffering people for whom trust in the physician was the primary instrument of treatment. We lose sight of everything Osler taught us.

V.

As if the challenges of "online professionalism" and Facebook "friending" don't complicate doctor-patient relationships enough, there is the additional strain of online rating services, where patients rate their physicians along several service-related parameters and then, if they choose, append brief evaluative comments. No less than the writings of 1980s bioethicists, who looked askance at the "friendship model" of physician-patient relationship, the physician rating websites that first appeared in the late 1990s—HealthGrades.com, RateMDs.com, WebMD.com, Vitals.com, et al.—are an outgrowth of the patient rights movement, with its associated demand for public accountability, that gained traction in the 1970s and blossomed in the 1980s. The ratings websites did not emerge *in vacuo*. Among their antecedents are the *U.S. News and World Report* annual "guide to hospitals" launched in 1990 and the innumerable "best doctors" listings for cities and regions that followed over the next several years. All these listings and guides were based on surveys in which large numbers of physicians were asked to identify the "best hospitals" or the "best physicians" in their respective specialties.[36] The online rating services, which invite individual patients to evaluate individual doctors, are another matter, and taken together, represent the apotheosis of the consumerist vision of health care: We are consumers, our doctors provide services, and we have every right to evaluate their performance in ways that matter to us and presumably to others "in the market" for medical services. And who is to say this is a bad thing? What is wrong with knowing that the wait time for one doctor is unacceptably long or that another spends most of an office visit making eye contact only with his tablet?

There is nothing at all wrong here, as long as we are content with a consumerist orientation toward health care. If doctors are merely the corporeal equivalents of home repair experts, then perusing their star gradings, reading their consumer feedback, and noting if they are "Recognized Doctors" are good things entirely. The problem arises for the many patients who persist in viewing their physicians as something more than body-maintenance tradesmen. For them, the rating websites, no less than Facebook and Twitter, have a downside.

For doctors, of course, ratings and comments can be damaging because—excepting only the review/scheduling service ZocDoc[37]—they are not vetted; they encourage impulsiveness and verbal "acting out" on the part of individuals who may bear a grudge and may not even be patients of the doctor in question. Rare is the physician who cheerfully accepts rating websites because, "though virtually useless for meaningful evaluation of an individual physician," they "make for refreshing reading" and, taken in the aggregate, may provide useful qualitative data on patients' needs and preferences.[38] One wonders how many physicians have the time and inclination to read and ponder patient ratings "in the aggregate" while remaining unconcerned with their own location on the totem pole of patient appraisal.

But my concern here is not for the doctor but for patients in search of more than body work. For them, the rating websites have an insidious long-term consequence, and this has to do with their impact on doctors' emotional availability to patients and willingness to make this availability the linchpin of the special friendships associated with medical caring. Never mind that, according to one 2012 study, online ratings of physicians are generally very positive, with rating variations deriving largely from evaluations of punctuality and staff.[39] To the extent that doctors feel vulnerable—both professionally and financially— to the vagaries of patient feedback, they are forced to devalue that aspect of their professional identities that, in the pre-Internet world, was integral to doctoring.

It is a matter, once more, of the caring aspect of care, which over time becomes embedded in meaningful human connections that resist decomposition into discrete units of bodily tune-up and repair, more or less conveniently rendered. This kind of personalized caring, with its procedurally driven, hands-on component, was integral to family medicine through the 1960s and lives on among a dwindling minority of generalists, especially those who care for underserved, often rural, communities. But for the vast majority of physicians, including frontline primary care physicians, the rating sites have put them on the defensive and, in so doing, rendered mutual the consumerist orientation toward medical treatment (not care) that makes doctors plumbers of the body.

Some doctors who have felt the sting of negative feedback—whether "fake reviews" by fired employees, diatribes by angry patients denied medications they sought but didn't need, or constructive comments on professional shortcomings—have gone on the offensive. Medical Justice, a member-based "medical identity management" firm launched in 2002, developed a contract to be signed by the patients of its client physicians. Via the contract, which came into use in 2007, patients assigned copyright to any subsequent online review of the physician to the physician being reviewed. In this manner, doctors who received less than flattering feedback could claim copyright infringement and have the offending patient review removed from the rating service. In exchange for the patient's assignment of copyright, doctors agreed, by contract, not to share the patient's medical data with marketers.

Unsurprisingly, the contracts neglected to inform patients that by law doctors cannot share their confidential data with marketers without their prior authorization. The "privacy blackmail" contracts were jettisoned at the end of 2011, subsequent to a lawsuit and then a complaint filed with the Federal Trade Commission by the Center for Democracy and Technology.[40]

Copyright law is no longer being misused to suppress patients' rights to evaluate doctors, but physicians and their advocates remain inventively proactive in coping with the prospect of negative ratings. Rather than absorbing body blows to their professional selves, and having learned that courts provide no redress, they have embraced the growing role of physician ratings in medical practice and begun soliciting patient feedback through their own websites. Patients may be contacted by staff and invited to provide positive feedback on one or more of the rating websites.[41] In 2012, in a dramatic about-face, Medical Justice began supplying client doctors with iPads to give to patients at the point of leaving the office. Patients are asked to write a review, and the firm makes sure that their comments (presumably positive, possibly coerced) are posted on a review site. In the medical free market, there apparently is no defense like a good offense.[42] This is an example of what the sociologists Wendy Espeland and Michael Sauder, in a study of law school rankings, termed "gaming the system" to improve rankings.[43]

Even when preemptive strategies for obtaining positive feedback fall short, there are things to do. In "Responding to Negative Online Comments," the featured article in a recent issue of *MCMS* [Montgomery County Medical Society] *Physician*, a risk management specialist takes physicians down the list. "Don't panic," he tells them, and don't respond immediately or impulsively to negative feedback. "Not all negative comments are worthy of your time to respond," he continues. "A response may start a chain reaction of negative slurs and comments, potentially leading to litigation." Clearly false or inflammatory feedback warrants contact with the website administrator in the hope that the site's content guidelines will lead to removal of the offensive posting. Suing a reviewer, he cautions, is a problematic affair, and physicians contemplating such action should consult their attorneys as soon as possible. And there is the otherwise proactive strategy given here as a postscript to negative feedback: "follow up with positive information about your practice," but never, he warns, resort to posting fake consumer reviews.[44]

What's wrong with this picture? The physician rating websites provide the kind of transparency in health care long urged by consumer groups and the federal government, especially through the Centers for Medicare and Medicaid Services. Such transparency, it has been held since the 1970s, will improve the quality and costs of care. But what is the *nature* of this transparency, and what exactly does it allow us to see? For the vast majority of doctors, those who receive a rating or two or none at all, we see very little. We do not see these men and women as human caregivers bound by professional ethics to reach out to other humans who come to them as needy "petitioners" hopeful that the doctor's care will restore their damaged humanity (Pellegrino). Less grandiloquently, we do not see how willingly these men and women embrace—or fail to embrace—the relational matrix in which care and caregiving traditionally came together. The ratings provide only a black-and-white, two-dimensional x-ray, often tendentiously rendered, of the "bones" that frame a doctor's activities: office appearance; wait times; staff friendliness; time spent with a particular patient; and the like. And the energy spent soliciting, monitoring, and worrying about patient ratings is energy that might otherwise be deployed caring for patients in conflict-free ways far removed from the commercial world of consumer feedback. By putting doctors on the defensive, by mobilizing a proactive sensibility lest they receive negative feedback, the ratings make it harder for them to follow in the footsteps of Osler by understanding the patient's illness experience and the moral basis for clinical care.[45]

Never mind the even grimmer predicament of emergency room (ER) physicians, whose hospitals are now obligated to survey discharged patients on their hospital experience. In some cases, a portion of ER physicians' compensation is tied to the "quality" of services they provide, which in turn is linked in part to the patient ratings they receive. Recent surveys document the readiness of many ER physicians to overprescribe and order unnecessary studies in order to send happier patients out of ER rooms and to the patient-satisfaction survey forms that await them.[46] The result? A growing tendency to inappropriate care and dramatically inflated costs to Medicare among patients who make ER visits. The irony is that high patient satisfaction ratings by patients have not been shown to correlate with measurable indices of higher quality care. A 2012 survey of 52,000 respondents to the national Medical Expenditure Panel Survey by researchers at the University of California, Davis, for example, showed that over a seven-year period (2000–2007) participants in the highest patient satisfaction quartile not only spent more on prescription drugs, but were 12% more likely to be admitted to the hospital and accounted for 9% more in total health care costs than survey participants who did not give their providers such stellar ratings.[47]

The kind of "patient satisfaction" associated with surveys is not the "satisfaction" associated with patient-centered care, much less long-term trusting relationships rooted in procedural and expressive touch. Rather, it is a commodified, point-of-service satisfaction associated, as noted, with ease of scheduling, wait times, staff courtesy, and pain management. Physicians in search of such satisfaction are, to their own dismay, becoming less concerned with their patients' compliance with medical directives (now "recommendations" or "suggestions") than with their own compliance with patients' expectations. Patients, for their part, may rely more on met expectations than objective medical outcomes in rating their doctors. In primary care, where office visits are brief and pressure on clinicians to maximize "throughput" (i.e., to see as many patients as possible during office hours) is intense, there is pressure to make patients happy by, for instance, prescribing dangerously addictive opioids rather than taking the time to discuss alternative treatments. Physicians who comply with unreasonable patient requests are in a bind, since their desire to satisfy patients and avoid poor satisfaction scores may trump medical judgment, in which case they "may find themselves in the role of 'customer service' providers rather than medical professionals or healers."[48] Unsurprisingly, preliminary survey data show an association between utilization of patient satisfaction surveys and job dissatisfaction and attrition among physicians, especially ER and primary care physicians.[49]

So here, finally, is the payoff: Between the Scylla of eviscerated Facebook "friending" and the Charybdis of point-of-service patient ratings (associated with excessive testing, overprescribing of controlled substances, and physician burnout), physicians are increasingly pulled away from a relational model of caregiving, a trend that all the patient-centered training and empathy workshops in the world cannot reverse. The fact is that the vast majority of private-practice physicians today have less energy and/or inclination to give patients in search of something more than body maintenance what physicians have traditionally offered them: a special kind of friendship.

VI.

And yet such friendships continue to blossom, and this is because friendship is not an elective connection to which one gives or denies assent in an electronic instant. It is a different kind of connection, one that grows slowly over time to the point that often its depth and meaning can only be identified in retrospect, as a fait accompli. This is why doctor-patient friendships are most customary between patients and their "personal" doctors, for here the relationship is continuing, with the potential of deepening into friendship as time passes and medical trials and tribulations come and go. Even now, in an era of patient empowerment, we read accounts of such friendship and how it changed the way this or that doctor practiced medicine, reshaped his medical identity, even transformed her.[50]

In the years following World War II, when diagnosis remained largely a hands-on affair relying on physical examination and history taking, doctor-patient friendship was not a singular event in a medical career worthy of journal publication. It remained an element of the physician's modus operandi and could be valued for a number of pragmatic reasons. In his Shattuck address of 1949, Paul Dudley White, the eminent cardiologist, discussed them one by one. Friendship, he held, enlarged and personalized history taking by encouraging patients to provide fuller accounts of their illness; in this manner doctor-patient friendship contributed to accurate diagnosis and ensured better compliance with treatment. It also contributed to the growth of medical knowledge, since it facilitated patients' cooperation in "special investigations of symptoms, signs, mechanisms of disease that involved physiologic and biochemical procedures, prognosis, and therapy." It also made patients willing partners in clinical teaching. "Some of the most important lessons that I have been able to present in my teaching to both undergraduates and graduates of medicine," White remarked, "have been made possible because some of my most articulate patients, who have taken an active part in the teaching of my students individually, in small groups, or even in large amphitheater clinics, have been warm friends of mine."[51]

White did not address systematically what others of the era did: that patients would be much more satisfied with their doctors if the latter, in the words of no less esteemed a consultant than Walter C. Alvarez, "simply showed any signs of liking them personally."[52] But White's brief gives one final reason for doctor-patient friendship, and it is the simplest and most telling: "there is a great personal satisfaction and joy in the establishment of human friendship, not wholly definable, both for the doctor and, I am sure, for his patients."[53] And this satisfaction and joy, White went on to observe, was typically experienced in the community in which doctor and patient met and became friends.

In the world of traditional family medicine, the kind of medicine that typified the first half of the twentieth century and that my father was able to practice through the 1970s, community medicine was intergenerational, with the medical challenges traversed by doctor and patient encompassing the trials and tribulations of other family members as well. Community-embedded caregiving both normalized and sustained the medically appropriate friendships that developed over time between family doctors and the families under their care. Becoming part of the community, accommodating the mindset of community members, earning the respect and trust and, yes, friendship of community leaders—these injunctions are sounded in countless valedictories and addresses, including those of Oliver Wendell Holmes in 1871, William Thayer in 1928, and Paul Dudley White in 1949.[54]

The scientific advances of World War II and recognizably modern medicine of the 1950s and '60s had not yet altered this reality: Medical care in smaller communities often remained medical care among friends.[55] In his President's Address to the American Medical Association in 1956, Dwight Murray, a general practitioner with 35 years of small city practice under his belt, made the point loud and clear. Paying tribute to the thousands of families he had served throughout his career, he remarked that, "Like thousands of my colleagues in general practice, I have gotten to know many of them intimately. I deem it a privilege to have had the opportunity of serving their medical needs, and I am convinced that I would be welcomed into their homes as a friend."[56]

Today, this tributary flowing into doctor-patient relationships remains wide and deep among those remaining physicians who practice "old style" medicine, especially in rural communities. But outside of them, and allowing for noteworthy exceptions, it has narrowed greatly. In an effort to widen the tributary anew, family medicine educators of the 1990s recommended special training in "psychosocial skills" in an effort to remedy the disinclination of family-doctors-in-the-making to address the psychosocial (read: community-embedded, friendship-promoting) aspects of medical care. Survey research of the time showed that most residents training to become primary care physicians not only devalued psychosocial care, but also doubted their competence to provide it. A 2009 report from the Department of Family Medicine and Community Health of the University of Massachusetts Medical School suggested that little had changed in the intervening years. It began by alerting readers to the fact that "the specialty of family medicine has committed to instruction in numerous community-related skills meant to complement clinical training." It then proceeded to a survey of graduates of a family medicine residency program over a 30-year period in order "to assess confidence in and participation in a range of community-related activities." Among recently trained family physicians, the researchers found, "predoctoral training in community skills" had not made them more likely to use those skills, leaving the researchers to ponder how "community skills training during medical school can be reinforced and extended through residency so that young physicians may engage with their communities earlier in their careers."

My father would probably have appreciated the need for such programs, but would also have viewed them as sadly remedial attempts to transform individuals with medical training into physicians. Gifted generalists of his generation did not require instruction "in numerous community-related skills" because their medicine, their care-giving, was actualized in community settings. They were community doctors who were drawn to general practice precisely because it promised them "participation in a range of community-related activities." Such participation was a sine qua non of their doctoring, not a skill set to be acquired over time. And it encouraged the development of friendships with patients that were no less authentic on account of being constrained by the fact that one party to the friendship was one's doctor and the other one's patient. Indeed, the asymmetry in the relationship attested to its special nature, since it was the physician's intelligence, his agreeableness, his amiability, his sympathy—in all his "traits of character"—that made him fit "to enter into the most intimate and confidential relations with the families of which you are the privileged friend and counselor." This is Oliver Wendell Holmes addressing the graduating class of Bellevue Hospital College in 1871.[57]

VII.

And this takes us back to Suzanne Koven, who imputes the "austere façade" she offered patients during her early years of practice to those imposing nineteenth-century role models "whose oil portraits lined the walls of the hospital [MGH] in which I did my medical training." Among the grim visages that stared down from on high was that of the illustrious James Jackson, Sr., who brought Jenner's technique of smallpox inoculation to the shores of Boston in 1800, became Harvard's second Hersey Professor of the Theory and Practice of Medicine in 1812, and was a driving force in the founding of MGH, which opened its doors in 1821. Koven cites a passage from the second of Jackson's *Letters to a Young Physician* (1855) in which he urges his young colleague to "abstain from all levity" and "never exact attention to himself."

But why should absence of levity and focal concern with the patient be tantamount to indifference, coolness, the withholding of *physicianly* friendship? Was Jackson really so forbidding a role model? Composing his *Letters* in the wake of the cholera epidemic of 1848, when the remedies of orthodox or "regular" medicine, especially bleeding and purging, proved futile and only heightened the suffering of thousands, Jackson cautioned modesty when it came to therapeutic pretensions. He abjured the use of drugs "as much as possible," and added that "the true physician takes care of his patient without claiming to control the disease in all cases." Indeed he sought to restore "cure" to its original Latin meaning, to *curare*, the sense in which "to cure meant to take care." "The physician," he instructed his protégé,

> may do very much for the welfare of the sick, more than others can do, although he does not, even in the major part of cases, undertake to control and overcome the disease by art. It was with these views that I never reported any patients *cured* at our hospital. Those who recovered their health before they left the house were reported as *well*, not implying that they were made so by the active treatment they had received there. But it was to be understood that all patients received in that house were to be cured, that is, taken care of.[58]

And then he moved on to the narrowing of vision that safeguarded the physician's caring values, his *cura*:

> You must not mistake me. We are not called upon to forget ourselves in our regard for others. We do not engage in practice merely from philanthropy. We are justified in looking for both profit and honor, if we give our best services to our patients; only we must not be thinking of these when at the bedside. There the welfare of the sick must occupy us entirely.[59]

Koven sees the Hippocratic commitment that lies beneath Jackson's stern glance and, with the benefit of hindsight, links it to her friendship with her patient Emma. "As mutually affectionate as our friendship was," she concludes, "her health and comfort were always its purpose." Indeed. For my father and generations of caring generalists before him, friendship of a special kind was foundational to clinical caring; it inhered in the medical calling. It was not extramural, not reserved for special patients, but a way of being with *all* patients. And it was precisely this way of being, this constancy of caring, that made his doctoring a kind of friendship-in-action. His way of being, shared by countless other doctors, calls to mind one of Montaigne's provisos, that "In friendship there is a general and universal warmth, temperate, moreover, and uniform, a constant and settled warmth, all gentleness and smoothness, with no roughness or sting about it."[60] And this general, settled warmth, orbiting around a sensibility of *cura* and a wide range of hands-on procedural activities, was not a heavy thing, leaden with solemnity. It was musical. It danced.

In the early 1960s, my father returns from a nursing home where he has just visited a convalescing patient. I am his traveling companion during afternoon house calls, and I greet him on his return to the car. He looks at me and with a sly grin remarks that he has just added "medicinal scotch" to the regimen of this elderly gentleman, who sorely missed his liquor and was certain a little imbibing would move his rehab right along. It was a warmly caring gesture worthy of Osler, that lover of humanity and inveterate practical joker. And a generation before Osler, the elder Jackson would have smiled. Immediately after cautioning the young physician to "abstain from all levity," he added: "He should, indeed, be cheerful, and, under proper circumstances, he may indulge in vivacity and in humor, if he has any. But all this should be done with reference to the actual state of feeling of the patient and of his friends." Just so.

CHAPTER 9

General Practice and Its Discontents

Take from scientific medicine the contributions made to it by the country doctor and you rob it of half its glory.
—Victor C. Vaughan, *A Doctor's Memories* (1926)

P ity the American general practitioner, whose imminent disappearance has been forecast since the late nineteenth century. Here is Andrew Smith writing about "The Family Physician" in *Harper's* in 1888:

> It will readily be seen that amid all these claimants for pathological territory there is scarcely standing-room left for the general practitioner.[1]

And here is Abraham Jacobi, the founder of modern pediatrics, in 1910:

> The time when every family, rich or poor, had its own family physician, who knew the illnesses and health of its members and enjoyed the confidence of the upgrowing boys and girls during two or three generations, is gone.[2]

Here is A. F. van Bibber, a small-town practitioner and popular writer from Maryland, in "The Swan Song of the Country Doctor" of 1929:

More recent investigation shows that almost one-third of the towns of 1,000 or less throughout the United States which had physicians in 1914 had none in 1925 . . . it will be seen at a glance that the present generation of country doctors will have practically disappeared in another ten years.[3]

For the pulmonologist and TB specialist Paul Dufault, who celebrated the glories of American medicine at midcentury, the general practitioner was little more than a relic, albeit an admirable relic about whom one might rhapsodize:

Those who have reached middle age still remember the general practitioner, now almost extinct in some localities. Closely resembling modern internists, they were a grand old type, freelancing in abscesses and phlegmons, shuttling between mother and baby, turning a hand at small repairs, amputating a finger, sewing a cut, making little incursions into allergic territory, encouraging the depressed wife, upbraiding the exuberant husband, looking into a roguish eye, peering into a deaf ear, holding down a rebellious stomach or extinguishing a fiery rash as the occasion arose. They knew much about many things and did much for many people. May fate be kind to those who remain![4]

Far more glum was David Rutstein, head of Harvard Medical School's department of preventive medicine, in 1960:

But complete medical care means more than the sum of the services provided by specialists, no matter how highly qualified. It must include acceptance by one doctor of complete responsibility for the care of the patient and for the coordination of specialist, laboratory, and other services. Within a generation, if the present situation continues, few Americans will have a personal physician do this for them.[5]

And finally, in our own time, here is the primary care educator Thomas Bodenheimer, speaking not only of family physicians (FPs) but of the entire category of "primary care physicians" (PCPs) that includes family physicians, general internists, and general pediatricians:

Whoever takes up the cause of primary care, one thing is clear: action is needed to calm the brewing storm before the levees break.[6]

In Great Britain, the provenance of such jeremiads is older still. In Scotland, Dr. John Brown, equally esteemed as physician and essayist, complained in 1858

> of what is now too rare—the old feeling of a family doctor—the familiar kindly welcoming face that has presided through generations at births and deaths; the old friend who bears about and keeps sacred, deadly secrets and who knows the kind of stuff his flock is made of; all this sort of thing is greatly gone.[7]

Traditionally, American historians in search of an explanation for the recurrently imminent demise of the family doctor in their own country have landed on medical specialization, which began in earnest after the Civil War, quickened in the 1880s and 1890s, and came to fruition in the years immediately following World War II. Over the course of some 70 years, from roughly 1880 to 1950, specialism replaced generalism, pure and simple. And yet family doctors, for all the dismal predictions and all the growth of specialism, are still with us. Indeed, many of us rely on them.

So what is wrong with the traditional account that pins the blame on medical specialization? For one thing, it overlooks the gradual manner in which specialism seeped into American medical practice over the course of the better part of a century. Medical specialties, like other professions, have their own structural requirements—the development of diagnostic procedures and treatment interventions specific to the specialty; extended residency training programs during which the diagnostic skills and procedural interventions are taught; and certifying examinations attesting to the fact that the skills and interventions have been well learned. And then there are the institutional correlates of these procedural developments: the creation of membership organizations for members of the specialty; the holding of annual conventions to keep members abreast of advances in their field; and the publication of specialty journals that disseminate the latest research and clinical findings of the specialists in question.

But these structural requirements came into being gradually, roughly between 1880 and 1950. Before the requirements were set in stone, before the specialty organizations became mature in the sociological sense, there was considerable room for generalists to maneuver, to declare themselves specialists of one type or another. This is readily apparent in internal medicine, the most generalist of the specialties and the specialty that lacked the limited domain of practice and specialized techniques and procedures of the surgical specialties.[8] It gained a nebulous foothold with the formation of the Association of American Physicians (AAP) by a small group of elite East Coast physician-researchers in 1885, but it was only a decade later that Osler, then AAP president, invoked the term "internal medicine" as a descriptor of the kind of physician the group represented. The founding members of the AAP were not only astute diagnosticians but scientific investigators with postgraduate study in European laboratories. Now, in 1895, Osler formalized the connection: He defined the internist of the future as a consultant to general physicians whose expertise derived from extensive laboratory training in chemistry, physiology, and pathology, and the resulting ability to bring laboratory science to bear at the patient's bedside. Internal medicine, for Osler, was not a specialty but a vocation that a scientifically oriented physician might embrace over the course of his career. A good consultative practice, he opined, would follow a full 20 years of study, research, and clinical experience.[9]

The American Board of Internal Medicine (ABIM), shorn of Osler's expansive claims and absent the cooperation of the AAP, was finally established in 1936. It was governed by an American pragmatism alien to Osler and had no desire that every internist be board certified; only a small number of outstanding consultants in the Oslerian mold, it was thought, would take the certifying examinations.[10] So the board did not prevent general practitioners from the late 1930s through the 1950s—often GPs of academic bent who had taken a second year of internship and/or learned pathology in hospital laboratories—from simply declaring themselves internists. Some of these GP-internists would take and pass the internal medicine boards and even achieve organizational prominence in the world of internal medicine. This was true of J. Dunbar Shields and Saul Jarcho, the two pioneering internists profiled by Sharon Kaufman in *The Healer's Tale: Transforming Medicine and Culture* (1993). Neither had residency training, but, on deciding to become internists, both took and passed the board certifying examinations in internal medicine in 1947 and 1950, respectively.[11] I recall my generalist father, William Stepansky, introducing me to a colleague who, he later told me, was a well-regarded internist, with attendant hospital privileges, who had never taken a residency. This was in the mid-1960s.

The declaratory path to specialization, the simple naming of oneself as a specialist, was entrenched in the surgical specialties a century before I met my father's residency-less internist colleague. There were enormously competent American surgeons throughout the nineteenth century, but the American College of Surgeons was only created in 1913. There were specialized eye doctors (oculists), nose doctors (rhinologists), and throat doctors (laryngologists) throughout the second half of the nineteenth century, but the American Board for Ophthalmic Examinations was only founded in 1915, followed by the National Board of Examiners of Otolaryngology in 1924. Operative gynecology and obstetrics were in full swing in the final decades of the nineteenth century, but the American Board of Obstetrics and Gynecology only came into being in 1930. The pace quickened with the formation of the Advisory Board for Medical Specialization in 1933, and by 1937 12 medical specialty boards had come into being. And yet in 1940, on the eve of America's entry into World War II, three out of four American physicians identified themselves as general practitioners.[12]

The resilience of general practitioners in the face of pre-World War II specialization also concerns the manner in which emergent specialty knowledge and procedures could be absorbed into general practice without declaring oneself an outright specialist. Through the Second World War and into the 1950s and '60s, we have seen, generalists had a baseline procedural competence that contemporary primary care physicians typically do not. This competence, this procedural orientation to practicing medicine, empowered them to add new specialty procedures to their armamentarium, with or without formal postgraduate training and without running into the brick wall of credentialing. Within certain parameters, generalism was able to envelop specialism, amoeba-like, according to the interests of the practitioner and the requirements of his or her practice.

After World War II, outside of smaller communities, the parameters were already shrinking, but the mindset of my father and other community generalists of the postwar decades still hearkens back to the hemmed-in manner in which generalists of the late nineteenth century accommodated specialism. This was the period when specialism typically bolstered generalism, when, in the words of Mary Putnam Jacobi, "the most useful functions of specialists are still exercised with tacit reference to the intelligent practitioner, who is compelled, not indeed to know all about all medicine, but to hold the key of admission to any of its branches, of which, at any moment, he may have practical need."[13]

Putnam offered her assessment in 1882, and Osler echoed it a decade later, when he wrote of "generalizing special knowledge" and lauded postgraduate schools for enabling practitioners to revive old technical skills and acquire new ones.[14] The belief that specialism would enlarge the scope of generalism was a recurrent theme in the literature of the early twentieth century, and it was still in evidence after World War II. Witness Reginald Fitz, the prominent Harvard-based internist of the 1930s and '40s, a leading light of the AMA's Section on Practice of Medicine and Council on Medical Education and member and one-time chairman (1944–1946) of the American Board of Internal Medicine. He mused in 1950 that the specialist of the future would have to be concerned with "discovering new technics that, when once established, can be used safely and expertly by doctors without highly special training."[15]

The conviction that specialist knowledge would be available to, and applied by, generalist physicians underscores the degree to which medical specialization through the 1930s was less a fact than a trend in medical practice. Until World War II, family physicians often developed what the medical educator Herman Weiskotten termed "a special interest in certain phases of medicine." Weiskotten, who surveyed at five-year intervals the graduates of American and Canadian medical colleges from 1915 through 1950, documented the large percentage of GPs with such "special interests," and the various ways in which they obtained the specialized competencies that went with them. Writing of the "early period of the trend toward specialization," he observed how

A number of these physicians [GPs] developed a special interest in certain phases of medical practice. As a result of their own initiative and frequently in association with older and more experienced physicians on more or less specialized hospital services, they developed special interests and abilities while continuing the family practice of medicine. Some took time off from their practice for variable periods of more intensive training at medical centers, either in this country or abroad. A number of these physicians, as they became recognized as having unusual ability in the field of their special interest, tended to limit their practice to it. However, as a rule many of these physicians with their previous experience in general medical care did not hesitate to continue to assume responsibility for the over-all medical care of patients, especially those they had previously served as family physicians.[16]

As hospital-based residency programs gained traction in the 1920s and '30s as the preferred route to specialty practice, the proportion of GPs who claimed specialty interests declined, a trend captured by Weiskotten's comparative statistics. Among graduates of the medical class of 1930, for example, 45% of those who entered practice without formal specialty training identified themselves as GPs five years after graduation, whereas 55% who gave "special attention" to one or another specialty still identified themselves as GPs. Among graduates of the class of 1945, on the other hand, the percentages were dramatically inverted: 76% of the postwar generalists later reported practicing general medicine, whereas only 24% claimed "special attention" to a specialty. What the percentages mask is the expansion of residency training programs, which equipped newly minted physicians not merely to give special attention to a specialty but actually to limit their practices to it. Whereas 30% of the 1930 graduates reported limiting their practice to a specialty, 74% of the class of 1945 reported being full-time specialists.[17]

Weiskotten's survey results quantify what historians have long understood: that World War II and the years immediately thereafter propelled medical specialization forward and jeopardized the status of the general practitioners. The acceleration of the trend began in the American military, where well-defined specialist groups were developed, especially under the auspices of the Army Specialized Training Program and the Navy V-12 program, the vast majority of whose trainees became specialists after the war. It was the U.S. Army that made board certification the sine qua non of specialty status, since it used it to classify physicians as medical specialists entitled to higher rank (captain instead of first lieutenant) and pay than the general medical officers (GMOs). The lesson was not lost on the general practitioners and incompletely trained (or self-named) specialists who entered the service: in 1945 over 13,000 returning medical officers were expected to seek board certification in one or another specialty.[18] Where were all these returning officers to complete their specialty training? The building of new hospitals, greatly aided by the subsidization provided by the Hill-Burton Act of 1946, supplied part of the answer. The growth of residency training programs—7,625 in 1945; 12,003 in 1947; 18,669 in 1950[19]—went hand in glove with the GI Bill of Rights, which subsidized up to four years of residency training for the returning medical officers.

But even these intertwined factors would have been insufficient to jeopardize the status of general practitioner if the scientific and clinical infrastructure of the specialties had not kept pace with the push supplied by the American military, the Hill-Burton Act, the growth of residency training programs, and the GI Bill. And here, once more, the war was the great catalyst. The range of advanced operative techniques developed by the military—in thoracic surgery, in orthopedics, in plastic and reconstructive surgery—called into question the long-held prerogative of generalists to practice major surgery in their community hospitals.

Even outside surgery, postwar diagnostic and treatment technologies available only in hospital settings bolstered the status of specialty medicine, both inside and outside the hospital. The gulf between generalists with special interests and specialists proper widened on account of these technologies, which increasingly required an expertise that was acquired during residency and fellowship training and, as such, was available to the specialists with hospital privileges but progressively less so to the generalists with specialty interests.

Consider cardiology, where postwar experiments in the use of countershock and direct current to treat ventricular fibrillation (irregular, rapid heartbeat); the development of closed-chest cardiac massage; and the introduction of continuous EKG monitoring in the

1960s all reduced deaths from cardiac arrest.[20] The opening of the first intensive care units (ICUs) in the early 1950s was responsive to the newly complex postsurgical management of cardiac patients and to the specialized skill sets of both the cardiologists and the ICU nurses who managed them.[21] These clinical developments, aided by the reorganization of the American Heart Association in 1946 to fund cardiovascular research and the founding of the American College of Cardiology in 1949,[22] established the bona fides of cardiology as a clinical subspecialty of internal medicine. Over the next two decades, cardiology would increasingly fall outside the operational domain of generalists in private practice. In community hospitals that lacked the services of fellowship-trained cardiologists, it fell to the general internists, not the GPs, to handle cardiac cases.

Or consider nephrology, the medical subspecialty dealing with kidney disease. It is not even included in Weiskotten's survey results published in 1956. The need for kidney specialists only arose in conjunction with diagnostic and treatment technologies that relied on specialized knowledge and training. Through the late 1950s, renal dialysis—the cycling of blood through a machine that filters out waste products when the patient's own kidneys are unable to do so—was available only as a short-term treatment for patients in acute renal failure. It could keep them alive for perhaps a few weeks, at which point their own kidneys would hopefully resume functioning.

The breakthrough came in 1960, when Belding Scribner, working at the University of Washington, designed a permanent indwelling Teflon shunt that allowed a patient in kidney failure to be connected to a dialysis machine for an extended period without a new surgical procedure each time.[23] Long-term dialysis became part of hospital medicine throughout the 1960s, and as the technology and concurrent medical management of dialysis patients improved, progressively more debilitated patients in kidney failure became eligible for dialysis. And so we needed more kidney specialists to treat them in the hospital and then to manage them at home. They gathered together in the American Society of Nephrology, founded in 1966; the specialized nephrology nurses followed suit three years later with the American Nephrology Nurses Association. Finally, in 1972, with passage of Section 2991 of the Social Security Act, Congress provided funding for all treatment costs associated with end-stage kidney disease, including long-term dialysis.[24] So now everyone with end-stage kidney disease could receive dialysis, and we needed even more nephrologists to care for them.

Concurrent with the refinement and expanded application of renal dialysis was the emergence of kidney transplantation as a viable alternative treatment for end-stage renal disease. A series of six successful kidney transplants between identical twins at Boston's Peter Bent Brigham Hospital in 1954 and 1955 was followed by successful transplants between nonidentical twins at Brigham in 1960 and then utilizing a cadaver kidney in 1963.[25] Of course, kidney transplants were anything but routine in the decade that followed, but the foregoing developments sufficed to mobilize a new breed of nephrologists, the "transplant nephrologists" who directed the nascent transplantation programs at major medical centers and came together in the American Society of Transplant Physicians in 1982. This kind of specialty practice was far beyond the realm of general practitioners and general internists.

The building of new hospitals; the availability of advanced technologies in the hospitals; the reliance on medical specialists to employ these technologies; and the complicated management issues that arose from them—taken together these postwar developments reframed the status of general practitioners in a way that the medical specialism of the 1920s and '30s could not. These several factors were preconditions for the crisis in general practice, but even taken together they did not make the crisis a reality. By the early 1950s, we had the hospitals; we had the specialists; and we had advanced diagnostic and treatment procedures to sustain specialty practice. But where were the patients? How did they learn about specialty medicine and the role of the modern hospital in providing care for acute illness? What led them to consider bypassing their family doctors when they became seriously ill and going directly to the cardiologist, the nephrologist, or the surgeon?

The fourth leg of the stool was the tremendous growth of voluntary health insurance after the Second World War. Bolstered by the Blue Cross advertising campaigns of the late 1930s and '40s, which stressed both the role of the hospital as the appropriate setting for treating acute illness and the prudent good sense of investing in group health policies,[26] enrollment in voluntary health insurance plans underwent explosive growth after the war. In 1946, 81 Blue Cross hospital plans and 44 Blue Shield medical plans were competing with commercial insurers, the latter able to offer uniform rates and benefits to national companies with branches in different states. The percentage of Americans with hospital coverage went from less than 10% in 1940 to nearly 70% in 1955.[27] The establishment of the Blue Cross Association as a national operating organization in 1956 and Congressional passage of the Federal Employees Health Benefits Program in 1959, with its smorgasbord of insurance options for federal employees, were sequelae to the explosion.

Who were all these Americans newly safeguarded from major illness by voluntary health insurance? They were middle-class, predominantly white, working Americans who received insurance through their employers. And the specialists came to them. Among the trends documented by Weiskotten in his periodic surveys was the diffusion of specialty medicine into smaller communities. Among medical school classes of 1935, 1940, and 1945, the percentage of full-time specialists practicing in communities of under 50,000 residents climbed from 26% to 29% to 35.4%. Grappling for an explanation for the spread of specialty medicine outside of large urban centers, Weiskotten found it "difficult to state how important recent hospital construction programs and the spread of group clinics have been in attracting more specialists to the smaller communities," and he underscored the trend by noting that fully 22% of 1945 graduates who were full-time specialists practiced in communities of fewer than 25,000.[28]

By 1950, everything seemed in place. Postwar building programs; the growth of specialty medicine as taught in three- to five-year residency training programs; the movement of younger specialists to smaller communities; and the expansion of health insurance among the middle class—the trends coalesced into storm clouds hovering over the time-honored institution of the family doctor.

But wait a minute. The storm never erupted; the specialist downpour never occurred. The clouds appeared to lighten—at least for a time. This is because the nation's generalists, among whom were the battle-tested general medical officers (GMOs) of World War II, refused to lay down their arms beneath the darkening skies of specialty medicine. They fought back organizationally, politically, and clinically. This is the counternarrative that reframes the dominant narrative about the triumph of specialty medicine after World War II. It begins with the formation of the American Academy of General Practice in 1947 and continues with the movement to transform old-style general practice into the new specialty of family practice in the mid-1960s.

II.

General practitioners of medicine were the medical heroes of World War II, but, for all the reasons given above, many of them returned home at war's end to find their medical standing at their local hospitals in jeopardy. Specialization had made great inroads during the war years, and, while the GPs were fighting the war in Europe, many hospitals reclassified their staff physicians on the basis of specialist qualifications. GPs of course were low men on the totem pole, and some found that the very hospitals where they had worked before the war had rescinded their surgical privileges after their return. Stanley R. Truman, the first secretary of the American Academy of General Practice and chronicler of its founding, recalled this very situation at his own Merritt Hospital in Oakland, California. "Some of these men had gone away with major surgical privileges," he later recalled, "and had been assigned leading surgical responsibilities here and overseas. They were furious when they came home and found themselves in 'Class A'." (Class A was the lowest rung of the hospital hierarchy, in which surgery could only be performed after consultation and under supervision.) One day in late 1945, Truman continued,

> I met Harold Maloney who had just come back. He was one of our lead-ing general practitioners; a fine doctor and surgeon; a member of the American College of Surgeons and in 'Class A.' We had previously talked about an organization of general practitioners; and this day, in talking the situation over again, we agreed that an organization was urgent.[29]

And so the GPs organized, first into the General Practitioners Asso-ciation of Truman's Alameda County; then in 1945 into the Section on General Practice of the American Medical Association; and finally in 1947 into the American Academy of General Practice (AAGP). The organizers and officers of the AAGP, who assumed the burden of promoting the new organization and encouraging the formation of local chapters, made no bones about the reason for its existence. It was not about "family practice," "comprehensive care," "total patient care," or any of the other buzzwords invoked two decades later in the discussions that led to the creation of the American Board of Family Practice in 1969. It was about power, pure and simple, and power in postwar America meant the power to treat one's own patients in the hospital, including patients who required operative obstetrics and major surgery.

Returning GPs, who, as general medical officers, had met wartime needs at both ends of the specialty spectrum—in psychiatry and in surgery—were aghast at rumors that certain stateside hospitals—perhaps their *own* hospitals—planned to limit their staffs to board-certified medical specialists by the early '50s. Was this their reward for exemplary service to the nation? "Since the Second World War," intoned the AAGP's first president, Paul Davis, in 1948, the GP "has been discriminated against in many cases, and had his professional standards encroached upon." In 1953, two of New York's leading GPs recollected: "It was as if the hospitals were about to put up signs reading: If you're a general practitioner, keep out!" A few years later, Eric Royston, another prominent AAGP booster, recalled the postwar feeling among GPs of being discriminated against in their medical associations "and being pushed to the periphery in the metropolitan hospitals."[30] The AAGP would come to the rescue; it would have the strength of numbers,[31] which meant it would have the power. The AAGP's resolve to keep GPs in the hospitals and put scalpels back in their hands was baldly stated in Article II of its constitution, which set forth this organizational objective: "To preserve the right of the general practitioner to engage in medical and surgical procedures for which he is qualified by training and experience."[32]

The notion that specialty competence in postwar America could be determined outside residency training by something as ambiguous as "training and experience" was the loose thread that ultimately caused the AAGP's appealing quilt of postwar medicine to unravel. Certainly, in the late '40s and early '50s, there were many GPs equipped by training and experience to perform general surgery and operative obstetrics, but they were the older GPs, many of whom had pursued surgical "interests" before the war and further honed operative skills during the war. Indeed, prior to the war, general practice was a perfectly acceptable conduit to surgical specialization. "In those days," recounts J. Dunbar Shields, the internist who, absent residency training, became governor of the New Hampshire chapter of the American College of Physicians, "people could teach themselves surgery to some degree." Shields himself was hired out of internship in 1933 to partner with a GP in rural Concord, New Hampshire, one Don McIvor. McIvor had "no special training in anything" but became a highly respected surgeon nonetheless:

> He did it by assisting others. He began to do minimal things—appendectomies and hernia repairs. Then he began to go to meetings and find out how to do surgery. He got to be good. He wanted to drop medicine and just do surgery. And he wanted somebody to come in and take over the medical part of his practice.[33]

But McIvor, like countless other surgeons serving smaller communities, became a surgeon in the 1920s and '30s, when informal "training and experience" carried more weight than after the war, even among generalists who had distinguished themselves as specialists-by-training-and-experience during the war. The notion that the medical staffs of postwar hospitals could be reorganized into coequal sections of medicine, surgery, and general practice, with members of the latter receiving privileges in internal medicine, pediatrics, obstetrics, and surgery "as determined for each applicant by the credentials committee of the staff"[34] was fanciful, a looking backward to the way specialty expertise had often been acquired before the war.

Equally backward was the AAGP's early notion that surgical privileges were necessary in order to give GPs interested in surgery the opportunity to improve themselves in the field, "to have the opportunity for such advancement to the same degree that he [or she] might anticipate it in other of the specialties."[35] The fact of the matter was that GPs were not formally trained in any of the specialties, and the

AAGP's position, as articulated in 1951 by John Boyd, chairman of the AAGP's Commission on Hospitals, failed to acknowledge the widening gap between "specialty interests" and full-time specialty practice, which fell back on skills that, for the younger generation, could only be acquired in post-internship residencies.

Boyd took the argument a step further, indeed to the point of reductio ad absurdum, by suggesting that residency training was only an "artificial prerequisite" for specialty practice, which should only be a matter of demonstrated ability. With the skill of a seasoned debater saddled with the losing side of a proposition, he reminded the readers of *JAMA* that the specialty boards themselves were established not by those with postgraduate hospital training but rather "by those who had served conscientious preceptorships in obtaining the proficiency that made possible the training of specialists now in these boards." That American medicine should now discard the "proved value of the preceptorship plan of training" was for Boyd "unthinkable." Indeed, the very notion "that long periods of prerequisite 'in residency' training should be required of all doctors" was "an impossibility and actually not desirable."[36]

The problem with Boyd's arguments and all such arguments of the time is that they froze the skill set required to specialize in one or another medical specialty at a decidedly prewar level. They ignored, that is, the growth of the specialties during and after the war, including the emergent technologies developed for, and recruited into, specialty practice. They also ignored the degree to which specialty training provided a baseline procedural competence, attested to by specialty board certification, that greatly abbreviated, if not obviating entirely, the time-consuming, politicized, and sometimes contentious process of determining an individual practitioner's "proficiency" in this or that specialty in this or that community at this or that point in time. Finally, Boyd's arguments ignored the fact that specialty medicine in postwar America was being consensually validated in ways that, despite disparities of access that remain with us to this day, served the public's interest. Americans had begun seeking out specialists after World War I, and the trend only accelerated after World War II.

Although the AAGP and its citywide precursors managed here and there to stabilize the older GPs' hospital status as it existed before the war, restoring, for example, their prerogative to perform minor surgeries such as tonsillectomy and adenoidectomy,[37] it could not insulate GPs from the continuing development of specialty medicine. And this development took place in hospitals and entailed ever more sophisticated procedures and interventions. Given this reality, specialty encroachment of GP hospital privileges might be slowed but never halted. And along with the organizational support came the stigma, which is exactly what the AAGP sought to avoid. In the late '40s, many GP-surgeons resisted joining the AAGP lest, publicly identified as GPs, they would have their surgical privileges rescinded. On the other hand, those few GP residency programs that proved successful in the early '60s, mostly in California, were those that taught surgery and permitted GP residents to perform major operations.[38] It was all about surgery, all about procedures, all about treatment-related prerogatives within the hospital.

The AAGP, for all its organizational muscle and marketing prowess, could not prevail because of what specialization had come to *mean* after the war. Hospital-based residency training of three to five years was fast becoming the sine qua non of medical practice per se. One-year internships, on the other hand, were becoming relics of a different time and place. They had arisen in post-Civil War America because late-nineteenth-century medical colleges, with only a few exceptions, were didactic and allowed students little if any contact with living, breathing (and dying) patients. Internships, which until the turn of the century were few in number and vigorously competed for, introduced students to patient care in the relatively controlled environment of the hospital before setting them loose on the public. As such, they were usually viewed as completing undergraduate medical training, nothing more.[39]

How applicable was this rationale in the world of post-World War II medicine, where students had four years of undergraduate training, two of which were entirely clinical? No sooner was the AAGP founded in 1948 than the American Medical Association's Council on Medical Education and Hospitals countered with its "Essentials of Approved Residencies in General Practice." By the mid-1950s, it was clear to all parties that the traditional postgraduate preparation for a career in general practice—the one-year "rotating internship" in which the intern spent a month or two, successively, in different hospital services—was simply inadequate.[40]

At the time of its founding, the AAGP had acknowledged the need for post-internship training by making membership contingent on continuing education in the form of 150 hours of approved postgraduate instruction every three years. The nature of these postgraduate courses was not stipulated; it was left to individual AAGP members to devise personal programs for "keeping up to date" by taking postgraduate courses according to their own interests. Here and there, innovative approaches to postgraduate training were developed. In Illinois and Kansas, respectively, instructional teams traveled throughout the state, conducting one- and two-day workshops at centralized locations. The postgraduate division of the Albany Medical College in New York went a step further. In a wonderful "analogue" anticipation of online learning, the college offered postgraduate instruction via two-way radio, enabling physicians within a 150-mile radius of the medical college's radio station to participate in conferences led by college faculty.[41] But postgraduate instruction, however useful, was never more than a stopgap measure that accommodated the resistance of the older AAGP members to a residency requirement. In truth, though, the three-year post-medical college residency was the only way to go; it was the "obvious solution to the problem" of providing adequate postgraduate training to the GPs of tomorrow.[42]

It did not take long for the AAGP to appreciate the inadequacy of its "continuing education" path to upgrading the status of the postwar GP. In 1955, it joined forces with the AMA's Council on Medical Education to create a Residency Review Committee, which proceeded to release a revised version of the council's "Essentials" document of 1948. And then, in 1955, the academy finally instituted its own residency requirement for new membership applicants. Henceforth, young GPs could only become active academy members at the time they entered practice if they had completed a two-year residency after their internship.[43]

By the early 1960s, the vision of the up-to-date GP who took postgraduate courses in lieu of a three-year residency remained credible, but only among the early cohort of AAGP members. My father was among them. Drawing on pharmacy training, wartime surgical experience, and postwar preceptorships and postgraduate courses, he provided sophisticated multispecialty care to his rural patients through the 1970s.[44] By the early 1960s, however, a new generation of medical school graduates viewed this pathway to broad-based competence as archaic, a final nod to the war-tested GPs of the 1940s and early '50s and, before them, to the old-style "consultant physicians" of the 1920s and '30s, those gifted Oslerian generalists for whom "general proficiency is simply special proficiency in many fields."[45]

Nor did the first generation of general practice residencies do anything to staunch the flow of postwar medical school graduates into the specialties. Initially termed "mixed residencies" or "general residencies" by the AMA's Council on Medical Education and Hospitals in 1948, these programs were, with the occasional exception, simple continuations of the internship for an additional year or two, absent educational standards or specific clinical goals. And medical school graduates realized as much. In the Council's 1950 annual report on internships and residencies, 32 programs offered a miniscule 92 positions for general practice residents, less than 0.5% of the 19,364 approved residency positions of all types available that year. Five years later, in 1955, 155 approved general practice programs offered 614 residency positions, now a shade more than 2% of the 25,486 approved residency positions of all types.[46] Adding insult to injury, in 1954–1955, only 66% of the tiny number of approved general practice residency positions were filled, and more than a third of those who filled them were graduates of foreign medical schools. In internal medicine, by way of contrast, 578 approved programs offered 4,828 residency slots, 81% of which were filled.[47] These realities led to the dim assessment of C. Wesley Eisele, the highly regarded director of the general practice residency program at the University of Colorado School of Medicine. Speaking to the Advisory Board for Medical Specialties at the 52nd Annual Congress on Medical Education and Licensure in Chicago on February 12, 1956, he acknowledged that "great numbers of prospective general practitioners continue to seek fragments of specialty residencies in preference to the general practice residency opportunities now available."[48]

Less than a decade after the AAGP's founding, then, it was clear to most GP educators and many of the Academy's own leading lights that the original plan of GP renewal was not working and that a different approach would have to be developed. In a sea of residency-trained specialists, they reasoned, why not swim with the big fish? When, in the mid-1960s, efforts to upgrade the status of the generalist centered on creation of a new residency-based specialty, "family practice," it was no longer a matter of surgical privileges within the hospital. This battle, outside of the smallest community hospitals where GPs formed the entire medical staff,[49] had already been lost. Witness the AMA Council on Medical Education/AAGP jointly prepared description of "The Essentials of a General Practice Residency" of 1955, where it was agreed that:

> Any time that is devoted to general surgery and to surgical special-ties should emphasize diagnosis, preoperative and postoperative care, minor surgery and emergency care. A program in which a majority of the resident's time is spent in the operating room cannot be considered as meeting the requirements of this type of residency.[50]

No, family practice would be a new and different *kind* of specialty, one less concerned with procedures and surgeries than with holis-tic, patient-centered, intergenerational caregiving. The retreat from proceduralism was codified in the "Core Content" of family practice adopted by the AAGP in 1966. The family practitioner (FP) of the future, it held, would assume "comprehensive and continuing respon-sibility" for his or her patients. This meant that family practice would be a "horizontal specialty" that cut across the other specialties. It would fall back on "function" rather than a "body of knowledge."[51]

What was lost in the new rhetoric of patient-centered caregiving was the very thing that mattered so much to the AAGP two decades earlier: safeguarding the GP's prerogative to perform those procedures and interventions that fell within the domain of the *practicing* (as opposed to the *caring*) generalist. The proponents of family practice could no longer hope to wrest control of a piece of the medical pie, so they elaborated a new and, so they hoped, specialized gloss on the pie in its entirety. This amounted to proposing a "sort of a focus"[52] for the FP of the future who, like his colleagues in pediatrics and general internal medicine, would complete a three-year hospital-based residency after completing medical school, upon which he or she would be eligible for specialty certification by the family practice specialty board. Then the FP, like the pediatrician and internist, would be a specialist, with responsibilities and respect commensurate with this elevated status. Or so the proponents of the FP movement hoped.

But there was a problem with this rescue operation. What FP proponents and educators failed to do was delineate in a conventional manner the *procedural correlates* of the FP's "focus"—the things that *all* FPs would be trained to do that qualified as specialist interventions, not just attitudinal correlates of caregiving that meshed with their person-centered ideology.

The question-begging nature of early definitions of family practice is nowhere more evident than in the matter of surgery. By the mid-1960s, the founders of family practice realized full well that the American College of Surgeons would never cede residency-trained family practitioners the prerogative to perform major operations in the hospital. To make matters still worse, the AAGP was beset with a schism within its own ranks: there were the predominantly older GPs who did considerable surgery (including operative obstetrics) and the predominantly younger GPs who did not. The former believed family practice should include a strong surgical component; the latter did not. The older GP-surgeons were sufficiently concerned about the exclusion of surgery from family practice to oppose the development of a family practice specialty board through the early '60s. How could the chasm be bridged? The pragmatic (non) solution adopted by AAGP officialdom was simply to leave the issue open. The AAGP's vision of the new family practice specialist, as spelled out in its "Core Content" position paper of 1966, assigned family practitioners the nebulous domain of "applicable surgery," meaning that "the physician in family practice should be trained to do the types and kinds of surgery he would be required to perform after graduation."

There is considerable irony in this manifesto: the very effort to transform old-style general practice into specialized family practice hinged on a willingness to fall back on a pre-1940s notion of specialization in which budding generalists would somehow know, in advance of practice, what kinds of techniques they would need to master for their future work. They would then "pick up" these techniques during residency or after residency in the world of everyday practice and occasional postgraduate courses.

But how were the young doctors to know what skills they would need? This was the very problem encountered by Wesley Eisele and his colleagues in the three-year GP residency program developed at the University of Colorado in 1948. Adopting a pre-1940s approach to trainees' use of the hospital setting, they allowed their postwar GP residents to opt out of a regular rotation across the major medical services so that they could tailor their postgraduate training to their personal needs and desires. The "serious disadvantages" of this training approach quickly became apparent. The plan, Eisele recounted,

> assumed unjustifiably that a young and inexperienced physician was in a position to know precisely what he required for practice. The fallacy was disclosed by the frequency with which residents asked to change their schedules. All too often, a [GP] resident would end up with an unbalanced program that was notably deficient in training for important segments of his future practice.[53]

In ignoring this lesson of the recent past, family practice educators of the mid-'60s fashioned a medical specialty that was not only "different," but virtually antithetical to the very *meaning* of specialization. That is, if family practice is a medical specialty of *any* kind, then *all* FP residents should receive common training in a range of diagnostic and treatment procedures that, in their totality, add up to *specialist interventional care*.

The willingness to localize procedural skills, to leave it to individual practitioners and/or training programs to determine which skills would be "appropriate" to family practice, was of course a nod to the surgical specialists, whose advanced training and control of hospitals were shored up by the postwar climate of opinion. But it had the paradoxical effect of marginalizing the family practitioner out of the gate: once you begin localizing the procedural, hands-on component of any specialty, medical or otherwise, you risk gutting the specialty, cutting away the shared procedural content that coalesces into expert knowledge and sustains a common professional identity. What kind of specialty leaves it to the individual to fill in the procedural content of the specialty as he or she proceeds through training and practice?

Here we arrive at a central dilemma of family medicine. I invoke it here in support of the need for a new kind of generalist physician who is procedurally empowered in the manner of older GPs of the 1940s and '50s. We need to oscillate back to generalists who can do many things and away from generalist physicians who *hypothetically* know their patients "better" but are increasingly content to "coordinate" their care. The family practice movement failed because it sought the impossible: to create a new kind of specialty that would not delimit expertise in treatment-specific ways.

The family practitioner of the 1970s was to be an interpersonally embedded, empathically attuned, total-patient provider. He or she was to provide comprehensive care that was intergenerational, mind-body care. Proponents of the movement spent years debating what "comprehensive care" meant and ultimately had to beg the question. The result was a medical specialty that, until very recently, lacked consensually agreed-on procedural requirements. The semantically strained, even oxymoronic, vision of a non-specialty specialty, a specialty that rejected specialist values, was an amalgam of 1960s counterculture, the social sciences, and a dash of psychoanalytic object relations theory (per Michael Balint), all abetted by the dearth of "personal physicians" and the emergence in the 1970s of the patient rights movement. In chapter 6, we saw this combination of idealism and naïveté play out in the writings of G. Gayle Stephens, one of the founders of the family practice movement. For Stephens, we recall, medical technology, the "mechanical appurtenances of healing," had already reached a point of diminishing returns in the early '70s, so that the need for the new-style family practitioner became a moral imperative. The residency-trained FP, he held, would liberate medicine from its "captivity" to a flawed mechanistic view of reality and medicine and, in so doing, "improve the total health of our nation."[54]

Family practice was of its time—it was entirely admirable and terribly ill-fated. This is why only 8% of non-osteopathic medical students now choose to "specialize" in it.[55] It is also why a number of top-tier medical schools—Harvard, Yale, Johns Hopkins, Columbia, and Cornell, among them—do not even have departments of family medicine.

This, then, is the historical baggage that we bring to the health care crisis before us now. We have (surprise!) a serious shortage of primary care physicians that can only get worse in the years immediately ahead. *Our* crisis is the culmination of 150 years of *their* crises, of one after another generational lament about the dying out of the family doctor. But now, perhaps, the family doctor really *is* dying out. So here we are, with the Patient Protection and Affordable Care Act of 2010 in place, and projections about the need for over 50,000 more primary care physicians by 2025 to cope with aging baby boomers and the newly insured coming into focus month by month. And here we are with emergency room visits and their associated costs continuing to climb, because many of the newly insured still do not have access to primary care doctors and because the Affordable Care Act has released a pent-up demand for medical care among them.[56]

The development of the family practice specialty in the late 1960s failed utterly to reduce the flow of medical school graduates into the specialties. Now we all fish for care in a sea of specialists. Even our primary care specialists, beset with the need to see a succession of patients in record-breaking, income-generating, productivity-maximizing time, have been forced to abandon the generalist values that persisted, despite the gloomy prognoses, into the postwar generation. Many of us are content—or not content—to manage ourselves with the aid of a coterie of specialist providers, whereas the uninsured and newly insured flood clinics and emergency rooms. The storm clouds hovering over generalist medicine appear as dark as ever. Has the family doctor's Armageddon finally arrived?

CHAPTER 10

A New Kind of Doctor

I have come to believe that it is the flesh alone that counts. The rest is that with which we distract ourselves when we are not hungry or cold, in pain or ecstasy.

—Richard Selzer, *Mortal Lessons* (1976)

"Potential access challenges"—that's the current way of putting the serious shortage of primary care physicians in our own time. Aggravated by the 33 million Americans now receiving or soon to receive health insurance through the Patient Protection and Affordable Care Act of 2010, the dearth of primary care physicians is seen as a looming crisis capable of dragging us back into the medical dark ages. Medical school graduates continue to veer away from the less remunerative primary care specialties, opting for the well-fertilized and debt-annihilating verdure of the subspecialties. Where then will we find the 51,880 additional primary care physicians that, according to the most recent published projections,[1] we will need by 2025 to keep up with an expanding, aging, and more universally insured American population?

Now the bleak scenarios are back in vogue, and they are more frightening than ever, foretelling a consumer purgatory of lengthy visits to emergency rooms for private primary care—or worse. Dr. Lee Green, chair of Family Medicine at the University of Alberta, offers this bleak vision of a near future where patients are barely able to see primary care physicians at all:

> Primary care will be past saturated with wait times longer and will not accept any new patients. There will be an increase in hospitalizations and increase in death rates for basic preventable things like hypertension that was not managed adequately.[2]

I have no intention of minimizing the urgency of a problem that, by all measurable indices, has grown worse in recent decades. But I do think that Dr. Green's vision is a tad over the top. It is premised on a traditional model of primary care in which a single physician assumes responsibility for a single patient. As soon as we look past the traditional model and take into account structural changes in the provision of primary care over the past four decades, we are able to forecast a different, if still troubling, future.

Beginning in the 1970s, and picking up steam in the 1980s and '90s, primary care medicine was enlarged by mainstream providers without medical degrees. I refer to physician assistants and nurse practitioners (often referred to as "mid-level" practitioners), psychiatric nurses, and clinical social workers who in many locales have collectively absorbed the traditional functions of primary care physicians. The role of these providers in American health care will only increase with implementation of the Patient Protection and Affordable Care Act and the innovative health delivery systems it promotes as solutions to the crisis in health care.

I refer specifically to the act's promotion of "Patient-Centered Medical Homes" (PCMHs) and "Accountable Care Organizations" (ACOs), both of which involve a collaborative melding of roles in the provision of care. PCMHs, in particular, seek to tilt the demographic and economic balance among medical providers back in the direction of primary care and, in the process, to render medical care more cost-effective through the use of information technology, evidence-based care (especially the population-based management of chronic illnesses), and performance measurement and improvement. To these ends, PCMHs equate primary care with "team-based care, in which physicians share responsibility with nurses, care coordinators, patient educators, clinical pharmacists, social workers, behavioral health specialists, and other team members."[3] Web-based education and email and phone contact with the Home's PCP and other team members, it is believed, will enhance the ability of patients to manage chronic conditions and identify new problems requiring medical assistance. And electronic communication will not only promote patient involvement in their care; it will also provide a venue for patient evaluation of the Home's "performance."

This, in any event, is the vision of the patient-centered medical home set forth jointly by the American Academy of Family Physicians, American Academy of Pediatrics, American College of Physicians, and American Osteopathic Association in a joint statement of 2007, revised and reissued in 2011.[4] The degree to which the overarching goals of these new models—reduced hospital admissions and readmissions and more integrated, cost-effective management of chronic illnesses—can be achieved will be seen in the years ahead. Skepticism about the ability of the models to transform primary care was well articulated before passage of the Patient Protection and Affordable Care Act.[5] Withal, it is clear that these developments, heralded by passage of the Health Information Technology for Economic and Clinical Health (HITECH) Act of 2009[6] and propelled by the Obama administration's investment of $19 billion to stimulate the use of information technology in medical practice, all point to the diminished role of the all-purpose primary care physician.

So we are entering a brave new world in which mid-level providers, all working under the supervision of generalist physicians in ever-larger health systems, will assume an increasing role in primary care. Indeed, PCMHs and ACOs, which attempt to redress the crisis in primary care through electronic information systems and additional payment to PCPs for care coordination, will have the paradoxical effect of relegating the traditional "caring" aspects of the doctor-patient relationship to nonphysician members of the health care team. The trend away from patient-centered care *on the part of physicians* is already discernible in the technical quality objectives (like mammography rates) and financial goals of ACOs that increasingly pull primary care physicians away from relational caregiving.

The culprit here is time. ACOs, for example, may direct PCPs to administer depression scales and fall risk assessments to all Medicare patients, the results of which must be recorded in the electronic record along with any "intervention" initiated. In all but the largest health systems (think Kaiser Permanente), such tasks currently fall to the physician him- or herself. The new delivery systems do not provide ancillary help for such tasks, which makes it harder still for overtaxed PCPs to keep on schedule and connect with their patients in more human, and less assessment-driven, ways.[7] The electronic dimension of "care coordination," be it noted, falls within the framework of 15-minute office visits, and the supplementary payments to PCPs and their staffs for such coordination and the technology implementation it entails will not bring PCP income up to the level of medical specialists—not by a long shot.[8] Still, the new delivery systems will build on a team approach to primary care that has been utilized to advantage for several decades now.

So, yes, we're going to need many more primary care physicians, but perhaps not as many as recent projections suggest. The estimate of 51,880 given by Petterson and his colleagues,[9] for example, is an extrapolation from "utilization data"—the number of PCPs we will need to accommodate the number of office visits made by a growing, aging, and better insured American population at a future point in time. But these data do not incorporate the growing reality of team-administered primary care. The latter already includes patient visits to physician assistants, nurse practitioners, and clinical social workers and is poised to include electronic office "visits" via the Internet. For health services researchers, this kind of distributed care suggests the reasonableness of equating "continuity of care" with "site continuity" (the place where we receive care) rather than "provider continuity" (the personal physician who provides that care).

Of course, we are still left with the massive and to date intractable problem of the uneven distribution of primary care physicians (or primary care "teams") across the population. Since the 1990s, attempts to pull PCPs to those areas where they are most needed have concentrated on the well-documented financial disincentives associated with primary care, especially in underserved, mainly rural areas. Unsurprisingly, these disincentives evoke financial solutions for newly trained physicians who agree to practice primary care for at least a few years in what the federal government's Health Resources and Services Administration designates "Health Professional Shortage Areas" (HPSAs). The benefit package currently in place includes medical school scholarships, loan repayment plans, and, beginning in 1987, a modest bonus payment program administered by Medicare Part B carriers.[10]

A recent, elaborate proposal to persuade primary care physicians to go where they are most needed adopts a two-pronged approach. It calls for creation of a national residency exchange that would determine the optimal number of residencies in different medical specialties for each state, and then "optimally redistribute" residency assignments state by state in the direction of underrepresented specialties, especially primary care specialties in underserved communities. This would be teamed with a federally funded primary care loan repayment program, administered by Medicare, that would gradually repay participants' loans over the course of their first eight years of post-residency primary care practice in an HPSA.[11]

But this and like-minded schemes will come to naught if medical students are not drawn to primary care medicine in the first place. There *was* such a draw in the late 1960s and early '70s; it followed the creation of "family practice" as a residency-based specialty and developed, as we have seen, in tandem with social activist movements of the period. But it did not last into the '80s and left many of its founding proponents, such as G. Gayle Stephens, disillusioned. Despite the financial incentives already in place (including those provided by the federal government's National Health Service Corps[12]) and the existence of "rural medicine" training programs,[13] there is no sense of gathering social forces that will pull a new generation of medical students into primary care. Nor is there any reason to suppose that the dwindling number of medical students whose sense of calling leads to careers among the underserved will be drawn to the emerging world of primary care in which the PCP assumes an increasingly administrative and data-driven role as coordinator of a health care team. It was the reduced scope of practice—their inability to go beyond coordination, administration, and routine management of uncomplicated acute illness and stable chronic illness—that was so disillusioning to the generalists interviewed by Timothy Hoff in *Practice Under Pressure*.[14]

In truth, I am skeptical that financial packages, even if greatly enlarged, can overcome the specialist mentality that emerged after World War II and was well entrenched by the 1970s. Financial incentives assume that medical students would opt for primary care if not for financial *disincentives* that make it harder for them to do so. Recent literature suggests that financial realities *do* play an important role in the choice of specialty.[15] But there is more to choice of specialty than debt management and long-term earning power. Specialism is not simply a veering away from generalism; it is a pathway to medicine with its own intrinsic satisfactions, among which are prestige, authority, procedural competence, problem-solving acuity, and lifestyle. These satisfactions are at present vastly greater in specialty medicine than in primary care. This is why primary care educators, health economists, and policy makers place us (yet again) in a state of crisis.

Financial incentives associated with primary care are important and probably need to be enlarged far beyond the status quo. But at the same time, we need to think outside the box in a number of ways. To wit, we need to rethink the meaning of generalism and its role in medical practice (including specialty practice). And we need to find and nurture (and financially support) more medical students who are drawn to primary care. And finally, and perhaps most radically, we need to rethink the three current primary care specialties (family medicine, general pediatrics, and general internal medicine) and the relationships among them. Perhaps this long-established tripartite division is no longer the best way to conceptualize primary care and to draw a larger percentage of medical students to it.

II.

Existing approaches to the crisis of primary care are like Congressional approaches to our fiscal crisis. They have been, and will continue to be, unavailing because they shy away from structural change that would promote equity. I suggest the time has come to think outside the financial box of subsidization and loan repayment for medical students and residents who agree to serve the medically underserved for a few years. And so I offer the following proposals.

1. We should redefine "primary care" in a way that gives primary care physicians (PCPs) a fighting chance of actually *functioning* as specialists. *This means eliminating "family medicine" altogether.* The effort to make the family physician (until 2003, the family practitioner) a specialist among specialists was tried in the 1970s and by and large failed—not for FP patients, certainly, but for FPs themselves, who failed to achieve the academic stature and clinical privileges associated with specialist standing. It is time to face this hard fact and acknowledge that the era of modern general practice/family medicine, as it took shape in the 1940s and came to fruition in the quarter century following World War II, is at an end. Yet another round of financial incentives that make it easier for medical students and residents to "specialize" in family medicine will fail. Making it *easier* will not make it *easy enough*, nor will it overcome the specialist mentality inculcated in students during medical school and residency training.[16] Further policy-related efforts to increase the tenability of family medicine, such as increasing Medicare reimbursement for primary care services or restructuring Medicare to do away with primary care billing costs, will be socioeconomic Band-Aids that cover over the professional, personal, familial, and, yes, financial strains associated with family medicine in the twenty-first century. Vague and unenforceable "mandates" by state legislatures directing public medical schools to "produce" more primary care physicians have been, and will continue to be, political Band-Aids.[17]

2. As a society, we must re-vision *generalist* practice as the province of general internists and general pediatricians. We must focus on developing incentives that encourage internists and pediatricians to practice general internal medicine and general pediatrics, respectively. This *reconfiguring* of primary care medicine will help advance the "specialty" claims of primary care physicians. Historically speaking, internal medicine and pediatrics *are* specialties, and the decision-making authority and case management prerogatives of internists and pediatricians are, in many locales, still those of specialists. General internists become "chief medical officers" of their hospitals; family physicians, with exceedingly rare exceptions, do not. For a host of pragmatic and ideological reasons, many more American medical students at this juncture in medical history will enter primary care as internists and pediatricians than as family physicians.

3. Part of this re-visioning and reconfiguring must entail recognition that generalist *values* are not synonymous with generalist *practice*. Generalist values can be cultivated (or neglected) in any type of postgraduate

medical training and implemented (or neglected) by physicians in any specialty. There are extraordinarily caring physicians among specialists, just as there are less-than-caring primary care physicians aplenty. Caring physicians make caring interventions, however narrow their gaze. My wonderfully caring dentist only observes the inside of my mouth, but he is no less concerned with my well-being on account of it. The claim of G. Gayle Stephens that internists, as a class, were zealous biologists who were committed to modern medicine's "mechanistic and flawed concept of disease," whereas family physicians, as a class, were humanistic, psychosocially embedded caregivers, was specious then and now.[18] A telling counterpoise comes from no less an authority than Alvan Feinstein, whose *Clinical Judgment* was published in 1967, preceding Stephens's tendentious claim by 11 years. "Since verbal data are more important in internal medicine than in any other specialty of organic disease," wrote Feinstein, "an internist's ability to communicate with sick people is as basic a tool of his craft as his knowledge of molecular biology."[19] General internists who practice clinical medicine, excepting those employed by hospitals as "hospitalists," *are* primary care physicians, and they can be expected to be no less caring (or, obversely, no *more* caring) of their patients than family physicians. This is truer still of general pediatrics, which, as far back as the late nineteenth century, provided a decidedly patient-centered agenda for a cohort of gifted researcher-clinicians, many women physicians among them, whose growth as specialists (and, by the 1920s and '30s, as pediatric subspecialists) went hand in hand with an abiding commitment to the "whole patient."[20]

4. We will not remedy the primary care crisis by eliminating family medicine and developing incentives to keep internists and pediatricians in the "general practice" of their root specialties. In addition, we need policy initiatives to encourage subspecialized internists and subspecialized pediatricians to continue to work as generalists. This has proven a workable solution in many developed countries, where the provision of primary care by specialists is a long-established norm.[21] And, in point of fact, it has long been a de facto reality in many smaller American communities, where medical and pediatric subspecialists in cardiology, gastroenterology, endocrinology, et al. continue to practice general internal medicine or general pediatrics. Perhaps we need a new kind of mandate: that board-certified internists and pediatricians practice general internal medicine and general pediatrics, respectively, for a stipulated period (say, two years) before beginning their subspecialty fellowships.

Can we remedy the shortage of primary care physicians through the conduits of internal medicine and pediatrics? No, absolutely not. Even if incentive programs and mandates increase the percentage of internists and pediatricians who practice primary care, they will hardly provide the more than 50,000 new primary care physicians we will need by 2025.[22] Nor will an increase in the percentage of medical students who choose primary care pull these new providers to the underserved communities where they are desperately needed. There is little evidence that increasing the supply of primary care physicians affects (mal)distribution of those providers across the country. Twenty percent of the American population lives in nonmetropolitan areas and is currently served by 9% of the nation's physicians; over one-third of these rural Americans live in what the Health Resources and Services Administration of the U.S. Department of Health and Human Services designates "Health Professional Shortage Areas" (HPSAs) in need of primary medical care.[23] Efforts to induce foreign-trained physicians to serve these communities by offering them J-1 visa waivers have barely made a dent in the problem and represent an unconscionable "brain drain" of the medical resources of developing countries.[24] The hope that expansion of rural medicine training programs at U.S. medical schools, taken in conjunction with increased medical school enrollment, would meet the need for thousands of new rural PCPs has not been borne out. Graduating rural primary care physicians has not been, and likely will not be, a high priority for most American medical schools, a reality acknowledged by proponents of rural medicine programs.[25]

Over and against the admirable but ill-fated initiatives on the table, I propose two focal strategies for addressing the primary care crisis as a crisis of uneven distribution of medical services across the population. First, we must expend political capital and economic resources to encourage people to become physician's assistants (PAs) and nurse practitioners (NPs), and then we must develop incentives to keep them in primary care. This need is more pressing than ever given evidence that mid-level practitioners are more likely to remain in underserved areas than physicians,[26] and the key role of mid-level providers in the Accountable Care Organizations and Patient-Centered Medical Homes promoted by the Affordable Care Act of 2010.

Unlike other health care providers, PAs change specialties over the course of their careers without additional training, and since the late 1990s, more PAs have left family medicine than have entered it. It has become incumbent on us as a society to follow the lead of the armed forces and the Veterans Health Administration in exploiting this health care resource.[27] To wit, we must provide incentives to attract newly graduated PAs to primary care in underserved communities and to pull specialty-changing "journeyman PAs" back to primary care.[28] We must also ease the path of military medics and corpsmen returning from Iraq and Afghanistan into PA programs by waiving college-degree eligibility requirements that have all but driven them away from these programs.[29] Although the physician assistant profession came into existence in the mid-1960s to capitalize on the skill set and experience of medical corpsman returning from Vietnam, contemporary PA programs, with few exceptions, no longer recruit military veterans into their programs.[30]

Secondly, and more controversially, we need a new primary care specialty aimed at providing comprehensive care to rural and underserved communities. I designate this new specialty *procedural care medicine* (PCM) and envision it as the most demanding, and potentially the most rewarding, of the primary care specialties. PCM would enlarge on the recruitment strategies employed by the handful of medical schools with rural medicine training programs.[31] But it would require a training curriculum, a residency program, and a broad system of incentives all its own.

III.

Current proposals to remedy the crisis in primary care, especially among those Americans living in small, rural communities, are politically correct (or, in the case of J-1 waivers for foreign-trained physicians, ethically unacceptable) gestures. Small adjustments in Medicare reimbursement schedules for physicians serving the underserved and unenforceable mandates by state legislatures that public medical schools "produce" more primary care physicians are all but meaningless. Rural medicine programs at a handful of medical colleges basically serve the tiny number of rural-based students who arrive at medical school already committed to serving the underserved. Such programs have had little if any impact on a crisis of systemic proportions. If we want to pull significant numbers of *typical* medical students into primary care, we must empower them and reward them—big time. So what exactly do we do?

I propose we phase out "family medicine" for reasons I have adduced and replace it with a new primary care specialty to supplement general internal medicine and general pediatrics. Physicians who train in *procedural care medicine* will become *procedural care specialists*. They will be equipped to care for underserved populations, many of whom live in rural areas and lack ready access to specialist care. Self-evidently, procedural care training will revalue the medical history and physical examination, which remain an essential basis for diagnosis in resource-poor settings.[32] And the care these doctors provide will be procedurally enlarged beyond the scope of contemporary family medicine. Like their predecessors, the modern general practitioners of the post-WWII generation, they will be trained to doctor their patients in hands-on ways, to perform a range of office-based diagnostic procedures and minor treatments that increasingly send patients to specialists and hospital outpatient departments.

Procedural care specialists will serve the underserved, whether in private practice or under the umbrella of Federally Qualified Health Centers, Rural Health Centers, or the National Health Service Corps. They will complete a four-year residency that equips *all* procedural care specialists to perform a range of diagnostic and treatment procedures that primary care physicians now *occasionally* perform in certain parts of the country (e.g., colposcopy, sigmoidoscopy, nasopharyngoscopy), but more often do not. It would equip them to do minor surgery, including basic dermatology and complicated wound management. I leave it to clinical educators to determine exactly which baseline procedures can be mastered within a general four-year procedural care residency, and I allow that it may be necessary to expand the residency to five years. I further allow for *procedural tracks* within the final year of a procedural care program, so that some board-certified procedural care specialists would be trained to perform operative obstetrics whereas others would be trained to perform colonoscopy.[33] The point is that *all* procedural care specialists would be trained to perform a range of *baseline procedures*. As such, they would be credentialed by hospitals as "specialists" trained to perform those procedures and would receive the same fee by Medicare and third-party insurers as the "root specialists" for particular procedures.

Procedural care specialists will train in hospitals but will spend a considerable portion of their residencies learning and practicing procedurally oriented primary care in community health centers. Such centers are the ideal venue for learning to perform "specialty procedures" under specialist supervision; they also inculcate the mindset associated with procedural rural medicine, since researchers have found that residents who have their "continuity clinic" in community health centers are more likely to practice in underserved areas following training.[34]

On completion of an approved four- or five-year residency in procedural care medicine and the passing of PCM specialty boards, procedural care specialists will have all medical school and residency-related loans wiped off the books. Period. This financial relief will be premised on a contractual commitment to work full time providing procedural primary care to an underserved community for no less than, say, eight years. Procedural care specialists who make this commitment should not only be relieved of all medical debt; they deserve a bonus as well, because they have become national resources in health care.

Aspiring big league baseball players who are drafted during the first eight rounds of the MLB draft, many right out of high school, typically receive signing bonuses in the $100,000 to $250,000 range. In 2014, the top 100 MLB draftees each received a cool half million or more, and the top 50 received from 1.6 million to six million.[35] I propose that we give each newly trained procedural care specialist a $250,000 signing bonus in exchange for his or her eight-year commitment to serve the underserved. Call me a wild-eyed radical, but I think physicians who have completed high school, four years of college, four years of medical school, and a four- or five-year residency program and committed themselves to bringing health care to underserved rural and urban Americans for eight years deserve the same financial consideration as journeymen ball players given a crack at the big leagues.

Taken together, the two foregoing proposals will make a start at decreasing the income gap between one group of primary care physicians and their colleagues in medical subspecialties and surgical specialties. This gap decreases the odds of choosing primary care by nearly 50%; it is also associated with the career dissatisfaction of PCPs relative to other physicians, which may prompt them to retire earlier than their specialist colleagues.[36] I am not especially concerned about funding the debt waiver and signing bonuses for board-certified procedural care specialists. These physicians will bring health care to over 60 million underserved Americans and, over time, they will be instrumental in saving the system, especially Medicare and Medicaid, billions of dollars. Initial costs will be a drop in the bucket in the context of American health care spending that consumed 17.4% of GDP in 2013 and is expected to reach 19.3% in 2023. Various funding mechanisms for primary care training—Title VII, Section 747 of the Public Health Service Act of 1963, the federal government's Health Resources and Services Administration, Medicare—have long been in place, with the express purpose of expanding geographic distribution of primary care physicians in order to bring care to the underserved. The Affordable Care Act of 2010 may be expected to increase their funding greatly.

IV.

These proposals offer an alternative vision for addressing the crisis in primary care that now draws only 3% of nonosteopathic physicians to federally designated health professional shortage areas and consigns over 20% of Americans to the care of 9% of its physicians. The mainstream approach moves in a different direction, and the 2010 Macy Foundation–sponsored conference, "Who Will Provide Primary Care and How Will They Be Trained?" typifies it. Academic physicians participating in the conference sought to address the crisis in primary care through what amounts to a technology-driven resuscitation of the "family practice" ideology of the late 1960s. For them, PCPs of the future will be systems-savvy coordinators/integrators with a panoply of administrative and coordinating skills. In this vision of things, the Patient-Centered Medical Home becomes the site of primary care, and effective practice within this setting obliges PCPs to acquire leadership skills that focus on "team building, system reengineering, and quality improvement."

To be sure, physicians remain leaders of the health care team, but their leadership veers away from procedural medicine and into the domain of "quality improvement techniques and 'system architecture' competencies to continuously improve the function and design of practice systems." The "systems" in question are health care teams, redubbed "integrated delivery systems." It follows that tomorrow's PCPs will be educated into a brave new world of "shared competencies" and interprofessional collaboration, both summoning "the integrative power of health information technology as the basis of preparation."[37]

When this daunting skill set is enlarged still further by curricula addressing prevention and health promotion, wellness and "life balance" counseling, patient self-management for chronic disease, and strategies for engaging patients in all manner of decision-making, we end up with new-style primary care physicians who look like information-age reincarnations of the "holistic" mind-body family practitioners of the 1970s. What exactly will be dropped from existing medical school curricula and residency training programs to make room for acquisition of these new skill sets remains unaddressed.

I have nothing against prevention, health promotion, wellness, "life balance" counseling, and the like. Three cheers for all of them—and for patient-centered care and shared decision-making as well. But I think health policy experts and medical academics have taken to theorizing about such matters—and the information-age skill sets they fall back on—in an existential vacuum, as if "new competencies in patient engagement and coaching"[38] can be taught didactically as opposed to being *earned* in the relational fulcrum of clinical encounter. "Tracking and assisting patients as they move across care settings," "coordinating services with other providers," providing wellness counseling, teaching self-management strategies, and the like—all these things finally fall back on a trusting doctor-patient relationship. In study after study, patient trust, a product of empathic doctoring, has been linked to issues of compliance, subjective well-being, and treatment outcome. Absent such trust, information-age "competencies" will have limited impact; they will briefly blossom but not take root in transformative ways. And patients do not develop trust in relation to medical homes or medical teams; they learn to trust their doctors.

I suggest we attend to first matters first. We must fortify patient trust by training primary care doctors to do more, procedurally speaking, and then reward them for caring for underserved Americans who urgently need to have more done for them. The rest—the tracking, assisting, coordinating, and counseling—will follow. And the patient-centered medical home of the future will have patient educators, physician assistants, nurse practitioners, and social workers to absorb physicians' counseling functions, just as it will have practice managers and care coordinators to guide physicians through the thicket of intertwining information technologies.

Returning to the issue of patient trust takes us back to procedural medicine, to the laying on of hands, and its future role in primary care. There is a large literature, both professional and lay, that documents the devaluation of primary care skills alongside the procedural skills of medical and surgical specialists. On the one hand, we have primary care physicians who (in principle at least) give their patients the time they need, understand them as vulnerable individuals, and then devise treatment approaches responsive to their personal needs and preferences. On the other hand, we have specialists who perform discrete procedures for which they receive considerably more remuneration than PCPs, whose diagnostic and interpersonal skills and investment of time brought the patient to the specialist in the first place, and whose post-procedure management of the patient may well be long term and demanding.

Among a plethora of illustrative examples, I choose a passage from the internist-geriatrician Jerald Winakur's moving memoir of his father's descent into Alzheimer's disease, which opens to a broader, often elegiac meditation on the caring generalist values that inform Winakur's geriatric practice. He writes, for example, of an 80-year-old woman who scheduled an appointment because she had experienced some kind of "spell." Winakur gave her all the time she required: a thorough physical examination followed by routine studies done in his office, followed by an explanation of additional tests to be performed as an outpatient, followed by alerting her to what symptoms she should be on the lookout for should he send her home, followed by a gentle explanation of why she might have to be hospitalized sooner rather than later, and so on. "We talk and talk," he writes.

"Nothing is written in stone. We can go about the evaluation in a different manner, another sequence. We can watch and wait. I will be available." The "comprehensive follow-up visit" that followed the initial visit, he recounts, took from 30 to 60 minutes. And then he invokes a comparative perspective to understand the perversity of a system that enshrines procedures and devalues time-consuming patient care:

> If I were in an ER and had just sutured a one-inch laceration—a technical act that takes minutes—I would get about the same amount I received for the patient visit I described, or "x" dollars for my efforts. If I had become a gastroenterologist, I could pass a scope through a colon and get 3x. Remove a mole and collect almost 3x. Interpret an echocardiogram (performed remotely by a technician)—as cardiologists do—and get 3x. Or do a stress test—another technician-performed procedure—and collect 6x from Medicare. Had I become a radiologist, I could sit in a darkened room and read MRI scans—and collect almost 9x per study. Believe it or not, my ear, nose, and throat colleague is reimbursed almost as much by Medicare to clean the wax out of my elderly patient's ear during an office visit as I receive for the above encounter I described.[39]

If we are to draw more medical students into primary care, we must redress these gross disparities and revalue the cognitive skills at the heart of primary care; we must pay proportionately more to the frontline clinicians who provide preventive care and manage chronic illnesses. We must recognize, as a society, that management of chronic illness frequently means management of intersecting chronic illness*es*, in the process of which PCPs are expected to manage risk, help patients cope with uncertainty, and determine treatment priorities in accord with a patient's values, preferences, and lifestyle.

But will this ever happen? Highly doubtful. The AMA's Resource-Based Relative Value Scale Update Committee (RUC), which establishes Medicare reimbursement rates for all medical services, cognitive and procedural, militates against anything more than incremental change. Twenty-one of its 31 members are appointed by medical specialty societies, its meetings are closed, and over 90% of its recommendations to the Centers for Medicare and Medicaid Services (CMS) are enacted by Medicare.[40] Equally important, the RUC's recommendations serve as industry-wide benchmarks used by private health insurers to negotiate fee schedules with providers. This means that a single specialty-dominated committee, which meets in secret and is not subject to oversight, not only determines how $70 billion in annual Medicare spending is distributed among physicians, but also structures reimbursement schedules in the private sector.

Can we realistically expect this committee, 17 of whose permanent seats are assigned to specialty societies that account for a tiny portion of Medicare billing—e.g., neurosurgery, plastic surgery, pathology—to come to the rescue of beleaguered PCPs? I think not. To be sure, minor concessions to generalists have been made. In 2012, for example, the AMA announced the creation of two new primary care seats on the committee, one of which was a permanent seat assigned to the American Geriatrics Society. But two additional seats are far short of what is required to remedy the drastic imbalance between the value of primary care services and those of the procedural specialties. The committee's periodic updates of its Resource-Based Relative Value Scale (RBRVS) remain based entirely on what the committee construes as physician work effort, i.e., the time involved in performing a cognitive or procedural service, which includes the purported technical skill and mental effort required along with the patient risk it entails. This notion of medical effort factors in neither the health outcome of a service nor its value to the patient.

There is little reason to believe this procedurally weighted system of valuation will change any time soon. The Harvard economist William Hsiao, who led the team that devised the Resource-Based Relative Value Scale (RBRVS) in the late 1980s, remarked in 2013 that the AMA "does not have the in-house technical expertise to produce objective and scientifically sound RBRVS updates," so that "the updating of RBRVS has become a tool for [the] AMA to gain the political support of selected specialties." The Accuracy in Medicare Physician Payment Act of 2013 (H.R. 2545), introduced in Congress by Representative Jim McDermott, would create a panel of independent experts (including patient representatives) within Medicare to identify distortions in Medicare fee schedules. But the bill was referred to the House's subcommittee of health in July 2013, where it has languished.[41]

Nor will the financial incentives built into the new models of primary care provide meaningful redress for PCPs. Additional payments for care coordination, patient education, and implementation of information technology are supplementary; they will at best prop up in the short term the system that has marginalized PCPs in the first place. Left untouched by the new models is what Hoff characterizes as "a high-patient volume, transaction-based model of primary care delivery" in which "overly complex, 'high maintenance,' or noncompliant patients become distractions derailing an otherwise efficiently planned workday."[42] Accountable Care Organizations and Patient-Centered Medical Homes reframe PCPs' role without enlarging their scope of practice or supplanting a fee-for-service system that devalues their services alongside the procedures performed by their specialist brethren.

The proposal to replace family medicine with a new primary care specialty, procedural care medicine, attacks the crisis of primary care from a different direction. It is at first glance an improbable notion, a radical restructuring of specialty medicine as it emerged in the decades following World War II and culminated in the founding of the American Board of Family Practice in 1969. But in important ways it is actually a more conservative, and hence realizable, approach to drawing significant new numbers of medical students into primary care and inducing them to go where they are most needed. It leaves in place, that is, the fee-for-service structure that, for many physicians and their organizations, not to mention their political allies, remains the ultimate expression of American medicine, the ne plus ultra of our collective freedom to choose (and of our doctors to bill) as we see fit. Primary care physicians whose procedural armamentarium has been bolstered by additional residency training and whose performance of procedures is reimbursable at specialist rates will enlarge the generalist's scope of practice. The financial incentives to procedural care specialists who commit to a lengthy period of serving the underserved—the elimination of all medical debt and a $250,000 bonus at the time of passing their specialty boards—will pull medical students to underserved communities like nothing before. In America, sadly, money talks. So why not let it talk to debt-burdened, ideal-drained medical students in socially constructive and ethically estimable ways?

Even outside a fee-for-service structure, among the growing percentage of primary care physicians who enter practice as salaried employees of hospitals, group practices, health plans, and other health care organizations, the return to procedural caregiving can only have a salutary effect. By enlarging the treatment prerogatives of these PCPs, by establishing a new balance between care coordination and hands-on doctoring, it will empower them and hopefully reduce their high risk of burnout.[43]

Procedural care medicine will come to the rescue of primary care in yet another way. By enabling a new generation of differently trained "family doctors" to return to their roots in procedural medicine, it will reinvigorate the role of touch in general medical care and, in so doing, widen a tributary that flows into a trusting relationship between patient and doctor. There is the notion in clinical medicine that cognitive skills and procedural skills are antipodal, that they represent radically different aspects of medical caregiving. But in primary care, why must this be the case? To be sure, the range of procedural interventions available to procedural care specialists will never be what it was in the postwar decades, when gifted GPs like my father practiced office surgery, dermatology, urology, and obgyn—all the while scheduling double sessions for psychotherapy. But there can still be general recognition among medical educators that procedural skills are integral to primary care, that the touch of hands and also of hand-held instruments can amplify the impact of "cognitive services" in meaningful and measurable ways.

In truth, absent some degree of procedural reinforcement, patient-centered medicine will remain little more than a sop to disenchanted patients and old-style primary care educators. There is no evidence that expressly "patient-centered" additions to the medical school curriculum have any effect on how physicians practice medicine. What we do have, on the other hand, is qualitative evidence that patient-centered PCPs who give patients additional time are frowned upon by productivity-driven colleagues. Empirical studies demonstrate that women physicians provide more patient-centered care to their patients than their male counterparts: they conduct longer office visits during which they discuss the larger context of the patient's condition in supportive, caring, and psychologically attuned ways. Researchers, never at a loss for devitalizing abstraction, refer to their "higher levels of psychosocial and socioemotional exchange."[44] And yet women physicians in primary care often feel *stigmatized* because their patient-centered approach to caregiving renders them less productive within their group practices. Some end up feeling like "second-class citizens" whose practice style invites "negative fallout." This is because patient-centered caregiving strains a business model predicated on high patient volume and quick patient visits. Small wonder then that, among Hoff's interviewees, patient-centered female PCPs were frustrated. They had learned that "taking longer with a patient gets viewed by practice colleagues as inefficiency threatening the bottom line, not something producing higher-quality care."[45]

The laying on of hands is a tangible expression of patient-centeredness. In the domain of human relations, centering, after all, is mediated through the senses; it is the conjoining of sensory modalities and channeling of sensory energy onto a person who, in the most primitive and perduring sense, is a *bodily* person. This is why Freud, in accounting for the genesis of mental life, termed the ego "first and foremost a bodily ego," an ego that "derived from bodily sensations."[46] Physicians who lay their hands on their patients, who do things to their patients' bodies, access primitive bodily egos in ways that care coordinators and wellness counselors cannot. This is because the same touch that is diagnostic to the physician is therapeutic to the patient.

Throughout history, physicians have realized as much and sought to deepen therapeutic touch when diagnosis is not the issue. In the ancient Egypt of the Edwin Smith Papyrus (circa 1500 BCE), the *swnw* (physician) at bedside placed his hand right into the patient's open wound, conveying in this ritualized act control, reassurance, and healing. In the Philadelphia of the early 1840s, Jefferson Medical College's pioneering surgeon Thomas Dent Mütter prepared his patients for the ordeal of anesthesia-less surgery with several days of gentle touch and massage of the body parts to go under his blade. And in the Baltimore of the early 1900s, Osler, walking the long wards of Johns Hopkins Hospital, periodically stopped to squeeze the toes—and thereby lift the spirits—of his ward patients.[47] Of course, Mütter had no empirical knowledge of the effectiveness of massage therapy for stress and pain reduction any more than Osler understood the complex neuroanatomy and neurophysiology of what researchers term "affectionate touch."[48] They did not require such knowledge. Like doctors past and present, they instinctively used their hands as instruments of caring.

Throughout the animal kingdom physical touch comforts; witness Jane Goodall's apes, who reassure one another by a hand touching a hand.[49] Asian elephants comfort distressed members of their group with reassuring trunk touches, even placing their trunks in the mouths of their unhappy companions.[50] I walk my gentle greyhound, Wynona, to the park where we encounter another greyhound, Violet, recently off track and shaking in fear. Wynona instinctively wraps her neck around Violet's neck and Violet is calmed. In medicine, there is more to it than comfort contact: medical touch communicates and conjoins; it reassures by conveying to physician and patient, from their complementary vantage points, that something is being done, that matters are being taken in hand.

Even Jerald Winakur, otherwise exasperated at the devaluation of generalist listening, pondering, and problem solving, returns finally to touch to convey his deep connection to his patients. Here is a generalist for whom the physical examination, in the manner of Osler, remains "a sacred rite," a conjoining of "intellect and muscle and memory—inspecting, palpating, percussing, auscultating, going back again when something seems amiss or different, remaining attentive to the task, postponing the probing of the tender area to the last." The men and women who entrust themselves to his care, he writes, "have allowed me to touch and probe their bodies and draw blood from their veins. They have, in their trust of me, undergone countless deeper probings, patiently suffered discomfort and pain and indignities in the belief that I would ease their travails, calm their fears, reassure them, treat their sicknesses, and sometimes even save their lives."[51]

Winakur is exemplary, a wonderfully caring old-school physician who embraces his patients as friends and fellow sufferers. But what he misses, perhaps, is the degree to which the touching and probing and drawing of blood communicate healing intent and, as such, are foundational to the trust bestowed on him. To be sure, trust over time renders more tolerable the touching and probing and piercing and draining and cutting. But trust also grows out of, and is sustained by, these very activities, as long as they are guided by a therapeutic intent that is, if not empathic, at least caring and supportive. Once beyond the range of simple observation and palpation, care and support entail explaining—making sure the patient understands why this or that procedure is being performed, what the doctor can learn from it, what relief can be expected from it, and why, all things considered, it is a good thing to do.

Of course, the nature and extent of procedural explanation are always relative to the needs of the patient, and such needs take as referent both the patient's personality and the historical moment at which the procedure is performed. There have always been patients who neither need to know, nor even want to know, very much. Some find it psychologically difficult to know more than they have to know, a predisposition less than tenable in an era of informed consent and patient rights. Other patients, perhaps a majority in this day and age, want to know it all.

Medical history sensitizes us to the relative valence of this or that procedure at a particular moment in time. A cold metal stethoscope on the chest of a female patient of the mid-nineteenth century was often a distasteful procedural act requiring reassurance and explanation—much less so a half century later and now not at all. Sticking an esophagoscope down the throat of a young patient with diphtheritic membranes or lye-induced strictures and ulceration in the early twentieth century had to have been more traumatizing to child and parents alike—even, or especially, if the child was hospitalized and "etherized"—than it was a half century later, when "modern" ENT and pediatric anesthesiology rendered such procedural invasions routine and safe, if still anxiety inducing. One can only imagine the anxiety and discomfort attendant to primitive sigmoidoscopy that followed the Berlin internist Hermann Krauss's development of the distally lighted sigmoidoscope in 1904—a far cry from the routine and only mildly unpleasant flexible sigmoidoscopy of our own time. More prosaically still, consider the procedural stress attendant to self-administered insulin injections before disposable syringes and then prefilled "pens" and ultra-thin pen needles made the task a minor nuisance. One can only imagine the anxiety of patients who

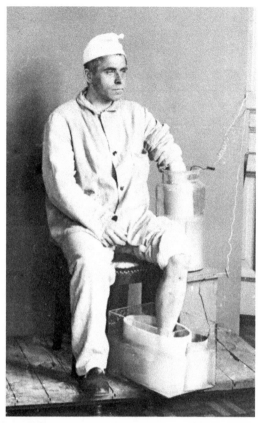

Figure 10.1 A patient sitting for an EKG in Willem Einthoven's Leiden laboratory, ca. 1905. (Image used with kind permission of Museum Boerhaave Leiden.)

received EKGs, via Einthoven's string galvanometer, in the second decade of the last century. They sat with an arm and a leg in separate buckets of saline solution that served as electrodes, amid imposing machinery that initially occupied two hospital rooms, weighed some 600 pounds, and required five operators.[52] Now an EKG takes a few minutes of technician time, with heart tracings printed out on a hand-held device. What, one wonders, were the early patients told by their doctors?

At the opposite end of the spectrum, it bears noting that for some patients even the simplest of procedures can be unnerving, even traumatizing. Here is one of my father's patients recounting in gory detail her martyrdom at the hands of the nurse who drew her blood in 1960:

> Dear Dr. Stepansky,
>
> Please don't ever recommend the same nurse to take blood from my arm again! My left arm has been hurting me ever since, and it was pain-ing me so much for two days after she took those 3 flasks of blood from my left arm, at the same time splattering some over the counter. THIS HAPPENS TO BE MY PRECIOUS BLOOD, which I have very little to spare, as far as I am concerned.
>
> You should have given me a pre-warning or told me you had inten-tions of taking that much. I am afraid I will not have as much faith in your judgement as I had before.
>
> I only hope to God, the money I have already spent will be of con-structive value to my health and purpose of my coming to you. Up to my last visit, you were doing fine. And after *all* that blood, it better prove something, or tell me something, in some way or another.[53]

And, as if this patient hadn't made herself clear, she added to her type-written missive a handwritten postscript: "There just won't *ever* be *another* blood test after this!" Here is a patient whose vulnerability is encircled by partnering bravado. She offers a candid evaluation of her doctor's "performance" that transcends the bloodletting, teamed with an imperious injunction that leaves no doubt who will be calling the shots (or needle pricks) henceforth. I imagine my father called her, apologized for the discomfort occasioned by the "procedure," and then calmly and supportively explained to her why the blood studies—all three flasks' worth—were necessary to help him understand and treat her condition. I can hear him promising to draw her blood himself in the future, as gently and sparingly as possible, if newly arising prob-lems caused her to reconsider her steely resolve of the moment.

When the physician takes the time to know her patients well enough to provide appropriately worded and toned explanations of what she is doing (or will be doing) and why she is doing it, she has become a patient-centered proceduralist whose care and support address the patient not only as a bodily ego but as a vulnerable person, a suppli-cant in search of wholeness.

CHAPTER 11

What Do Nurse Practitioners Practice?

A common question was 'Are you a nurse, or are you a mini-doc?' My answer was, is, and will always be: 'I am a nurse with primary care skills. I take care of my patients within a nursing framework. . . . my values lie in nursing, not in the medical model.

—J. A. Berg & M. E. Roberts,
"Recognition, Regulation, Scope of Practice:
Nurse Practitioners' Growing Pains" (2012)

We agree certified nurse practitioners can provide many core primary care services, but it is important that this not be misunderstood as suggesting that nurses are interchangeable with physicians in providing the full depth and breadth of services that primary care physicians provide.

—J. F. Ralston & S. E. Weinberger,
"Nurses' Scope of Practice" (2011)

Whatever the fate of primary care medicine in America—whatever the role of Accountable Care Organizations, Patient-Centered Medical Homes, or other kinds of electronically driven delivery systems—the role of nurse practitioners (NPs) and physician assistants (PAs) will only increase. This is because the paucity of primary care physicians, especially among the underserved, is a structural reality of American health care as it took shape after World War II. The structure in question—the historical pull to specialty medicine; the emergence of specialty-specific technologies and procedural interventions; the public's expectation of specialty care; and the different career trajectories of generalist and specialist physicians—has deep, intertwined roots among legislators, insurers, organized medicine, physicians, and the public. Perhaps a structural revamping of the primary care specialties, such as my proposal for a new kind of procedurally oriented provider, can loosen some of these all but petrified roots and promote change. But the political forces allied against such revamping are formidable. The shortage of generalist physicians is not going away any time soon, certainly not in our lifetimes. And this reality leaves us with an ever-increasing reliance, as both individuals and a society, on mid-level providers trained in the mainstream model of medical care. Nurse practitioners are, and will continue to be, the most important group of nonphysician generalist providers. As of March 2015, there were more than 205,000 NPs licensed in the United States, with 86.5% of them trained in primary care, and over half of them (54.5%) trained as family NPs.[1]

In addition to their critical role in team-based medicine, NPs staff the nurse-led health centers and "retail clinics" now found in pharmacies (e.g., CVS Caremark Corporation's MinuteClinic), supermarkets, and big box stores like Target and Walmart. The clinics in particular provide cost-effective and virtually wait-free care for increasing numbers of Americans.[2] In an effort to integrate with the medical mainstream, retail clinics have recently begun to coordinate care with other health systems by implementing and sharing electronic health records. In 2014, for example, CVS's MinuteClinic signed more than 30 affiliation agreements with large health care systems.[3] This is an auspicious development, to be sure, but the new reliance on mid-level providers in these clinics has come at a price. It opens a can of worms that has been with us since the 1960s and is very much with us today. It concerns the relationships between nonphysician mainstream providers and medical doctors.

There is no question that primary care of the near future will revolve around team-based medicine. Even today, high-performing primary care practices rely on care teams to which patients are assigned (or "empaneled"). For these forward-looking group practices, the team approach is viewed "as a necessity for the survival of adult primary care."[4] It not only promotes routine screenings, health coaching, and complex care management, but also adds capacity to group practices; it has given rise to a new mantra: "sharing the care."[5] Nurse practitioners already play a key role in team medicine, and that role will become more vital still in the years ahead. But this secure socioeconomic forecast leaves unaddressed the critical interprofessional challenge: How exactly do nurse practitioners collaborate with their physician colleagues, and how will this collaboration change in the years ahead? The most important dimension of these questions involves what is referred to as "scope of practice," i.e., the range of diagnostic, treatment, and prescribing prerogatives allowed by state law. To wit, what will the mid-level provider's scope of practice be, and how autonomously will he or she be allowed to "practice" within that scope? A half century after the first advanced training programs brought nurses into the ranks of clinical providers, these two questions continue to bedevil nursing, medicine, insurance companies, and state legislatures.

The crucial role of nurse practitioners in modern health care delivery is well established and, for me at least, beyond dispute. But questions of scope of practice and practice prerogatives (including, as we shall see, the prescribing of medication) remain contentious, and different state legislatures have codified different answers. It is with some trepidation that I wade into debates that will likely continue at medical, nursing, and legislative levels for some time to come. But, throwing caution to the winds, let me offer one historian's perspective on a few aspects of these knotty issues, framed by the history of nursing in the decades following World War II.

II.

The service of American nurses during the war was no less distinguished and no less essential to victory than that of American general practitioners, the General Medical Officers of the Army Medical Corps. Nurses—59,000 in the Army Nurse Corps and 18,000 in the Navy Nurse Corps—did heroic duty both abroad and at home, and their stories continue to edify and inspire. In 1940, only 340,025 Americans, all but 12,561 of them women, identified themselves as professional nurses. This was far short of what the nation at war would require, especially on the home front.[6] In response to an urgent need for more trained nurses, the Public Health Service created a Division of Nursing Education to administer a Cadet Nurse Corps. Funded by the Bolton Act of 1943, the corps recruited 179,000 high school graduates between July 1, 1943, and October 15, 1945. After an accelerated certificate program of 30 months, senior nurse cadets spent the final six months of their training working full time, mainly at U.S. hospitals and rehabilitation centers, both of which they kept going in the face of the massive loss of graduate nurses to the armed forces.[7] By all accounts, they performed splendidly and selflessly. By the time the program ended in 1948, over 127,000 young women, 3,000 of whom were black, had completed corps training and become professional nurses.[8]

It was also during the war that psychiatric nursing and nurse-midwifery gained traction as nursing specialties. Acceptance of the need for graduate education beyond hospital training programs went hand in hand with these developments. Beginning in 1945, the Nursing Division of the Kellogg Foundation, under the leadership of Margaret Tuttle, funded university-based nursing programs at 10 handpicked universities. A year later, in 1946, Congress passed the Hill-Burton Act, which provided matching funds for the construction of new hospitals, especially in the South and Midwest. New hospital construction, teamed with the skyrocketing number of insured Americans able to avail themselves of hospital care, greatly increased the need for trained hospital nurses. Ironically, the same factors that imperiled the professional status of the returning general practitioners, who feared being locked out of their hospitals entirely, gave returning and freshly minted R.N.s a cornucopia of hospital-based employment opportunities. Nurses were in short supply and needed everywhere. The American Hospital Association sent out an alarm as early as 1944, when 23% of its member hospitals reported closing wards and operating rooms because they lacked nurses to staff them. And then in 1950 it reported over 22,000 unfilled nursing positions among its member hospitals.[9]

Nursing opportunities received a further boost in 1946 through passage of the National Mental Health Act, which fueled the growth of psychiatric nursing. By 1951, practicing psychiatric nurses numbered around 12,000;[10] four years later the nurse-midwives achieved professional autonomy with the establishment of the American College of Nurse Midwifery, which set its own educational practice standards independently of the American Nursing Association.[11] Even institutionalized racism, which had long gained expression in segregated nurse training programs for white and black nurses, seemed in retreat after the war. Optimism ruled the day. In 1951, the National Association of Colored Graduate Nurses dissolved and was absorbed into the American Nursing Association.[12]

But if things were looking up for nurses after World War II, they were looking up in very traditional ways. Postwar hospital nurses remained poorly paid; their wages and benefits, according to a U.S. Department of Labor report of 1947, fell behind those of many other women workers.[13] Nor were hospital administrators inclined to accommodate their demands for higher salaries. Typically, they shored up their nursing staffs by hiring aides and practical nurses, a trend that R.N.s were powerless to oppose and in fact often supported.[14]

And despite the Kellogg Foundation's foray into university-based nursing programs and the creation of the first advanced training program in psychiatric nursing at Teachers College of Columbia University in 1946,[15] the overwhelming majority of nurses remained generalists who staffed the nation's hospitals. Eleven hundred hospital-based schools provided their training in the late 1940s.[16] An increasingly complex patient population found its way into these hospitals, which meant that nurses were forced to master emergent technologies and new treatment protocols while learning to manage patients with conditions that rarely brought them to the hospital before the war: stroke, inflammatory bowel disease, advanced kidney disease.[17] They were obliged to know more and expected to do more, and yet their professional identity was essentially unchanged: They were underpaid physicians' helpmates to whom increasingly demanding tasks were relegated absent any prerogative to diagnose and treat.

This remained the situation of professional nurses at the dawn of the 1960s. Beginning in 1960 the Kellogg Foundation's Nursing

Advisory Committee threw its weight behind the idea of a master's-degree-level clinical nurse specialist, but there were no training programs at the time to implement the vision. Nor, finally, did the federal Nurse Training Act of 1964, which grew out of the Advisory Committee's influence with the surgeon general, promote professional self-transformation. Indeed, the act, which poured over four billion dollars into nursing education over the next 10 years, served only to sustain what the nursing historian Joan Lynaugh terms "long-standing ambivalence about higher education for nurses." The ambivalence derived from the act's support of three separate levels of nurse training: two-year community college programs, three-year hospital R.N. programs, and four-year university-based bachelor's degree programs.[18]

Given these postwar realities, the expansion of nursing's role in the direction of specialized clinical expertise occurred in a remarkably brief stretch of time. In 1955, the American Nurses Association (ANA) approved a legal definition of nursing practice that prohibited "acts of diagnosis and prescription of therapeutic or corrective measures," and it was only seven years later, in 1962, that the ANA began holding clinical sessions at its annual convention.[19] Even then, until 1968, the ANA's Code for Professional Nurses framed the nurse's professional responsibilities in terms of the nurse's relationship to physicians.[20] It was in the mid-'60s, spearheaded by reforms in nursing education then underway, that the term "nurse practitioner" came into use. It conveyed a nurse with "specialized expertise," often in hospital settings, that grew out of additional training beyond the three years of hospital-based training that led to state licensure as a registered nurse.

"Specialized expertise" is an evocative but imprecise term. In nursing, it initially conveyed expertise in one or another aspect of hospital-based care. In the early 1900s, nurses acquired expertise as x-ray technicians and microscopists, and then again in the 1930s, they "specialized" in monitoring polio patients in their iron lungs. During World War II, nurses both on the front lines and in stateside hospitals began to perform venipunctures to administer fluids intravenously; after the war, they continued to do so, and some became specialized IV therapists, performing and monitoring IVs all along their units. So there had been nurses with specialized expertise for more than a half century when the expertise was finally acknowledged by hospital administrators and physicians. It was only in the mid-'60s, one might say, that nurses' specialized expertise, long normalized, was finally formalized.

III.

In postwar America, as noted, new technologies brought to bear in treating acutely ill hospitalized patients elicited an ever greater degree of nurse specialization—and the "degree" now came to entail independent clinical judgment. Self-evidently, we needed critical care nurses, obstetrical nurses, and dialysis nurses able to decide, in a doctor's absence, when to initiate or discontinue treatments in what the historian Margarete Sandelowski terms "emergent life-threatening conditions." By the 1960s, Sandelowski observes, the new "machinery of care" had fostered a more collegial and collaborative relationship between physicians and nurses.[21] But there was never any question that the machinery—vital function monitors, cardiac monitors, electronic fetal monitors, and the like—was integral to *medical* care in the hospital. The monitors were not invented by nursing scientists as extensions of nursing care; they were instruments of improved hospital care whose design, manufacture, and intended use fell within the domain of physicians and the medical model.

The nomenclatural challenge proved even greater when advanced nursing practice left the hospital setting and became office-based, especially in the realm of primary care. Historians of nursing such as Julie Fairman tend to collapse the distinction between hospital-based specialty nursing and independent "nursing practice" in a global narrative of nursing's coming of age in the four decades following the end of World War II. The storyline of professional self-becoming involves new forms of collegial collaboration between individual nurses and physicians, which, over time, empowered the nursing *profession* to liberate itself from the bondage of *organized* medicine, with its long-held belief in the subordinate role of nurses as "physician extenders." What tends to be glossed over is the phenomenology of expertise in relation to different professional activities. Expertise in the implementation of technologically driven, hospital-based monitoring—with the diagnostic and treatment prerogatives associated with it—is not the same as the expertise that inheres in being a "practitioner" of medicine.

Or does the latter expertise inhere in being a "practitioner" of nursing? In her illuminating history of the nurse practitioner movement in America, Fairman delineates the inter-professional tensions congealed in this question. Even Loretta Ford and Henry Silver, who collaboratively developed the first (pediatric) nurse practitioner training program at the University of Colorado in the mid-1960s, used different, politically laden terminology to describe exactly what kind of non-medical practitioner they were training. For the pediatrician Silver, the new provider would be a "nurse *associate*"; for the nurse educator Ford, she or he would be a "nurse *practitioner*."[22]

The linguistic-cum-political tension was played out in different pairs of descriptors. Nurse practitioners saw themselves as "taking on" diagnostic and treatment activities traditionally reserved for physicians, whereas physicians saw themselves as "delegating" certain medical tasks to nurses.[23] The need to define the nurse specialist's prerogative to diagnose and treat illness as something other than "medical" was at the heart of the American Nurses Association's need to distance itself from another nonmedically trained practitioner who emerged at this same moment in American history: the physician assistant. PAs, the first generation of whom were medical corpsman back from Vietnam, were precisely what newly empowered clinical care nurses, at least in the eyes of their professional organization, did not want to be: a *physician* assistant rather than an autonomous *nurse* practitioner.[24]

In the realm of independent practice, this claim was problematic, since diagnosis and treatment of illness is not nursing "practice" in any historically meaningful sense of the term. Rather, diagnosis and treatment have always fallen to the physician, as the word "physician" has been understood since the beginning of the thirteenth century, when Anglo-Normans gathered the Latin "physicus" and the French "physic" into the English "physic," from which the word "physician" as a medical practitioner came in to use later in the century. It is easy to see how nursing practice can envelop sophisticated technological skills that are teachable and learnable. But the art of diagnosis and treatment—and the qualities of learned judgment[25] that fall to this task—have always been the province of the physician.

The historical claim enfolds an epistemic claim, a claim about the nature of different kinds of knowledge. Nursing knowledge, as codified in Florence Nightingale's *Notes on Nursing: What It Is and What It Is Not* (1859) and the British and American training programs that adopted her model in the 1870s and thereafter, has never been *coextensive* with medical knowledge. For Nightingale and her cohort of nursing educators, it remained a "gendered" (read: womanly) knowledge of cleanliness and comfort care that drew on sanitary science and scientifically informed bedside observation, both infused with a maternalistic sensibility.[26] Indeed, the professionalization of nursing was authorized *by men* as an extension of women's domestic sphere: Nurses in field hospitals off the battlefields of Crimea and the American South during the Civil War were accepted as surrogate mothers, wives, and sisters of wounded and dying soldiers.

A generation later, when Isabel Hampton Robb published her influential textbooks on nursing practice and nursing ethics, comfort care had been enlarged by more sophisticated interventions associated with the growth of scientific medicine, especially bacteriology, during the final decade of the nineteenth century. But the gendered assumptions of mid-century pioneers like Nightingale and Clara Barton were left untouched. Nursing care, as Robb understood it, was still woman's work, the difference being that by the 1890s the rigorous demands of hospital care meant that nurse training schools sought "a higher order of woman to meet these requirements." Only by enrolling young women of the highest standards in nursing schools, she opined, would the institutions and communities in which trained nurses toiled "show forth the influence of that 'sweet ordering, arrangement and decision' that are woman's chief prerogatives."[27]

Whether or not the knowledge base that subtends the patient-centered and technology-related caring of nurses is something other than medical knowledge (as Nightingale and her contemporaries believed) or a neglected subset of medical knowledge, is beside the point. And the point is this: The *kind* of "knowledge and skills"[28] that enter into independent clinical practice—knowledge and skills that, to be sure, nurse practitioners and other nonmedical providers can acquire—are by their nature medical. This is one reason why the struggle of nurse practitioners to obtain state licensure that permits them to "practice" without medical oversight has been halting and may never succeed entirely.

It is not simply a matter of power in the sense of Foucault, of organized medicine's ability to withhold, control, and/or regulate entry into the world of practice. It is because the science of clinical evaluation, diagnosis, and treatment that emerged in postbellum America was *vested* in the medical profession, not in the nascent nursing profession. In the final three decades of the nineteenth century, we behold the paradigm shift that historians continue to write about: Medicine became scientific medicine, and this shift, with its associated educational and organizational changes, coincided with the emergence of a "profession" in the modern sense of the term. The physician, not his helpmate nurse, was part of the profession vested with the scientific understanding of illness and the cultural authorization to act on this understanding by diagnosing and treating it.[29] Nurses partook of this understanding and authorization through their connection to doctors and medicine. But nursing *science*, such as it was, did not provide them with an alternative to *medical* science.

The foregoing helps explain why, in retrospect, the ANA's insistence that pediatric nurse practitioners—the initial cohort of nurse practitioners—retain the prerogative to delineate their own scope of practice was foredoomed. ANA leaders sought to contest a medicalized notion of "practice" that, by the early 1970s, was incontestable. And the pediatric nurse practitioners of the time knew as much. Like their nurse anesthetist forebears, who formed the National Association of Nurse Anesthetists in 1932, and their nurse-midwife forebears, who formed the American College of Nurse-Midwifery in 1955,[30] they left the ANA and formed their own professional organization, the National Association of Pediatric Nurse Associates and Practitioners (NAPNAP) in 1973. And the NAPNAP, without further ado, accepted affiliation with the American Academy of Pediatrics. The pediatric nurses, if not the ANA leaders, realized that ANA insistence on complete nursing autonomy militated against the very idea of team practice—of a pediatrician, pediatric nurse practitioner, and nurse working together—and the reality that the pediatrician would ipso facto be the leader of the team.[31]

The dilemma for nurse practitioners is that they have spent over a half century trying to define themselves by what they are not. They are not physicians. They are not physician assistants or associates. They are not simply nurses with postgraduate training and master's degrees or doctorates. They practice primary care but they are not primary care physicians working within a medical model.[32] So what exactly are they?

In the late 1950s and 1960s, nurse educators like Esther Brown and Hildegard Peplau sought an answer by articulating a new basis for nurse practitioner expertise. In so doing, they adopted an orientation similar to that of the founders of the "family practice" specialty movement during the same time. They sought, that is, to equate the nurse practitioner's "expert clinical practice" with a psychotherapeutic sensibility and the ability to provide holistic psychosocial care. Social science course work and psychodynamic training, they hoped, would move the nursing practitioner away from medicine and toward this new kind of nursing expertise.

That Brown and Peplau spearheaded this effort in nurse education is hardly surprising, given their respective backgrounds. Brown, a social anthropologist on the staff of the Russell Sage Foundation, authored *Nursing for the Future* (1948), a foundation report that advocated university-based nurse training schools in the service of a vague psychosocial vision of nursing care. The nurse of the future, she wrote, would "complement the patient by supplying what he needs in knowledge, will, or strength to perform his daily activities and also to carry out the treatment prescribed for him by the physician." Peplau, widely considered the founder of psychiatric nursing, followed an M.A. at Columbia's Teachers College, where she completed the first course in advanced psychiatric nursing, with psychoanalytic training at New York's William Alanson White Institute.[33] She believed that psychiatric nurses would function as psychotherapists, and, implicitly, that all nurses would bring a broad psychosocial, really a psychotherapeutic, orientation to their work. Were Brown, Peplau, and their associates successful in reforming nursing training in a manner that subserved a new kind of nursing identity? No, certainly not in the manner they envisioned. And further, at the time their educational reforms were introduced in the nursing schools of large public universities, there were serious problems. Graduates overfed with the new social science curriculum, it was found, were simply unprepared to assume the responsibilities of hospital nursing *practice*.[34]

IV.

My father, William Stepansky, whose remarkable postwar career in family medicine has been woven into many of these chapters, was a pharmacist before he was a physician. He entered Philadelphia College of Pharmacy and Science in 1940, but his education was interrupted by induction into the army in March 1943, several months before he completed his junior year. He had not begun pharmacy college with the intention of attending medical school—this seemed an utterly far-fetched dream for the son of poor Russian émigrés who fled the Ukrainian pogroms in 1921 and struggled to raise a family in the Jewish enclave of South Philadelphia. His own mother thought him foolish for entering college and crazy (*meshuga*) when he mentioned his interest in medicine. In 1946, after two years of service as a surgical technician on the battlefields of France, Belgium, and Germany, and an additional six months as a laboratory technician in Pilzen, Czechoslovakia, he returned to Philadelphia, where he completed his pharmacy training in 1947. Only then, with the G.I. Bill in place, did he allow himself to envision a career in medicine, and following an inventive series of initiatives, he gained admittance to Jefferson Medical College, where he joined the freshman class in the fall of 1948.[35]

My father not only retained an active pharmacy license throughout his career but actually "practiced" pharmacy out of his office in Trappe, a small, rural borough 30 miles west of Philadelphia. He maintained an impressive inventory of basic and not-so-basic drugs, and he concocted, among other things, the marvelous "red medicine" of which I have written.[36] He became a staff research clinician for McNeil Labs and later participated in clinical drug trials with the Psychopharmacology Research Unit of the University of Pennsylvania. Pharmacy training certainly proved helpful to him and his rural patients, but it was not at the core of his professional identity. He was not a "pharmacist practitioner" or an "advanced practice pharmacist." He was a physician, a general practitioner of medicine.

Perhaps it is time for the nurse practitioner profession to dispense with the "nurse" appellation altogether. These men and women are not nurses as the notion of nurse professionalism has taken shape over the past century and a half, even if they come to their provider status through nursing training and the patient-centered values it instills. NPs extol the benefits of their nursing background but claim a professional role that all but severs their connection to a nursing tradition with its own remarkable exemplars of nursing *care*: Florence Nightingale, Clara Barton; the American and Filipino nurses caring for the ill and injured in the jungle hospitals of Bataan and the Malinta tunnel hospital wings of Corregidor in 1942; the Jewish nurses, exhausted, starving, and ill with malaria and dysentery, providing care and comfort to a remnant of Jewry in Berlin's Jewish Hospital between 1942 and 1945.[37] These nurses are extraordinary role models, but they are not the role models of independent practitioners who achieve their provider status through nursing training, any more than the leading lights of pharmacology remained my father's role models when he went from pharmacy into medicine.

To be sure, there were nurse providers long before there were nurse practitioners, but their care derived from a reformist activism that sought out immigrants and the rural underserved. One thinks, for example, of Lillian Wald, an early resident of Jane Addams's Hull House, whose nursing troops, beginning in 1893, fanned out from her Henry Street Settlement in Manhattan's Lower East Side to the New York City public schools, to the homes of ill school students, and, beginning in 1909, to the homes of working-class immigrants insured by Met Life's Industrial Department. Or one thinks of Mary Breckinridge, whose Frontier Nursing Service, beginning in 1928, brought professional nurse-midwives to Kentucky's eastern mountains to provide prenatal, obstetrical, and postnatal care.

Are Wald and Breckinridge models for contemporary nurse practitioners? Only in a limited sense. Their treatment skills were selective and in the service of social welfare reform. What they brought to their charges was *medical* care—vaccination, antibiotics, obstetrical care under the supervision of physicians—not a nursing-specific variant of primary care. For better or worse, *nurse* practitioners are *medical* providers, and they must parse out their professional raison d'être from a tradition that encompasses *medical* caregiving. Late-nineteenth-century pediatricians; physicians (mainly female) associated with the Settlement movement; physicians serving rural communities in the first half of the twentieth century and, more occasionally, in the decades that followed—these providers are among their role models, their exemplars of primary care informed—is it really so paradoxical?—by nursing values.

So I conclude this section with another modest proposal: I suggest that clinical training of several years duration beyond the R.N. or B.S.N. level takes NPs out of the realm of *nursing* practice altogether. With a nod to perduring intra- and inter-professional politics, let's cast aside the terms "medical," "physician," "nurse," and "nursing" altogether, and come up with something less saturated with polemics. Advanced practice nurses should henceforth be designated "licensed clinical providers" or "licensed clinical practitioners," with the appropriate specialty designation appended to their licenses, e.g., "licensed clinical provider—primary care" or "licensed clinical provider—nephrology" or "licensed clinical provider—oncology." These designations are accurate and neutral and therefore certain to please no one.

V.

"Yes," physicians will reply, "call them something other than nurse practitioners if you will. They are indeed clinical providers. But the fact remains that they have become clinical providers through nursing and the limited training it provides. There is still the matter of defining their role and differentiating it from that of providers with medical training." So we are back to the can of worms with which we began, the matter of determining the nursing-trained clinical provider's "scope of practice," the range of his or her activities and the autonomy with which she or he may practice them. The issue is most salient in the realm of primary care, and here the chasm between NPs (I revert to existing nomenclature for economy of expression) and primary care physicians is deep and perhaps unbridgeable.

And it has grown ugly as well. Indeed, entering the debate on the "scope of practice" between NPs and physicians is like parachuting onto a battlefield strewn with semantic landmines and decaying verbiage, while overhead one hears the whistle of incoming word-tipped artillery fire. For the opposing forces, the NPs and the MDs, negotiation about the scope of NPs' "doctoring" activities all too often gives way to incendiary propaganda and explosive metaphors. It has become, sad to say, a matter of logistics, planning, grand strategy, tactical advance and retreat.

When the nursing historian Julie Fairman and her colleagues argue that "physicians' additional training has not been shown to result in a measurable difference from that of nurse practitioners in the quality of *basic primary care services*,"[38] they leave unexamined the meaning of "basic primary care services." Someone, after all, has to do the defining, and in so doing, to differentiate basic services from services that, in given circumstances, are not so basic. Someone also has to stipulate how exactly "quality" is being assessed, qualitatively and quantitatively, in both the short and long term.

It is fine to make the commonsensical point that nurse practitioners should be permitted to practice "to the fullest extent of their skills and knowledge," as recommended by the authors of the Institute of Medicine (IOM) report of 2010, *The Future of Nursing*.[39] But who decides what "fullest extent" actually means in relation to specific clinical contingencies and management challenges? Is there even consensus on the meaning of NP "knowledge and competence" in contradistinction to the "knowledge and competence" of those who receive medical training? Literally, then, what are Fairman and her colleagues talking about?

NP advocates make tactical use of the word "partnership" in framing debates about NP expansion. And yes, certainly we need NPs and physicians to be collaborative partners in providing quality health care. But the notion of "partnership" also subserves polemics. Partnership, after all, need not entail parity among partners. In law and business, for example, there are senior partners and junior partners, name partners and equity partners, voting partners and nonvoting partners. In medicine, there are any number of procedures (e.g., colposcopy, sigmoidoscopy, colonoscopy) that fall within the domain of adult primary care, but that many primary care physicians no longer perform, even if they are competent to do so, owing to issues of liability and lack of third-party coverage. This does not mean that primary care physicians, gynecologists, and gastroenterologists are not "full partners" in care, but rather that "partnership" does not abrogate the need for a division of labor, with the differing responsibilities, obligations, and entitlements such division entails.

Many NP advocates repudiate a hierarchical division of labor entirely, since what they mean by "full partnership" is parity with physicians as primary care providers. They endorse the recommendation of the IOS report of 2010 that NP-physician collaboration jettison the notion of the physician as "captain of the ship" entirely and replace it with a notion of "situational leadership" in which "A physician, nurse, social worker or other provider may take the lead in a given situation."[40] (Left unsaid, of course, is how to decide, and who decides, when a "situation" requires the expertise of the physician.) The repudiation of physician oversight in toto has given rise to alarmist claims, like the notion that the failure to designate NPs as independent primary care providers not only "challenges NP practice and affects the quality and continuity of patient care" but militates against NPs' ability to participate fully in primary care teams.[41] Such concern is, to put it mildly, overblown. It flies in the face of successfully integrated systems (such as those of Geisinger Health System, Kaiser Permanente, and the Department of Veterans Affairs) in which NPs play a key role in physician-led teams. NPs who insist on parity, which is also expressed as the "equivalence" of NPs and physicians, see licensed NPs, of whom there are now over 205,000 in the U.S., as powering the "reinvention" of primary care in America, remedying gaps in quality and workforce shortages with high-value, high-quality, patient-centered care across the primary care spectrum.[42]

Physician groups threatened by the legislative incursions of non-medical providers like NPs are no better and probably worse. The Physicians Foundation is a nonprofit organization of medical groups formed to fight back against nonmedical invaders, especially nurse practitioners. Their report of November 2012, *Accept No Substitute: A Report on Scope of Practice*, brims with military metaphors. The authors, Stephen Isaacs and Paul Jellinek, write of "holding the line" on "expansionary forays" and summarize bulletins "fresh from the front lines." "What is the score so far?" they ask. "Who is winning these scope of practice battles?" And the military metaphors segue into sports metaphors, with the authors' dour acknowledgment that physicians "are usually playing defense on scope of practice," a reality brightened by occasional successes in eliminating nonphysician licensing. In the latter cases, they rejoice, physicians "are in fact able to move the ball up the field."[43]

What is one to make of such sophomoric posturing in the face of a serious and growing shortage of primary care physicians? Where will we find the more than 50,000 additional primary care physicians we will need by 2025?[44] It is easy to appreciate the exasperation of primary care NPs who face such opposition in the face of well-established facts. To wit: Only 15–20% of today's medical students will choose a primary care specialty; NPs provide more cost-effective care than their physician counterparts; patient surveys reveal overall satisfaction with the care provided by NPs; and half of all physicians in office practice already work with NPs, certified nurse-midwives, and/or physician assistants. All such facts are ceded by the authors of *The Physicians Foundation Report*.[45]

It is time for physicians to accept not only the reality but also the socioethical necessity of nonphysician providers. By the same token, it is time for nurse practitioners to accept the reasonableness of practice limits. An *expanded* scope of practice is not a scope of practice *coextensive* with that of physicians. There are indications for which physician consultation and supervision should be mandatory; there will probably be procedures that only physicians, including primary care physicians, are legally authorized to perform. Establishing boundaries will always be shaped by power politics and economic self-interest, but it need not be deformed by them. The process can be elevated by concern for public safety and prudent good sense. By way of identifying two areas in need of further dialogue informed by complementary needs for patient access and patient safety, consider the topics of chronic disease management and prescriptive authority.

VI.

Nurse practitioner advocates tout the important role of NPs in managing chronic disease, and type 2 diabetes is typically given as a case in point.[46] Certainly NPs can manage diabetics whose glucose levels must be monitored and insulin dosages adjusted. There is already evidence that specialized NPs are highly effective in collaborative practice with primary care physicians, where they serve as diabetic care coordinators.[47] What then is the problem? It arises from the fact that management of chronic disease, especially among the elderly, is rarely a matter of managing a single stable disease according to evidence-based protocols.

Before Frederick Banting isolated insulin in his Toronto laboratory in 1922, juvenile diabetes was a death sentence; its young victims were consigned to starvation diets and early deaths. Banting knew next to nothing of the complex pathophysiology of diabetes, but owing to his laboratory breakthrough, young diabetics now grow into adult diabetics and type 2 diabetics live to become old diabetics. Lifelong management of what has become a chronic disease will take them through a dizzying array of testing supplies, meters, pumps, and short- and long-term insulins. It will also put them at risk for the onerous sequelae of long-term diabetes: heart disease, kidney failure, neuropathy, retinopathy. Of course all the associated conditions of adult diabetes can be managed more or less well with their own technologically driven treatments (e.g., hemodialysis for kidney failure) and long-term medications.

The chronicity of diabetes is both a blessing and curse. Chris Feudtner, the author of the outstanding study of its transformation, characterizes it as a "cyclical transmuted disease" that no longer has a stable "natural" history. "Defying any simple synopsis," he writes, "the metamorphosis of diabetes wrought by insulin, like a Greek myth of rebirth turned ironic and macabre, has led patients to fates both blessed and baleful."[48] He simply means that what he terms the "miraculous therapy" of insulin only prolongs life at the expense of serious long-term problems that did not exist, that *could not* exist, before the availability of insulin. So depending on the patient, insulin signifies a partial victory or a foredoomed victory, but even in the best of cases, to borrow the title of Feudtner's book, a victory that is "bittersweet."

And the bittersweet nature of insulin therapy—the likelihood of intersystemic complications and intercurrent disease processes in later life—takes us back to the issue of "management" and what it entails across the life cycle. A 2011 cross-sectional study of over 104,000 patients at VA treatment sites in four Midwestern states found that NPs provided care for hypertension and diabetes comparable to that of primary care physicians. But it also found that more complex patients with both hypertension *and* diabetes tended to be cared for by physicians.[49] Is this finding surprising? To consider it so is to call into question the need for medical training per se.

Consider another example. Perhaps an NP with graduate training in nephrology (the physiology and diseases of kidneys) can manage end-stage renal disease (ESRD), a chronic disease that can be stabilized for long periods with dialysis. But what happens when such management, and the prolongation of life it entails, leads to diabetes and heart disease, as it often does? Over the past century, medical progress has time and again converted terminal disease into chronic disease, and with this shift, the historian Charles Rosenberg has observed, "we no longer die of old age but of a chronic disease that has been managed for years or decades and runs its course."[50] To which I add a critical proviso: Chronic disease rarely runs its course in glorious pathophysiological isolation. All but inevitably, one chronic disease pulls other chronic diseases into the running. Newly emergent chronic disease begins as collateral damage of chronic disease long-established and well-managed. Chronicities cluster; discrete treatment technologies leach together; medication needs multiply. And as chronic conditions multiply, especially among the elderly, evidence-based treatment guidelines, which generally have a single-disease focus, become less relevant to clinical management decisions.[51]

It is the inevitability of such collateral damage, especially among the elderly, that calls into question the appealingly commonsensical claim that nurse practitioners are perfectly competent to manage chronic disease. NPs who treat chronic disease in retail clinics and nurse-managed health centers typically do so on the basis of evidence-based protocols that are usually formulated for one disease process in isolation from others.[52] Such protocols are less relevant to the integrated management of multiple chronic conditions within individuals.[53] Nor can such protocols teach what Osler and his contemporaries understood as the variational biology of disease, i.e., the manner in which diseases and treatments vary according to the individuating biology of the patient.[54] I am not suggesting that NPs' expertise ends with single-disease management, but that their management skills have limits different from those of primary care physicians. And it is precisely the nature of these limits that needs to be addressed more concretely in scope-of-practice discussions.

Is it unreasonable to suggest that management of multiple coexistent conditions, what the Canadian researcher Ross Upshur terms "confluent morbidity," may not be reducible to the "skill set" of NPs, even as this set is enlarged by the medley of nonmedical skills inculcated by "nursing education and its particular ideology and professional identity"?[55] Chronic disease management, that is, often entails complexity of a distinctly medical sort. Diabetes is no longer a disease with a stable natural history,[56] but then neither is kidney disease, heart disease, or many types of cancer. So the question of what NPs can and cannot do needs to be fleshed out in a more clinically concrete manner. We need to know whether NP-generalists are as capable as primary care physicians of managing chronic illness in the context of life span issues and specific dimensions of patient care. They may not be as capable as primary care physicians, for example, at prioritizing interventions among older patients with multiple chronic diseases, especially when preservation of the patient's functional status must be weighed against efforts to reverse the "cause" of one or another disease through powerful treatments.[57]

VII.

Another "fullest extent" problematic concerns prescribing privileges. NPs and other advanced practice registered nurses or APRNs (licensed nurse anesthetists, licensed nurse-midwives, and clinical nurse specialists) demand the same authorization to prescribe medications as physicians. This insistence, globally formulated, masks the fact that prescriptive authority is always qualified in various ways. Perhaps physicians, NPs and APRNs, and legislatures should set the all-or-nothing rhetoric aside and wrestle with the far knottier, real-world question of "prescriptive authority of various levels" that gets codified in state law.[58] Should it be within the NP's scope of practice, for example, to change antibiotics without physician consultation for a child who comes to the pediatrician with fever, sore throat, and pain, and whose symptoms have not abated with first-line antibiotics prescribed by the NP?[59] To begin to get a handle on this kind of issue, one must at present read the law on NP scope of practice in a particular state, which is just what NPs are enjoined to do.[60]

Here is the point: Primary care NPs in *all* states deserve—and now have—"prescriptive authority," but reasonable people will differ on the breadth of this authority. Here is an issue that *can* be subject to empirical research and meaningful negotiation among all the stakeholders, including the public. To wit, what kinds of drugs are NPs *trained* to prescribe and, based on survey data, what kinds of drugs do they *actually* prescribe? Several studies from the 1980s showed "that NPs prescribe a very limited number of relatively simple medications to predominantly healthy populations."[61] Perhaps these studies have been superseded by more recent studies attesting to the broadened range of drugs now that primary care NPs are trained to, and do in fact, prescribe. Well and good. Then the "prescriptive authority" granted to NPs by legislatures should be broader rather than narrower.

But, normatively speaking, should it be equivalent to the prescriptive authority of primary care physicians? Should NPs, for example, be granted authority to prescribe major narcotics without collaborative arrangements with physicians and without limiting stipulations as to dosage and length of use? In managing patients with multiple coexisting conditions, where the signs and symptoms of multiple diseases and their treatments interact, can we rely on NPs to separate the effects of diseases from the adverse effects of prescribed medications? Here is another set of issues ripe for further negotiation informed by empirical research and considerations of patient safety. I bring no special expertise to the table beyond noting that NPs, however great their knowledge and competence, do not receive the same training in physiology, pathophysiology, and pharmacology that physicians do. I do not find it unreasonable that NP-issued scripts for certain classes of drugs should require some degree of physician involvement, as is now the case in 32 states.[62]

VIII.

The power differential between organized medicine and organized nursing, including medical specialty societies and NP/APRN societies, has made matters worse for highly trained nurse practitioners seeking to practice to the full extent of their knowledge and competence. But it has also led some NP representatives to demonize medical groups that seek *any* drawing of lines, since the very act of drawing a line, in their view, can only derive from the economic imperative to hold the line on NP rights. Consider the reaction of the editor of *Policy Politics Nursing Practice* in 2006 to the insistence of medical groups that the difference between nurse practitioners with doctorates and physicians be clarified for the benefit of patients. "Does anyone," he wrote, "seriously see it as part of a conspiracy to mislead patients by having APRNs refer to themselves as *doctor*? And are physical therapists (who are moving toward a requirement for doctoral-level education), psychologists, and pharmacists in on the conspiracy, too?"[63]

Well, no, hardly. But the issue here, shorn of polarizing rhetoric, isn't about willful misleading; it's about the cultural *valence* of the title "doctor" and the everyday meanings people impute to it in connection with health care. A patient who seeks treatment from a licensed primary care provider who is referred to and addressed as "doctor" will, absent some kind of a priori clarification, likely assume the doctor in question is a physician. This reality was borne out by the AMA's patient opinion survey of 2010, which found that 26% of patients identified NPs in general as medical doctors and an additional 5% were unsure. When the NP him- or herself was a "doctor," the confusion increased: 35% of respondents thought the DNP was a medical doctor, and another 19% were unsure.[64] It is hardly unreasonable to advocate patient education that clarifies the different roles and orientations of different kinds of providers. And nothing prevents NP groups from adopting and implementing their own strategy of patient education. What prevents them from developing and publicizing endorsements of the "doctor of nursing practice" degree that plays to the latter's "doctoring" strengths in contradistinction to those of physicians?

If there is a conspiracy out there, it is one perpetrated on the public by both physicians *and* NPs. It is a conspiracy of partial explanations. It is the conspiracy of those physicians who refuse to cede that nurse practitioners have arrived, that they are licensed clinical providers who are perfectly capable of providing a great deal of what has traditionally been the province of primary care medicine. But it is also the conspiracy of NP advocates whose rhetoric obscures a key issue: whether "fullest extent" of NP/APRN practice should be coextensive with the full extent of care that primary care physicians are trained to provide. I think not, and my skepticism follows from various considerations, not least of which is that family physicians train a total of 21,000 hours whereas NPs train between 3,500 and 6,000 hours.[65]

The yield of all these additional hours of training is not simply a matter of formal knowledge. It is foundational to what physicians of a philosophical bent have long referred to as "tacit knowledge"—a knowledge at the edge of awareness that cannot be codified or described or didactically taught. The role of tacit knowledge in the development of clinical expertise is well documented,[66] and its function in day-to-day clinical decision-making belies—or at least mitigates—the "equivalency argument" put forth by NPs unhappy with state nurse practice acts that, as they see it, "keep NPs from providing the comprehensive primary care services permitted by their licenses and educational preparation."[67] Their argument falls back on small-scale population studies that impute similar care by primary care physicians and NPs to comparable blood pressure readings and blood glucose control, as well as broadly comparable rates of emergency room visits and hospitalization.[68] But such measures barely touch on the complex nature of clinical judgment and the manner in which the physician's far lengthier training sustains what Alvan Feinstein, a half century ago, termed the "maze of multiple sequential inferences" that permit clinical evidence to be converted into an "anatomic diagnostic deduction." As Feinstein explained, medical training, with its extensive exposure to normal anatomy and physiology, provides the epidemiologic background that sustains standards of judgment for determining the range of "normal" in nondimensional clinical observation and for deciding which abnormality or collection of abnormalities should be regarded as diagnostic.[69] "Diagnostic," in this context, includes the ability to change focus, to reconsider what to accept and amplify, what to reject and ignore—in all to resist premature closure, often in the face of seemingly "common" symptoms that point to "common" ailments. To suggest that NPs possess this ability to the same degree as physicians is effectively to claim that medical and nursing training are not only coextensive but clinically indistinguishable.

None of which is to deny that NPs' scope of practice should be expanded commensurate with their training and experience. Nor that they have a key role to play in monitoring patients with chronic disease(s). Nor that they will be centrally involved in team-based models of health care, where their role will only be enlarged in the years ahead. With respect to the roles of physician and NPs in retail clinics (or "convenience care clinics") and nurse-managed health centers, there is room for discussion. There is consensus that NPs should be the main providers in such clinics, which doubled in number between 2012 and 2015 to over 2,800. The cost savings associated with patient visits to these clinics, as opposed to hospital emergency rooms or doctors' offices, are well documented.[70] But the question of whether NPs should manage these clinics without physician oversight of any sort reprises in yet another context ongoing debates about scope of practice.

Whether in the realm of retail clinics and health centers or traditional office practice, terms like "supervision," "collaboration," and "oversight," it should be remembered, are no less elastic than expressions like "scope of practice" and "fullest extent." Physician oversight of NP practice can be relaxed without being eliminated entirely, as evidenced by legislation signed into law by Virginia governor Robert McDonnell on March 10, 2012. The product of two years of discussion between the Medical Society of Virginia and the Virginia Council of Nurse Practitioners, Virginia House Bill 346 struck a compromise acceptable to both organizations: It requires NPs to work as part of a patient-care team led by a physician, but increases the number of NPs who can partner with a single physician from four to six. More importantly, it recognizes telemedicine as a legal form of oversight, which means that NPs in Virginia can work at different locations than their team physician, such as nursing homes and free clinics in medically underserved areas. Finally, it dispenses entirely with the language of supervision: Physicians lead health care teams; they do not "supervise" nurse practitioners.[71]

Virginia HB 346 is a scope-of-practice compromise that expands care in a state where more care *of any kind* is critically needed: Nearly two-thirds of Virginia has been designated Health Care Professional Shortage Areas. Other statewide agendas may elicit different kinds of compromise. Sadly, in a scope-of-practice literature riven by overheated rhetoric, there are few examples of creative compromise in the public's interest. One such example, which circles back to the management of chronic disease, comes from a survey of 200 NPs and 200 primary care physicians in the Philadelphia area conducted a decade ago. Both PCPs and NPs, the researchers found, were supportive of a collaborative approach to the management of patients with chronic conditions in which NPs, aided by an "encounter form" specific to each chronic condition, provided most ongoing care in routine visits. The physician's role was limited to seeing the patients for acute problems and "flare-ups" of their chronic conditions.[72]

Until there is a general willingness on the part of NPs, physicians, and their respective organizations to accept such compromises—compromises that may be no more than *tolerable* to either profession but that make things *better* by extending coverage to the uninsured and newly insured—then we can only expect continuation of the polemical warfare. Physicians need to accept that NPs deserve an expanded scope of practice commensurate with their training and experience and demonstrated ability to provide safe and effective primary care. But NPs need to accept that their scope of practice will necessarily fall short of what physicians are trained and legally authorized to do. Some form of physician oversight, however attenuated, is in the public's best interest. Until both warring camps accept (not embrace, just accept) the need for compromise, we the public will be getting the short end of the stick, whoever wields it.

Home Is Where Our Health Is

How nice if we could go to the doctor and feel at home. Sometimes, albeit more rarely these days, this is indeed the case. When we visit doctors we know and trust—especially doctors who are kind and reassuring and have cared for us for some time—we are at peace in their offices. For routine care, comfortable discomforts, non-worrisome seasonal maladies, the monitoring of stable chronic conditions—for such things going to the doctor can be pleasant, even a pleasure. It can become a part of social life, especially in the later years. Depending on our rapport with the office staff and our familiarity with the doctor, it can even be a medicalized version of a homecoming. We know we are in good hands.

What then of the Patient-Centered Medical Home (PCMH), where we are welcomed into a practice by a medical team comprising primary care physicians (PCPs), nurse practitioners (NPs), physician assistants (PAs), nurses, a care coordinator, perhaps a social worker, and an office staff, all working together harmoniously to provide "whole person" care. Whole person care, according to the *Guidelines for Patient-Centered Medical Home (PCMH) Recognition and Accreditation Programs* jointly released by the American Academy of Family Physicians, American Academy of Pediatrics, American College of Physicians, and American Osteopathic Association in February 2011, means taking responsibility for coordinating each patient's full array of health care services using a team-based approach—i.e., delivering care for all stages and ages of life, acute care, chronic care, behavioral and mental health care, preventive services, and end of life care—and coordinating and/or integrating care for services not provided by the PCMH across all elements of the complex health care system (e.g., subspecialty care, hospitals, home health agencies, nursing homes) and the patient's community (e.g., family public and private community-based services). . . . Primary care is the provision of integrated, accessible health care services by clinicians who are accountable for addressing a large majority of personal health care needs, developing a sustained partnership with patients, and practicing in the context of family and community.[1]

This pleasing vision of the medical home is hardly new. It originated in the 1960s among general pediatricians caring for children with serious chronic illness. For such children, the "home" would be a repository for clinical data and coordinate the work of specialists participating in the children's care.[2] In the 1970s, with the cost-cutting impetus of managed care systems, the pediatric chronic care model was extended to adult medicine, with generalists assigned the role of care coordinators for all their patients. Continuous, patient-centered care was integral to what was meant by "care coordination,"[3] so it was natural that the notion of the medical home, headed by the primary care physician, would be linked to the whole patient values of the emergent family practice movement. Here is G. Gayle Stephens, whom we encountered in chapter 6, making the case for the new specialty of family practice in 1973:

What is needed is an emphasis on wholes rather than parts, for that is what the clinician deals with—the illness as well as the disease, the person as well as the body or the mind, the family as well as the individual, the community as well as the group. Knowledge of wholes implies knowledge of parts, but the latter is not the only focus of concern. Being clinical does not require that one be also anti-intellectual, uncritically empirical, antitechnological, sentimental, or utopian. It is not tantamount to dealing in intuition, mysticism, folk wisdom, armchair philosophy, or magic. It is simply an extension of clinical competence to see people and illnesses in context.[4]

Stephens made the case for "family practice" during the same time that George Engel proposed the biopsychosocial model of illness (chapter 4), in which a hierarchy of explanatory levels—the biological, the personal, and the transpersonal—had to be factored in to the clinical understanding of each individual's illness experience. The contemporary PCMH is little more than Engel's model of illness distributed among team members whose collective efforts are fortified by information age technology. But Engel, for all the originality of his "systems theory" approach to illness, was hardly the first modern exponent of whole patient medicine. Why not go back to George Canby Robinson, whose *The Patient as a Person* of 1939 outlined a whole patient program with three components: (1) the integration of psychiatry into general medical care; (2) the restoration of the family physician in modern form to a position of prominence in managing patients and coordinating their care; and (3) the physician's recruitment of medical social workers into the practice to aid in the assessment of personality, home environment, and work relations.[5]

And why stop with Robinson? Elements of the medical home were in place long before the team approach to patient-centered medicine came together in formal models of total patient care. We see them in the child guidance clinics of the 1920s, where troubled children, together with their parents, were evaluated by a team comprising a social worker, psychologist, and psychiatrist. And we see them earlier still in Richard Cabot's introduction of medical social service into the outpatient department of Massachusetts General Hospital in 1905. Cabot, who was especially concerned that tubercular patients follow treatment recommendations at home, saw the medical social worker as essential to the development of preventive medicine; his insistence led to a one-year training program in medical social work at Boston School of Social Work beginning in 1912, with programs in New York and Philadelphia following shortly thereafter.[6]

So the turn to patient-centered care in the form of a medical home is really a return to whole patient values, implemented through a team approach, that are more than a century old. We have come full circle, except that the circle has been redrawn with the tools of a digital age. In the PCMH of today and tomorrow, we will receive electronic reminders of when we need preventive checkups and blood tests; an enhanced patient portal through which to access information and even receive care via email, web-based education, and phone contact. Team members, led by our primary care physician, will work in concert to provide us with "a satisfactory care experience, from the point of the patient walking into the practice to checking out after an exam-room visit."[7]

In this beneficent vision of things to come, the PCMH turns the gatekeeper model of primary care fashionable in the heyday of managed care on its head. Under the aegis of the gatekeeping model, insurers paid PCPs a capitation fee—a fixed, upfront payment for each patient under their care—that promoted cost savings by rewarding doctors for, in effect, keeping patients out of the office. Less care, less money. The PCMH, on the other hand, is ostensibly about "quality outcomes," where such outcomes not only provide patients with all the services they require, but provide them in a homelike environment of cooperative providers, all huddling around the latest evidence-based medical home treatment standards in order to provide the best treatment to each and every member of the medical family.

Never mind the structural impediments to implementing the vision—the continuation of fee-for-service billing and escalating imaging and medication costs—or the concern among PCPs themselves that the medical home is yet another passing fad. Never mind that the various stakeholders in the medical home concept have disparate, even incommensurable reasons for supporting the model. Never mind that the additional payments contemplated for medical home PCPs for care coordination and implementation of information technology will fail to bring their incomes up to the level of specialist providers and thereby fail to pull more medical students into the ranks of PCPs. And never mind, finally, that physicians are not trained to work as members of a team, and that many of them continue to view NPs and PAs as cost-effective extenders rather than partners in care.[8] Let us place all these reality concerns to the side and simply enjoy the soothing ring of a "patient-centered medical *home*."

We all want to feel at home in our homes. And we all want homes that are comfortably centered, if not *on* us then at least *around* us and *with* us. But all homes are not created equal; not all provide security, comfort, and a sense of belonging. The leper colony or "lazar house" common in Europe in the Middle Ages—that too was a home. Throughout its history, America has sanctioned and subsidized homes where security and a sense of belonging were incomplete, fragilely maintained, or missing altogether. Beginning in the 1820s, asylums were home to the "unworthy," to the unemployed, to criminals, to orphans. Veterans Homes, where a measure of belonging went hand in hand with disability and penury, date back to the United States Naval Home of 1834 and the National Soldiers Home of 1851. At the prompting of President Lincoln, the federal government established a system of national homes for disabled Civil War veterans, 11 of which were established between 1865 and 1930. Renaming almshouses "Homes for the Aged and Infirm" or "Homes for Aged Women" in the second half of the century hardly made these institutions more livable for their residents. Often the very name of the "home" gave the game away: Consider the "Home for the Friendless" opened by New York's American Female Guardian Society in 1848, or the countless "Homes for Homeless Girls" that sprouted up in cities in the decades following the Civil War. By the early twentieth century, the American landscape was dotted with homes for those deemed mentally unfit, for "idiots" and the "feeble-minded," for "moral imbeciles" and "fallen" young women, for epileptics. All such homes were merely the institutional setting for aiding the poor, the marginalized, the sexually corrupted (or corruptible), and the physically incapacitated.[9] They were not exactly happy homes in which residents could feel at home.[10] Now, of course, we have foster homes, group homes, and rehab homes aplenty.

The wealth of ambivalence congealed in the word "home" extends to the medical realm as well. From 1846 to 1849, Marion Sims's clinic in Montgomery, Alabama, was "home" to the African American slaves—as many as 11 at a time—on whom he conducted surgical experiments, absent anesthesia, en route to devising a surgical cure for obstetric (i.e., vesico-vaginal) fistulas. This was the period during which middle-class girls who refused to eat began being sent to private "hysterical homes," where they could be force fed and otherwise humiliated by authoritarian doctors. "Homes" are where victims of contagious diseases—especially immigrants with cholera, typhoid fever, and typhus—were quarantined during the late nineteenth and early twentieth centuries. Closer to our own time, nursing homes became home to the half million mentally ill persons deprived of institutional care following passage of Medicare in 1965.

These and countless other particulars help us keep in mind the uncertain human foundations of a home. In health care, terming a group of health care providers working under one roof a "home" hardly guarantees a homelike environment. Consider the range of possibilities captured by Robert Frost's remark: "Home is the place where, when you have to go there, they have to take you in." If and when we arrive at the threshold of a fully digitized, team-based, evidence-based, whole-patient-oriented, and, yes, patient-centered medical home, we will still sense the different possibilities and feel uncertain about the kind of reception that awaits us. Will we be invited to pass through the scheduling portal into a welcoming office environment, or will we merely be taken in?

Whatever the future of primary care medicine in America, connecting with a new doctor will for many of us remain a fraught enterprise, a matter of trial and error and occasionally a bona fide trial. Of course, we can sanitize the process through the Internet and let our fingers do the walking and the talking. More and more medical practices offer electronic portals through which prospective patients can make first contact and schedule an initial appointment. The portal is the electronic door to the medical home. The website ZocDoc, founded in 2007, widens the portal still further. Patients and doctors alike register on the site, and registered patients are then guided to registered providers in their vicinity who accept their insurance, at which point the patient simply schedules an appointment with a nearby ZocDoc provider in the desired specialty.[11] It's quick, it's clean, and it's utterly impersonal. With electronic scheduling, we accept human detachment in exchange for the ease and instantaneity of electronic connection. We make an online appointment and in a digital instant, voila, we are "in the system," connected to an unknown doctor and unknown staff members, to all of whom we are merely a digitized face in the crowd. Unsurprisingly, many of us still prefer to make contact with a prospective doctor the old-fashioned way: We pick up the phone and hope for a welcoming voice on the other end.

II.

Looking for a new primary care physician some time back, I received a referral from one of my specialists and called the office. "Doctor's office . . ." Thus began my nonconversation with the office receptionist. We never progressed beyond the generic opening, as the receptionist was inarticulate, insensitive, unable to answer basic questions in a direct, professional manner, and dismally unable, after repeated attempts, to pronounce my three-syllable name. When I asked directly whether the doctor was accepting new patients, the receptionist groped for a reply, which eventually took the form of "well, yes, sometimes, under certain circumstances, it all depends, but it would be a long time before you could see him." When I suggested that the first order of business was to determine whether or not the practice accepted my health insurance, the receptionist, audibly discomfited, replied that someone else would have to call me back to discuss insurance.

After the receptionist mangled my name four times trying to take down a message for another staff member, with blood pressure rising and anger management kicking in, I decided I had had enough. I injected through her Darwinian approach to name pronunciation—keep trying variants until one of them elicits the adaptive "that's it!"—that I wanted no part of a practice that made her the point of patient contact and hung up.

Now a brief letter from a former patient to my father, William Stepansky, at the time of his retirement in 1990 after 40 years of practicing family medicine in Trappe, Pennsylvania: "One only has to sit in the waiting area for a short while to see the care and respect shown to each and every patient by yourself and your staff." And this from another former patient on the occasion of his eightieth birthday in 2002:

I heard that you are celebrating a special birthday—your 80th. I wanted to send a note to a very special person to wish you a happy birthday and hope that this finds you and Mrs. Stepansky in good health. We continue to see your son, David, as our primary doctor and are so glad that we stayed with him. He is as nice as you are. I'm sure you know that the entire practice changed. I have to admit that I really miss the days of you in your other office with Shirley [the receptionist] and Connie [the nurse]. I have fond memories of bringing the children in and knowing that they were getting great care and attention.[12]

Here in microcosm is one aspect of the devolution of American primary care over the past half century. Between my own upset and the nostalgia of my father's former patient, there is the burgeoning business of practice management, which is simply a euphemism for the commercialization of medicine. There is a small literature on the division of labor that follows this commercialization, including articles on the role of new-style, techno-savvy office managers with business backgrounds. But there is very little devoted to the role of medical receptionists, and what there is comes mainly from Britain and New Zealand and the world of older style general practice. Two articles deal with practice efficiency, providing "never-fail strategies" for saving time and avoiding phone tag along with "practice rules" for managing appointments.[13] Two additional articles, one from Great Britain and one from New Zealand, deal more focally with the role of the receptionist in managing "space" and modulating stress as the maligned gateway to the practice. The British study from 1985 documents the usually justifiable hostility of patients toward officious receptionists who proffer medical advice and act as barrier between overextended GPs and their patients. The New Zealand study, published in 2015, is a more nuanced examination of the complex role of provincial clinic receptionists who must manage the "public space" of the waiting room from their highly visible and hence vulnerable space behind their desk.[14]

These studies are concerned with the receptionist's role in office settings where they must deal with disruptive children, ethnically marginalized patients, and anger about appointment delays for which they bear no responsibility. None of these sociologists train their sights on a different role assigned to the medical receptionist: that of phone receptionist, The One Who Answers The Phone. And that is my focus here. My experience with the Great Noncommunicator left me befuddled both about what this person was trained to do and, equally important, how she was trained to *be*. If a phone receptionist cannot tell a prospective patient courteously and professionally (a) whether or not the practice is accepting new patients; (b) whether or not the practice accepts specific insurance plans; and (c) whether or not the doctor grants appointments to prospective patients who wish to introduce themselves, then what exactly *is* he or she being trained to do?

There should be a literature on the interpersonal aspects of receptionist phone talk. Let me initiate it here. Many people—especially prospective patients unknown to doctor and staff—experience mild stress when they call the doctor's office. Sometimes it is the prospect of placing the call, and not the call itself, that is stressful. In either (or both) cases, prospective patients may be subject to a situational variant of what communications scholars term "telephone apprehension," a subtype of the larger category of communication apprehension.[15] Self-evidently, then, it is important to reassure the prospective patient on the phone that the doctor is a competent and caring provider who has surrounded him- or herself with coworkers who share his or her values and welcome patient queries. If group medical practices are to evolve into patient-centered medical "homes," then the doctor gives way to the medical team, with competence and caring distributed all around. In either case, there should be some effort to greet prospective patients on the phone in a friendly and receptive, if not exactly homey, way. There is a world of connotative difference between answering the phone with "Doctor's office," "Doctor Jones's office," "Doctor Jones's office; Marge speaking,"[16] and "Good morning, Doctor Jones's office; Marge speaking." The differences concern the attitudinal and affective signals that are embedded in all interpersonal transactions, even a simple phone query. Each of the aforementioned options has a different interpersonal valence; each, to borrow the terminology of J. L. Austin, the author of speech act theory, has its own *perlocutionary effect*. Each, that is, makes the recipient of the utterance think and feel and possibly act in a certain way apart from the dry content of the communication.[17]

"Doctor's office" is generic, impersonal, and blatantly commercial; it suggests that the doctor is simply a member of a class of faceless providers whose services comfortably nestle within a business model. "Doctor Jones's office" at least personalizes the business setting to the extent of identifying a particular doctor who provides the services. Whether she is warm and caring, whether she likes her work, and whether she is happy (or simply willing) to meet and take on new patients—these things remain to be determined. But at least the prospective patient's intent of seeing one particular doctor (or becoming part of one particular practice or one particular medical home) and not merely a recipient of generic doctoring services is acknowledged.

"Doctor Jones's office; Marge speaking" is a much more humanizing variant. The prospective patient not only receives confirmation that he has sought out one particular doctor (or practice), but also feels that his reaching out has elicited a human response, that his query has landed him in a human community of providers. It is not only that Dr. Jones is one doctor among many, but also that she has among her employees a person comfortable enough in her role to identify herself by name and thereby invite the caller to so identify her—even if he is unknown to her and to the doctor. The two simple words "Marge speaking" establish a bond, which may or may not outlast the initial communication. But for the duration of the phone transaction, at least, "Marge speaking" holds out the promise of what Mary Ainsworth and the legions of attachment researchers who followed her term a "secure attachment."[18] Prefacing the communication with "Good morning" or "Good afternoon" amplifies the personal connection through simple conviviality, the notion that this receptionist may be a friendly person standing in for a friendly provider or team.

Of course, even "Good morning; Marge speaking" is a promissory note. It rewards the prospective patient for taking the first step and encourages him to take a second, which may or may not prove satisfactory. If Marge cannot answer reasonable questions ("Is the doctor a board-certified internist?" "Is the doctor taking new patients?") in a courteous, professional manner, the promissory note may come to naught. On the other hand, the more knowledgeable and/or friendly Marge is, the greater the invitation to a preliminary attachment.

Doctors are always free to strengthen the invitation personally, though few have the time or inclination to do so. My internist brother, David Stepansky, told me that when his group practice consolidated offices and replaced the familiar staff that had worked with him (and before him, our father) for many years, patients' unhappiness at losing the comfortable familiarity of well-liked receptionists was keen and spurred him to action. He prevailed on the office manager to add his personal voicemail to the list of phone options offered to patients who called the practice. Patients unhappy with the new system and personnel could hear his voice and then leave a message that he himself would listen to. Despite the initial concern of the office manager, he continued with this arrangement for many years and never found it taxing. His patients seemed genuinely appreciative of the personal touch and, as a result, never abused the privilege of leaving messages for him. The mere knowledge that they could, if necessary, hear his voice and leave a message for him successfully bridged the transition to a new location and a new staff.

Physicians should impress on their phone receptionists that they not only make appointments but also provide new patients with their initial, and perhaps durable, sense of the physician and the staff. Phone receptionists should understand that patients—especially new patients—are not merely consumers buying a service, but individuals who may be, variously, vulnerable, anxious, and/or in pain. There is a gravity, however subliminal, in that first phone call and in those first words offered the would-be patient. Totally apart from the structure of a patient-centered medical home, the phone receptionist has it in his or her power to invite the caller into a welcoming environment that will be responsive to the patient's needs and appreciative of the patient's person. This is not an especially tall order, and it hardly summons forth the Rockwellian notion of a home. Nor, for that matter, does it encourage an expectation of empathic care by doctor and staff. What it does convey to the caller, however preliminarily, is an expectation of opening a real door (and not accessing an electronic portal) into a caring environment where the *patient's* disease will be diagnosed and treated, certainly, but also where the *person's* dis-ease at being ill (or at the prospect of being ill) will be contained and, as psychoanalysts like to say, "detoxified." And, make no mistake, this latter expectation matters. Many patients still cling to the notion that a medical practice—especially a primary care practice—will provide something beyond a business address for human body maintenance and repair. They still want the doctor's office to serve as a safe place, as what the pediatrician-psychoanalyst Donald Winnicott termed a "holding environment," if only in the minimal sense that they take the leap and schedule an appointment in the reasonable hope of landing in good and caring hands.

Journal Abbreviations in Notes

Acad. Med.	Academic Medicine
Acad. Psychiat.	Academic Psychiatry
Am. J. Bioethics	American Journal of Bioethics
Am. J. Cardiol.	American Journal of Cardiology
Am. J. Dis. Child.	American Journal of Diseases of Children
Am. J. Gastroenterol.	American Journal of Gastroenterology
Am. J. Law Med.	American Journal of Law and Medicine
Am. J. Med.	American Journal of Medicine
Am. J. Med. Qual.	American Journal of Medical Quality
Am. J. Med. Sci.	American Journal of Medical Science
Am. J. Nurs.	American Journal of Nursing
Am. J. Pharm. Educ.	American Journal of Pharmaceutical Education
Am. J. Psychiat.	American Journal of Psychiatry
Am. J. Public Health	American Journal of Public Health
Am. J. Sociol.	American Journal of Sociology
Am. J. Surg.	American Journal of Surgery
Am. Quart.	American Quarterly
AMA J. Ethics	American Medical Association Journal of Ethics
Amer. J. Nurs.	American Journal of Nursing
Amer. J. Pub. Health	American Journal of Public Health
Amer. Stud.	American Studies
Anesth. Prog.	Anesthesia Progress

Anesthesiology   Anesthesiology
Ann. Fam. Med.   Annals of Family Medicine
Ann. Intern. Med.   Annals of Internal Medicine
Annu. Rev. Neurosci.   Annual Review of Neuroscience
Annu. Rev. Publ. Health   Annual Review of Public Health
Appl. Ergon.   Applied Ergonomics
Arch. Intern. Med.   Archives of Internal Medicine
Arch. Med.   Archives of Medicine
Arch. Otolaryngol.   Archives of Otolaryngology

Behav. Inform. Tech.   Behavior and Information Technology
Behav. Res. Ther.   Behaviour Research and Therapy
Bioethics   Bioethics
BMC Fam. Pract.   BMC Family Practice
BMC Med. Educ.   BMC Medical Education
BMJ Open   BMJ Open
Bost. Med. Surg. J.   Boston Medical and Surgical Journal
Br. J. Gen. Pract.   British Journal of General Practice
Br. J. Pharmacol. Chemother.   British Journal of Pharmacology and
                                  Chemotherapy
Brit. Heart J.   British Heart Journal
Brit. J. Psychiat.   British Journal of Psychiatry
Brit. Med. J.   British Medical Journal
Bull. Hist. Med.   Bulletin of the History of Medicine
Bull. NY Acad. Med.   Bulletin of the New York Academy of
                                  Medicine
Bull. Parenter. Drug Assoc.   Bulletin of the Parenteral Drug
                                  Association

Can. Fam. Physician   Canadian Family Physician
Can. Med. Assoc. J.   Canadian Medical Association Journal
Card. Electrophysiol. Rev.   Cardiac Electrophysiology Review
Circulation   Circulation
Clin. Child Psychol. Psychiatry   Clinical Child Psychology and Psychiatry
Clin. Effective. Nurs.   Clinical Effectiveness in Nursing
Clin. Geriatr. Med.   Clinics in Geriatric Medicine
Clin. J. Am. Soc. Nephrol.   Clinical Journal of the American Society
                                  of Nephrology
Clin. Orthop. Relat. R.   Clinical Orthopedics and Related
                                  Research

Comp. Psychiat.	Comprehensive Psychiatry
Crit. Care Nurs. Q.	Critical Care Nursing Quarterly
Curr. Ther. Res. Clin. E.	Current Therapeutic Research-Clinical and Experimental
Dev. Psychol.	Developmental Psychology
Diabetes Care	Diabetes Care
Diabetes Res. Clin. Pr.	Diabetes Research and Clinical Practice
Edinb. Med. Surg. J.	Edinburgh Medical and Surgical Journal
Educ. Health	Education for Health
Ergonomics	Ergonomics
Fam. Med.	Family Medicine
Fam. Pract. News	Family Practice News
Health Affairs	Health Affairs
Health Care Anal.	Health Care Analysis
Health Educ. Behav.	Health Education and Behavior
Heart Lung	Heart and Lung
Holist. Nurs. Pract.	Holistic Nursing Practice
Image J. Nurs. Sch.	Image: The Journal of Nursing Scholarship
Int. J. Cardiol.	International Journal of Cardiology
Int. J. Psychoanal.	International Journal of Psychoanalysis
Int. J. Technol. Assess.	International Journal of Technology Assessment in Health Care
Issues Ment. Health Nurs.	Issues in Mental Health Nursing
J. Abnorm. Psychol.	Journal of Abnormal Psychology
J. Adv. Nurs.	Journal of Advanced Nursing
J. Am. Acad. Nurse Pract.	Journal of the American Academy of Nurse Practitioners
J. Am. Acad. Physician Assist.	Journal of the American Academy of Physician Assistants
J. Am. Acad. Psychoanal.	Journal of the American Academy of Psychoanalysis
J. Am. Dent. Assoc.	Journal of the American Dental Association

JAMA	Journal of the American Medical Association
J. Am. Psychoanal. Assn.	Journal of the American Psychoanalytic Association
J. Assn. Amer. Med. Coll.	Journal of the Association of American Medical Colleges
J. Child Psychother.	Journal of Child Psychotherapy
J. Clin. Nurs.	Journal of Clinical Nursing
J. Clin. Psychoanal.	Journal of Clinical Psychoanalysis
J. Contemp. Hist.	Journal of Contemporary History
J. Fam. Practice	Journal of Family Practice
J. Gen. Intern. Med.	Journal of General Internal Medicine
J. Health Biomed. L.	Journal of Health and Biomedical Law
J. Health Hum. Serv. Adm.	Journal of Health and Human Services Administration
J. Health Polit. Policy Law	Journal of Health Politics, Policy and Law
J. Hist. Behav. Sci.	Journal of the History of the Behavioral Sciences
J. Hist. Biol.	Journal of the History of Biology
J. Hist. Med.	Journal of the History of Medicine
J. Hist. Med. All. Sci.	Journal of the History of Medicine and Allied Sciences
J. Hosp. Med.	Journal of Hospital Medicine
J. Interprof. Care	Journal of Interprofessional Care
J. Invest. Surg.	Journal of Investigative Surgery
J. Med. Educ.	Journal of Medical Education
J. Med. Ethics	Journal of Medical Ethics
J. Med. Humanit.	Journal of Medical Humanities
J. Med. Internet. Res.	Journal of Medical Internet Research
J. Med. Philos.	Journal of Medicine and Philosophy
J. Med. Pract. Manage.	Journal of Medical Practice Management
J. Midwifery Womens Health	Journal of Midwifery and Women's Health
J. Nerv. Ment. Dis.	Journal of Nervous and Mental Disease
J. Nonverbal Behav.	Journal of Nonverbal Behavior
J. Nurs. Care Qual.	Journal of Nursing Care Quality
J. Nurs. Educ.	Journal of Nursing Education
J. Nurs. Hist.	Journal of Nursing History
J. Nurs. Pract.	Journal for Nurse Practitioners
J. Pediatr.	Journal of Pediatrics
J. Prof. Nurs.	Journal of Professional Nursing

J. Psychosoc. Nurs.	Journal of Psychosocial Nursing and
Ment. Health Serv.	Mental Health Services
J. Pub. Health Pol.	Journal of Public Health Policy
J. Roy. Coll. Gen. Pract.	Journal of the Royal College of General Practitioners
J. Soc. Hist.	Journal of Social History
J. Surg. Educ.	Journal of Surgical Education
J. Urology	Journal of Urology
Lancet	The Lancet
Lit. Med.	Literature and Medicine
Med. Care	Medical Care
Med. Econ.	Medical Economics
Med. Educ.	Medical Education
Med. Educ. Online	Medical Education Online
Med. Hist.	Medical History
Med. Humanit.	Medical Humanities
Med. Teach.	Medical Teacher
Men Nurs.	Men in Nursing
Milbank Q.	Milbank Quarterly
Mil. Med.	Military Medicine
N. Am. Rev.	North American Review
New Engl. J. Med.	New England Journal of Medicine
New York State J. Med.	New York State Journal of Medicine
Nurs. Hist. Rev.	Nursing History Review
Nurs. Inq.	Nursing Inquiry
Nurs. Philos.	Nursing Philosophy
Nurs. Pract.	The Nurse Practitioner
Nurs. Res.	Nursing Research
Nurs. Stand.	Nursing Standard
Ophthalmology Times	Ophthalmology Times
P. Natl. Acad. Sci. USA	Proceedings of the National Academy of Sciences of the United States of America
P. Roy. Soc. Med.	Proceedings of the Royal Society of Medicine
Patient Educ. Couns.	Patient Education and Counseling

Patient Pref. Adherence	Patient Preference and Adherence
Pediatr. Ann.	Pediatric Annals
Pediatrics	Pediatrics
Perm. J.	Permanente Journal
Perspect. Biol. Med.	Perspectives on Biology and Medicine
Pharos	The Pharos
Policy Polit. Nurs. Pract.	Policy, Politics and Nursing Practice
Proc. (Bayl. Univ. Med. Cent.)	Proceedings of the Baylor University Medical Center
Psychoanal. Quart.	Psychoanalytic Quarterly
Psychoanal. Stud. Child	Psychoanalytic Study of the Child
Psychopathology	Psychopathology
Psychosom. Med.	Psychosomatic Medicine
Public Health Ethics	Public Health Ethics
Representations	Representations
Rev. Med. Chile	Revista Medica de Chile
RN J.	RN Journal
Rutgers Law Rev.	Rutgers Law Review
Science	Science
Scien. Amer.	Scientific American
Signs	Signs: Journal of Women in Culture and Society
Sociol. Health Ill.	Sociology of Health and Illness
Soc. Sci. Med.	Social Science and Medicine
Soc. Stud. Sci.	Social Studies of Science
South Afr. Med. J.	South African Medical Journal
Southern Med. J.	Southern Medical Journal
Stud. High. Educ.	Studies in Higher Education
Technol. Cult.	Technology and Culture
Theor. Med. Bioeth.	Theoretical Medicine and Bioethics
Tubercle	Tubercle
Urology Times	Urology Times
Western J. Nurs. Res.	Western Journal of Nursing Research
Yale J. Biol. Med.	Yale Journal of Biology and Medicine

Notes

CHAPTER 1—INTRODUCTION: MEDICAL CARING, PAST AND PRESENT

1. E. D. Pellegrino, *Humanism and the Physician* (Knoxville: University of Tennessee Press, 1979), 124, 146, 184, and passim.

2. After writing this passage, I discovered Abraham Verghese's beautiful rendering of this very point in his encomium to the physical examination, "A Doctor's Touch," a recorded TED talk of July 14, 2011 (http://www.cnn.com/2011/10/02/opinion/verghese-doctors-touch/).

3. See R. Wachter, *The Digital Doctor: Hope, Hype, and Harm at the Dawn of Medicine's Computer Age* (New York: McGraw Hill, 2015), 71–90, for a dismal catalogue of the harm done to patients, physicians, and the public (via the Medicare overbilling facilitated by EHR data entry) by the current crop of EHR systems. Wachter quotes from a 2013 interview with Steven J. Stack, current president of the AMA, on the "clunky, confusing, and complex" nature of EHRs. According to Stack: "EHRs have been and largely remain clunky, confusing, and complex. Though an 18-month-old child can operate an iPhone, physicians with seven to ten years of postcollegiate education are brought to their knees by their electronic health records" (73).

4. W. E. Osmun, et al., "Patients' Attitudes to Comforting Touch in Family Practice," *Can. Fam. Physician*, 46:2411–2416, 2000. To be sure, one can hardly generalize from a single small-scale study, but I am aware of no other patient survey like it, and the results are, at the least, highly suggestive. Osmun and his researchers found, unsurprisingly, that patients

were more comfortable with "distal touch" (i.e., the physician touching the patient's hand or patting the patient's shoulder) than with "proximal touch" (i.e., the physician holding the patient's hand or putting an arm around the patient). There is a literature that examines the relational meanings of a richer phenomenology of touch (e.g., handshake, handholding, touch to the forearm, arm around the shoulder, arm around the waist, touch to the face), but it is based on subject responses to photographs of two people in non-medical settings. See especially the work of J. K. Burgoon, e.g., "Relational Message Interpretations of Touch, Conversational Distance, and Posture," *J. Nonverbal Behav.*, 15:233–259, 1991.

5. J. Bendix, "Can the Doctor-Patient Relationship Survive?", *Medical Economics*, 90:19–23, 2013; S. Jauhar, "Why Doctors Are Sick of Their Profession," *Wall Street Journal*, August 29, 2014 (http://www.wsj.com/articles/the-u-s-s-ailing-medical-system-a-doctors-perspective-1409325361). Jauhar elaborates his perspective on physician disenchantment in *Doctored: The Disillusionment of an American Physician* (New York: Farrar, Straus and Giroux, 2014).

6. J. Groopman, *How Doctors Think* (Boston: Houghton Mifflin, 2007), e.g., 54–58.

7. This is the approach of Jack Cochran and Charles Kenney in *The Doctor Crisis: How Physicians Can, and Must, Lead the Way to Better Health Care* (New York: PublicAffairs, 2014). Quoted phrases from 135, 183, 185.

8. Two books, *Freud, Surgery, and the Surgeons* (New York: Routledge, 1999) and *Psychoanalysis at the Margins* (New York: Other Press, 2009) mark this transitional phase of my intellectual journey.

9. P. E. Stepansky, *The Last Family Doctor: Remembering My Father's Medicine* (Montclair, NJ: Keynote Books, 2011).

10. I elaborated this claim in P. E. Stepansky, "When Generalist Values Meant General Practice: Family Medicine in Post-World War II Medicine," presented at the annual conference of the American Association for the History of Medicine, Atlanta, May 16–19, 2013.

11. See, e.g., M. Joy, "William Osler: Then and Now," *Am. J. Med.*, 79:5–9, 1985; H. B. Wheeler, "Healing and Heroism," *New Engl. J. Med.*, 322:1540–1548, 1990; R. L. Golden, "William Osler at 150: An Overview of a Life," *JAMA*, 282:2252–2258, 1999; J. A. Barondess, "Is Osler Dead?", *Perspect. Biol. Med.*, 45:65–84, 2002; and M. W. Millard, "Can Osler Teach Us About 21st-century Ethics?" *Proc. (Bayl. Univ. Med. Cent.)*, 24:227–235, 2011.

12. The notion of the Compleat Physician pertains not only to the range and depth of a physician's knowledge, but to his or her ability to use that knowledge compassionately and wisely. Pellegrino defines the Compleat

Physician formulaically as one who is capable in three separate dimensions: "he is a competent practitioner; he is compassionate; and he is an educated man" (*Humanism and the Physician*, 157). My father calls to mind this passage from the late-nineteenth-century neurologist S. Weir Mitchell: "There is a potent combination of alertness in observation, with a never-satisfied desire to know even the trifles of a case, which, with sagacity, gives a medical mental character as rare as it is valuable" (S. W. Mitchell, *Doctor and Patient*, 2nd ed. [Philadelphia: Lippincott, 1888], 38).

13. C. E. Schorske, *Thinking with History: Explorations in the Passage to Modernism* (Princeton: Princeton University Press, 1998), 3.

14. K. Hoyt, "Vaccine Innovation: Lessons from World War II," *J. Pub. Health Policy*, 27:38–57, 2006, at 38.

15. On the development of cortisone, see especially the account of E. C. Kendall, the Mayo Clinic biochemist who isolated Compound E and other steroids from the adrenal cortex (the outer portion of the adrenal gland) in the mid-1930s, "The Development of Cortisone as a Therapeutic Agent," Nobel Lecture, December 11, 1950 (http://www.nobelprize.org/nobel_prizes /medicine/laureates/1950/kendall-lecture.pdf) and the later accounts of H. M. Marks "Cortisone, 1949: A Year in the Political Life of a Drug," *Bull. Hist. Med.*, 66:419–439, 1992 and N. Rasmussen, "Steroids in Arms: Science, Government, Industry, and the Hormones of the Adrenal Cortex in the United States, 1930–1950," *Med. Hist.*, 46:299–324, 2002. The military's investigation of Compound E to relieve stress and fatigue, incidentally, produced "equivocal and unimpressive evidence," and its physiological research on adrenal hormones was declassified in late 1943. The seemingly miraculous anti-inflammatory properties of cortisone were demonstrated in a famed 1948 clinical trial at the Mayo Clinic "in which patients long crippled by rheumatoid arthritis walked (indeed, danced) with ease again" (Rasmussen, 317, 320).

16. The medical achievements of World War II were catalogued shortly after the cessation of hostilities by A. N. Richards, "The Impact of the War on Medicine," *Science*, 103:575–578, 1946. A half century later, these modernizing developments were ably surveyed by K. M. Ludmerer, *Time to Heal: American Medical Education from the Turn of the Century to the Era of Managed Care* (New York: Oxford University Press, 1999), chapter 7, "World War II and Medical Education." For references to war-related advances in specific medical specialties, see P. E. Stepansky, *The Last Family Doctor: Remembering My Father's Medicine* (Montclair, NJ: Keynote Books, 2011), 168. World War II advances in surgical specialties are given in detail in M. M. Manring, "Treatment of War Wounds: A Historical Survey," *Clin Orthop. Relat. Res.*, 467:2168–2191, 2009. For retrospectives on the wartime clinical trial of

nitrogen mustard as an anticancer drug for patients with leukemia, Hodgkin's disease, and other lymphomas, see A. Gilman, "The Initial Clinical Trial of Nitrogen Mustard," *Am. J. Surg.*, 105:574–578, 1963 and E. Freireich, "Nitrogen Mustard Therapy," *JAMA*, 251:2262–2263, 1984.

17. N. Rasmussen, "Making the First Anti-Depressant: Amphetamine in American Medicine, 1929–1950," *J. Hist. Med. All. Sci.*, 61:288–323, 2006; N. Rasmussen, "America's First Amphetamine Epidemic, 1929–1971," *Amer. J. Pub. Health*, 98:974–985, 2008.

18. F. M. Berger & W. Bradley, "The Pharmacological Properties of α:β dihdroxy (2-methylphenoxy)-γ-propane (Myanesin)," *Br. J. Pharmacol. Chemother.*, 1:265–272, 1946, at 265.

19. See P. R. Carter, "The Embryogenesis of the Specialty of Hand Surgery: A Story of Three Great Americans—a Politician, a General, and a Duck Hunter," *J. Hand Surg.*, 28:185–198, 2003 and S. A. Green, "Giants in Orthopaedic Surgery: Sterling Bunnell, M.D.," *Clin. Orthop. Relat. R.*, 47: 3750–3754, 2013. Specialized surgical centers were hardly limited to the hand. By 1944 there were 18 centers for neurosurgery; seven for amputations; six for chest surgery; five for plastic and ophthalmologic surgery; and three for vascular surgery. It was at these stateside centers, according to Fred Rankin, the army's chief consulting surgeon, that "the wounded soldier receives the final phases of definitive surgical care." See F. W. Rankin, "American Surgeons at War," in M. Fishbein, ed., *Doctors at War* (New York: Dutton, 1945), 173–193, at 188–189.

20. On the wide-ranging medical research supported by the Committee on Medical Research and its chairman, A. N. Richards, see C. S. Keefer, "Dr. Richards as Chairman of the Committee on Medical Research," *Ann. Intern. Med.*, 71:61–70, 1965.

21. In 1989, concerned that the flagship diagnostic technologies of his day (the CAT scan, MRI, echocardiograms, and sonogram) were eroding the diagnostic skills of younger physicians, David E. Rogers, then Walsh McDermott University Professor of Medicine at Cornell University Medical College, opined in the *Wall Street Journal* that "Clearly, the amount of 'hands-on' physician time with patients has been sharply reduced. No one can quantify the precious bonding between physician and patient that begins during the touching-feeling-looking-smelling process, but I tend to feel that it was—and still is— vital." D. E. Rogers, "Out of Touch: Is Technology Widening the Emotional Moat Between Doctors and their Patients?", *Wall Street Journal*, November 13, 1989, R38.

22. S. M. Petterson, et al., "Projecting U.S. Primary Care Physician Workforce Needs: 2010–2025," *Ann. Fam. Med.*, 10:503–509, 2012.

CHAPTER 2—DOES YOUR DOCTOR CARE?

1. My reference here is to the Edwin Smith Papyrus, the Ancient Egyptian scroll on the practical management of trauma wounds that dates to around 1600 BCE, but was copied from a text several hundred years older. See W. Moore, "The Edwin Smith Papyrus," *Brit. Med. J.*, 342:d1598, 2011 and A. Vargas, et al., "El Papiro de Edwin Smith y su Trascendencià medica y Odontológica," *Rev. Med. Chile*, 140:1357–1362, 2012. The document was acquired by the American Egyptologist Edwin Smith in 1862 but only published in translation (by the historian James Breasted) in 1930. In 2012, it was reissued in a new translation as G. M. Sanchez and E. S. Meltzer, *The Edwin Smith Papyrus: Updated Translation of the Trauma Treatise and Modern Medical Commentaries* (Atlanta: Lockwood Press, 2012).

2. Quoted in J. E. Bailey, "Asklepius: Ancient Hero of Medical Caring," *Ann. Intern. Med.*, 124:257–263, 1996, at 257, 258.

3. Plato, *Phaedrus* (ca. 370 BCE), transl. B. Jowett, 85; many editions, online at http://sparks.eserver.org/books/plato-phaedrus.pdf.

4. E. D. Pellegrino, "The Virtuous Physician and the Ethics of Medicine," in E. E. Shelp, ed., *Virtue and Medicine: Explorations in the Character of Medicine* (Dordrecht: Reidel, 1985), 243–255, at 246. I endorse Pellegrino over and against Robert Veatch, for whom patient "autonomy" robs the physician of any humanistic obligation to care for the patient in ways that transcend the mere conveyance of diagnostic "facts" and treatment options, from among which the patient alone, relying on his or her own values, must decide. See R. Veatch, *Patient, Heal Thyself: How the New Medicine Puts the Patient in Charge* (New York: Oxford University Press, 2008). Small wonder that the pediatrician and bioethicist John Lantos titled his review of Veatch's book, "Veatch Hates Hippocrates." See J. D. Lantos, "Veatch Hates Hippocrates," *Hastings Center Report*, 40:46–47, 2010.

5. E. D. Pellegrino & A. A. Pellegrino, "Humanism and Ethics in Roman Medicine: Translation and Commentary on a Text of Scribonius Largus," *Lit. Med.*, 7:22–38, 1988; E. D. Pellegrino, "Medical Ethics in an Era of Bioethics: Resetting the Medical Profession's Compass," *Theor. Med. Bioeth.*, 33:21–24, 2012.

6. P. E. Stepansky, *The Last Family Doctor: Remembering My Father's Medicine* (Montclair, NJ: Keynote Books, 2011).

7. P. E. Stepansky, "When Generalist Values Meant General Practice: Family Medicine in Post-WWII America." Paper presented at American Association for the History of Medicine, Atlanta, May 16–19, 2013.

8. S. A. Schroeder, "Primary Care at a Crossroads," *Acad. Med.*, 77:767–773, 2002, at 771.

9. R. L. Ferrer, S. J. Hambridge, & R. C. Maly, "The Essential Role of Generalists in Health Care Systems, *Ann. Intern. Med.*, 142:691–699, 2005, at 695.

10. D. H. Thom, et al., "Further Validation and Reliability Testing of the Trust in Physician Scale," *Med. Care*, 37:510–517, 1999; M. A. Hall, et al., "Trust in Physicians and Medical Institutions: What Is It, Can It Be Measured, and Does It Matter?", *Milbank Q.*, 79:613–639, 2001, at 631.

11. R. P. Caterinicchio, "Testing Plausible Path Models of Interpersonal Trust in Patient-Physician Treatment," *Soc. Sci. Med.*, 13A:81–99, 1979.

12. G. Lakoff & M. Johnson, *Metaphors We Live By* (Chicago: University of Chicago Press, 1980).

13. B. F. Kelly, et al., "Advanced Procedural Training in Family Medicine: A Group Consensus Statement," *Fam. Med.*, 41:398–404, 2009, at 403.

14. C. Rivet & S. Wetmore, "Evaluation of Procedural Skills in Family Medicine Training," *Can. Fam. Physician*, 52:561–562, 2006.

15. M. S. MacKenzie & J. Berkowitz, "Do Procedural Skills Workshops During Family Practice Residency Work?", *Can. Fam. Physician*, 56e: 296–301, 2010; J. Sturmberg, "Procedural Skills in General Practice: Are We Going to Lose This Facet of General Practice Care?", *Aust. Fam. Physician*, 28:1211–1212, 1999; I. P. Sempowski, A. A. Rungi, & R. Sequin, "A Cross-Sectional Survey of Urban Canadian Family Physicians' Provision of Minor Office Procedures," *BMC Fam. Pract.*, 7:18, 2006.

16. T. Hoff, *Practice Under Pressure: Primary Care Physicians and Their Medicine in the Twenty-First Century* (New Brunswick: Rutgers University Press, 2010), 88.

17. Kelly, "Advanced Procedural Training in Family Medicine," 402; Mackenzie & Berkowitz, "Do Procedural Skills Workshops Work?", 296.

18. Mackenzie & Berkowitz, "Do Procedural Skills Workshops Work?" 296; R. J. Ackermann, R. P. J. Pierzchajlo, & R. L. Vogel, "Colonoscopy Performed by a Family Physician: A Case Series of 751 Procedures," *J. Fam. Practice*, 44:473–480, 1997.

19. M. M. Chen, et al., "The Use of New Technologies by Rural Family Physicians," *J. Fam. Practice*, 38:479–485, 1994.

20. D. W. Stepansky, "My Father's Medicine and My Medicine: An Afterword," in P. E. Stepansky, *Last Family Doctor*, 144.

21. MacKenzie & Berkowitz, "Do Procedural Skills Workshops Work?", 298.

22. Hoff, *Practice Under Pressure*, 83, 108–110.

23. H. K. Rabinowitz, *Caring for the Country: Family Doctors in Small Rural Towns* (New York: Springer, 2004).

24. W. R. Houston, "The Doctor Himself as a Therapeutic Agent," *Ann. Intern. Med.*, 11:1416–1425, 1938, at 1419.

25. N. S. Lehrman, "Pleasure Heals: The Role of Social Pleasure—Love in Its Broadest Sense—in Medical Practice," *Arch. Intern. Med.*, 153:929–934, 1993.

26. E. Balint, "The Possibilities of Patient-Centered Medicine," *J. Roy. Coll. Gen. Practit.*, 17:269–276, 1969.

27. M. C. Beach, T. Inui, and the Relationship-Centered Care Research Network, "Relationship-Centered Care: A Constructive Reframing," *J. Gen. Intern. Med.*, 21:S3–S8, 2006, at S4.

28. K. E. Fletcher, et al., "The Composition of Intern Work While on Call," *J. Gen. Intern. Med.*, 27:1432–1437, 2012; L. Block, et al., "In the Wake of the 2003 and 2011 Duty Hours Regulations, How Do Internal Medicine Interns Spend Their Time?", *J. Gen. Intern. Med.*, 28:1042–1047, 2013; L. Block, et al., "Do Internal Medicine Interns Practice Etiquette-Based Communication? A Critical Look at the Inpatient Encounter," *J. Hosp. Med.*, 8:631–634, 2013.

29. P. W. Chen, "For New Doctors, 8 Minutes Per Patient," *New York Times*, May 30, 2013 (http://well.blogs.nytimes.com/2013/05/30/for-new-doctors-8-minutes-per-patient/).

30. E. A Rider, "Advanced Communication Strategies for Relationship-Centered Care," *Pediatr. Ann.*, 40:447–453, 2011, at 450.

31. W. B. Ventres & R. M. Frankel, "Patient-Centered Care and Electronic Health Records: It's Still About the Relationship," *Fam. Med.*, 42:364–366, 2010; I. Gaboury, et al., "Interprofessional Collaboration within Integrative Healthcare Clinics through the Lens of the Relationship-Centered Care Model," *J. Interprof. Care*, 25:124–130, 2011; W. L. Miller, et al., "Primary Care Practice Development: A Relationship-Centered Approach," *Ann. Fam. Med.*, 8:S68–S78, 2010.

32. S. D. Nightingdale, P. R. Yarnold, & M. S. Greenberg, "Sympathy, Empathy, and Physician Resource Utilization," *J. Gen. Intern. Med.*, 6:420–423, 1991; E. Rider, "Advanced Communication Strategies," 452.

33. L. Dyche & D. Swiderski, "The Effect of Physician Solicitation Approaches on Ability to Identify Patient Concerns," *J. Gen. Intern. Med.*, 20:267–270, 2005.

34. F. W. Peabody, "The Care of the Patient," *JAMA*, 88:877–882, 1927; G. Draper, "The Education of a Physician," *J. Nerv. Ment. Dis.*, 76:452–462, 1932; L. J. Henderson, "Physician and Patient as a Social System," *N. Engl. J. Med.*, 212:819–823, 1935; Houston, "The Doctor Himself as a Therapeutic Agent," op. cit.; W. Osler, *Aequanimitas, With other Addresses to Medical*

Students, Nurses and Practitioners of Medicine, 3rd ed. (New York: McGraw-Hill, 1932 [1904]).

35. O. Sacks, *A Leg to Stand On* (New York: Harper & Row, 1984); D. Newman, *Talking with Doctors*, 2nd ed. (Montclair, NJ: Keynote Books, 2011 [2006]).

36. W. C. Menninger, "Psychiatric Experience in the War, 1941–1946," *Am. J. Psychiat.*, 103:577–586, 1947, at 580.

37. J. M. Murray, "Accomplishments of Psychiatry in the Army Air Forces," *Am. J. Psychiat.*, 103:594–599, 1947, at 594.

38. R. R. Grinker & J. P. Spiegel, *Men Under Stress* (Philadelphia: Blakiston, 1945), 450; R. R. Grinker, "Brief Psychotherapy in Psychosomatic Problems," *Psychosom. Med.*, 9:98–103, 1947, at 100–101.

39. W. Menninger, "Psychiatric Experience in the War," 584; L. H. Smith & H. C. Wood, "The General Practitioner and the Returning Veteran," *JAMA*, 129:190–193, 1945, at 192.

40. C. C. Burlingame, "Psychiatry in 1950," *JAMA*, 144:1365–1368, 1950, at 1367.

41. D. L. Wilbur, "Treatment of 'Functional' Disorders, *JAMA*, 152:1192–1197, 1953.

42. M. B. Casebolt, "Fertile Fields for the General Practitioner," *JAMA*, 144:599–600, 1950; R. J. Needles, "Functional Illness—Medical Enigma," *JAMA*, 156:585–589, 1954, at 586.

43. W. Stepansky, "A Clinical Study in the Use of Valmethamide, an Anxiety-Reducing Drug," *Curr. Ther. Res. Clin. E.*, 2:144–147, 1960.

44. Stepansky, *Last Family Doctor*, 74.

45. H. Brody, "'My Story Is Broken; Can You Help Me Fix It? Medical Ethics and the Joint Construction of Narrative," *Lit. Med.*, 13:79–92, 1994, at 88, emphasis added.

46. C. M. Callahan, et al., "Depression of Elderly Outpatients: Primary Care Physicians' Attitudes and Practice Patterns," *J. Gen. Intern. Med.*, 7:26–31, 1992; E. S. Stoeckle, "Orientation of Medical Residents to the Psychosocial Aspects of Primary Care: Influence of Training Program," *Acad. Med.*, 69:48–54, 1994.

CHAPTER 3—THE HUNT FOR CARING DOCTORS

1. P. E. Stepansky, "*Humanitas*: Nineteenth-Century Physicians and the Classics," presented to the Richardson History of Psychiatry Research Seminar, Weill Cornell Medical College, New York, NY, October 3, 2007.

2. C. Lawrence, "Incommunicable Knowledge: Science, Technology and the Clinical Art in Britain, 1850–1914," *J. Contemp. Hist.*, 20:503–520, 1985, quoted at 504–505, 507.

3. S. Flexner & J. T. Flexner, *William Henry Welch and the Heroic Age of American Medicine* (Baltimore: Johns Hopkins University Press, 1968 [1941]), 63–65, 419–420; H. Cushing, *The Life of Sir William Osler* (London: Oxford University Press, 1940), 25, 39, 52.

4. W. Osler, *Aequanimitas, with other Addresses to Medical Students, Nurses and Practitioners of Medicine*, 3rd ed. (New York: McGraw-Hill, 1932 [1904]), 367, 463; L. F. Barker, *Time and the Physician* (New York: Putnam, 1942), 86.

5. A. W. Davis, *Dr. Kelly of Hopkins: Surgeon, Scientist, Christian* (Baltimore: Johns Hopkins University Press, 1959), 17, 21.

6. David Linn Edsall, who, as dean of Harvard Medical School and of the Harvard School of Public Health during the 1920s, engineered Harvard's progressive transformation, entered Princeton the same year (1887) Cushing entered Yale. Edsall came to Princeton "a serious-minded young classicist" intent on a career in the classics. See J. C. Aub & R. K. Hapgood, *Pioneer in Modern Medicine: David Linn Edsall of Harvard* (Cambridge: Harvard Medical Alumni Association, 1970), 7. On Cushing and the classics, see E. H. Thomson, *Harvey Cushing: Surgeon, Author, Artist* (New York: Schuman, 1950), 20.

7. K. M. Ludmerer, *Learning to Heal: The Development of American Medical Education* (New York: Basic Books, 1985), 256–257, 262.

8. V. A. McKusick, "The Minutes of the Johns Hopkins Medical History Club, 1890 to 1894," *Bull. Hist. Med.*, 27:177–181, 1953.

9. H. A. Christian, "Osler: Recollections of an Undergraduate Medical Student at Johns Hopkins," *JAMA*, 84:77–83, 1949, at 83.

10. W. Osler, "On the Educational Value of the Medical Society," *Bost. Med.Surg. J.*, 148:275–279, 1903, at 278.

11. F. W. Hafferty, "Beyond Curriculum Reform: Confronting Medicine's Hidden Curriculum," *Acad. Med.*, 73:403–407, 1998; J. Coulehan, "Today's Professionalism: Engaging the Mind but Not the Heart," *Acad. Med.*, 80:892–898, 2005; P. Haldet & H. F. Stein, "The Role of the Student-Teacher Relationship in the Formation of Physicians: The Hidden Curriculum as Process," *J. Gen. Intern. Med.*, 21(suppl):S16–S20, 2005; S. Weissman, "Faculty Empathy and the Hidden Curriculum" [letter to the editor], *Acad. Med.*, 87:389, 2012.

12. First published in 1903, *The Medical Library and Historical Journal* was renamed *The Aesculapian: A Quarterly Journal of Medical History,*

Literature and Art in 1908. It lives on as the *Journal of the Medical Library Association.*

13. N. Allison, "Transactions of the St. Louis Medical History Club, *Aesculapian,* 1:53–58, 1908, at 56.

14. N.A., "A Medical History Club: The Proceedings of The Charaka Club, Vol. V, 1919," *Brit. Med. J.,* 1:16, 1920; O. Temkin, "The Johns Hopkins Medical History Club," *Bull. Hist. Med.,* 7:809, 1939; W. R. B., "Johns Hopkins Medical History Club," *Brit. Med. J,* 1:1036, 1939.

15. K. M. Markakis, et al., "The Path to Professionalism: Cultivating Humanistic Values and Attitudes in Residency Training," *Acad. Med.,* 75:141–150, 2000; M. Hojat, "Ten Approaches for Enhancing Empathy in Health and Human Services Cultures," *J. Health Hum. Serv. Adm.,* 31:412–450, 2009; K. Treadway & N. Chatterjee, "Into the Water—The Clinical Clerkships," *New Engl. J. Med.,* 364:1190–1193, 2011. On contemporary Balint groups, see A. L. Turner & P. L. Malm, "A Preliminary Investigation of Balint and Non-Balint Behavioral Medicine Training," *Fam. Med.,* 36:114–117, 2004; D. Kjeldmand, et al., "Balint Training Makes GPs Thrive Better in Their Job," *Patient Educ. Couns.,* 55:230–235, 2004; and K. P. Cataldo, et al., "Association Between Balint Training and Physician Empathy and Work Satisfaction," *Fam. Med.,* 37:328–331, 2005.

16. On Moss's intriguing career, see L. W. Shaw, "Story of an Extraordinary Mountain Man," in the *Asheville [NC] Citizen Times,* December 19, 1965, reprinted on the website of the Fred A. Moss Charity Trust (http://www.fredmosstrust.org/asheville-citizen-times-19651219.php).

17. F. A. Moss, "Scholastic Aptitude Tests for Medical Students," *J. Assn. Amer. Med. Coll.,* 5:90–110, 1930, at 90.

18. See Moss, "Scholastic Aptitude Tests," 90–91 and F. A. Moss, "Report of the Committee on Aptitude Tests for Medical Schools," *J. Assn. Amer. Med. Coll.,* 16:234–243, 1941, at 234–235.

19. R. D. Powers, "The MCAT Revisited," *New Engl. J. Med.,* 310:398–401, 1984, at 399.

20. W. C. McGaghie, "Assessing Readiness for Medical Education: Evolution of the Medical College Admission Test," *JAMA,* 288:1085–1090, 2002, at 1090.

21. E. Rosenthal, "Molding a New Med Student," Education/Life Supplement, *New York Times,* April 15, 2012, 20–22.

22. J. L. Dienstag, "The Medical College Admission Test—Toward a New Balance," *N. Engl. J. Med.,* 365:1955–1957, 2011; J. L. Dienstag, "The Case for the New MCAT," *N. Engl. J. Med.,* 367:280–281, 2012.

23. L. J. Van Winkle, N. Fjortoft, & M. Hojat, "Impact of a Workshop about Aging on the Empathy Scores of Pharmacy and Medical Students," *Am. J. Pharm. Educ.*, 76:1–5, 2012.

24. S. E. Wilson, J. Prescott, & G. Becket, "Empathy Levels in First- and Third-Year Students in Health and Non-Health Disciplines," *Am. J. Pharm. Educ.*, 76:1–4, 2012.

25. E. R. Marcus, "Empathy, Humanism, and the Professionalization Process of Medical Education," *Acad. Med.*, 74:1211–1215, 1999; M. Hojat, et al., "The Devil Is in the Third Year: A Longitudinal Study of Erosion of Empathy in Medical School," *Acad. Med.*, 84:1182–1191, 2009.

26. This is the Heideggerian language used by Jodi Halpern in *From Detached Concern to Empathy: Humanizing Medical Practice* (New York: Oxford University Press), 77.

27. B. Woodward, "Confidentiality, Consent and Autonomy in the Physician-Patient Relationship," *Health Care Anal.*, 9:337–351, 2001.

28. E. J. Cassell, "Diagnosing Suffering: A Perspective," *Ann. Intern. Med.*, 131:531–534, 1999.

29. J. White, et al., "'What Do They Want Me to Say?' The Hidden Curriculum at Work in the Medical School Selection Process: A Qualitative Study," *BMC Med. Educ.*, 12:1–9, 2012; U. H. Lindström, et al., "Medical Students' Experiences of Shame in Professional Enculturation," *Med. Educ.*, 45:1016–1024, 2011; A. H. Brainard & H. C. Brislen, "Learning Professionalism: A View from the Trenches," *Acad. Med.*, 82:1010–1014, 2007; P. Haidet & H. F. Stein, "The Role of the Student-Teacher Relationship in the Formation of Physicians," *J. Gen. Intern. Med.*, 21:S16–20, 2006; M. Seabrook, "Intimidation in Medical Education: Students' and Teachers' Perspectives," *Stud. High. Educ.*, 29:59–74, 2004.

30. Haidet & Stein, "Role of the Student-Teacher Relationship," op. cit.; N. Ratanawongsa, et al., "Residents' Perceptions of Professionalism in Training and Practice: Barriers, Promoters, and Duty Hour Requirements," *J. Gen Intern. Med.*, 21:758–763, 2006; J. Coulehan, "Today's Professionalism: Engaging the Mind but Not the Heart," *Acad. Med.*, 80:892–898, 2005; B. Maheux, et al., "Medical Faculty as Humanistic Physicians and Teachers: The Perceptions of Students at Innovative and Traditional Medical Schools, *Med. Educ.*, 34:630–634, 2000; J. H. Burack, et al., "Teaching Compassion and Respect: Attending Physicians' Responses to Problematic Behaviors," *J. Gen. Intern. Med.*, 14:49–55, 1999.

31. See further Burack, "Teaching Compassion and Respect," 54.

32. B. H. Lerner, *The Good Doctor: A Father, a Son, and the Evolution of Medical Ethics* (Boston: Beacon Press, 2014).

33. M. Marinker, "Myth, Paradox and the Hidden Curriculum," *Med. Educ.*, 31:293–298, 1997, at 293; cf. Haidet & Stein, "Role of Student-Teacher Relationship," 3: "The *relational processes* of the hidden curriculum assure the *perpetuation* of its content" (emphasis in original).

34. P. E. Stepansky, *The Last Family Doctor: Remembering My Father's Medicine* (Montclair, NJ: Keynote Books, 2011), 114.

35. Brainard & Brislen, "Learning Professionalism," 1011.

36. Coulehan, "Today's Professionalism," 896.

37. For examples of such physicians and their role in the revitalization of primary care medicine in the 1970s, see Stepansky, *Last Family Doctor*, 130–133.

CHAPTER 4—IS YOUR DOCTOR EMPATHIC?

1. I have written about the rise and fall of Freud's surgical metaphor in relation to the psychoanalytic method in P. E. Stepansky, *Freud, Surgery, and the Surgeon* (New York: Routledge, 1999).

2. H. Kohut, *How Does Analysis Cure?*, edited by A. Goldberg with the collaboration of P. E. Stepansky (Chicago: University of Chicago Press, 1984).

3. D. A. Schön, *The Reflective Practitioner: How Professionals Think in Action* (New York: Basic Books, 1983); D. A. Schön, *Educating the Reflective Practitioner* (San Francisco: Jossey-Bass, 1987).

4. S. J. Crowe, *Halsted of Johns Hopkins: The Man and His Men* (Springfield, IL: Thomas, 1957), 130–131.

5. The goal of this thought experiment, psychoanalytically understood, is emotional oneness with the patient, so it is not tantamount to the "detached insight" model of empathy critiqued by Jodi Halpern in *From Detached Concern to Empathy: Humanizing Medical Practice* (New York: Oxford University Press, 2001), 68–74.

6. The imaginative component of empathy, which is more relevant to its function in psychotherapy than in medicine, is especially stressed by Alfred Margulies, "Toward Empathy: The Uses of Wonder," *Amer. J. Psychiat.*, 141:1025–1033, 1984.

7. G. L. Engel, "The Need for a New Medical Model: A Challenge for Biomedicine," *Science*, 196:129–136, 1977; G. L. Engel, "The Clinical Application of the Biopsychosocial Model," *Amer. J. Psychiat.*, 137:535–544, 1980 [1979]. For an appreciation of the biopsychosocial model, which has largely been supplanted by evidence-based medicine, see the essays collected in R. Frankel, et al., eds., *The Biopsychosocial Approach: Past, Present, Future* (Rochester, NY: University of Rochester Press, 2003).

8. S. R. Waldstein, et al., "Teaching Psychosomatic (Biopsychosocial) Medicine in United States Medical Schools: Survey Findings," *Psychosom. Med.*, 63:335–343, 2001.

9. J. Z. Sadler, "Knowing, Valuing, Acting: Clues to Revising the Biopsychosocial Model," *Comp. Psychiat.*, 31:185–195, 1990; Waldstein, "Teaching Psychosomatic (Biopsychosocial) Medicine," op. cit.; T. McClain, P. S. O'Sullivan, & J. A. Clardy, "Biopsychosocial Formulations: Recognizing Educational Shortcomings," *Acad. Psychiat.*, 28:88–94, 2004.

10. F. W. Peabody, "The Care of the Patient, *JAMA*, 88:877–882, 1927, at 888.

11. L. Thomas, *The Youngest Science: Notes of a Medicine-Watcher* (New York: Viking, 1983), 14–15, 13.

12. Quoted in P. E. Stepansky, *The Last Family Doctor: Remembering My Father's Medicine* (Montclair, NJ: Keynote Books, 2011), 58–59.

13. W. Stepansky, "A General Practitioner Looks at Medicine," Lecture to the Junior Class of Jefferson Medical College, Philadelphia, November 24, 1965 (original emphasis).

14. D. C. Ransom & H. E. Vandervoort, "The Development of Family Medicine: Problematic Trends," *JAMA*, 225:1098–1102, 1973. Four years later, the Canadian family medicine educator Walter Spitzer also identified "the concept of family systems" as "often neglected in the description or characterization of the discipline [of family medicine]," adducing the notion of a "clinical parish" to capture the FP's "obligation to an aggregate of people and families for whom he has ongoing responsibility." See W. O. Spitzer, "The Intellectual Worthiness of Family Medicine," *Pharos*, 40:2–12, 1977, at 8–9.

15. W. Stepansky, "A General Practitioner Looks at Medicine," op. cit.

16. N. M. Theriot, "Diagnosing Unnatural Motherhood: Nineteenth-Century Physicians and 'Puerperal Insanity'," *Amer. Stud.*, 26:69–88, 1990; N. M. Theriot, "Women's Voices in Nineteenth-Century Medical Discourse: A Step Toward Deconstructing Science," *Signs*, 19:1–31, 1993; N. M. Theriot, "Negotiating Illness: Doctors, Patients, and Families in the Nineteenth Century," *J. Hist. Behav. Sci.*, 37:349–368, 2001. For a complementary perspective that emphasizes how the social class of postpartum women affected physicians' attitudes toward their nervousness, see F. G. Gosling & J. M. Ray, "The Right to Be Sick: American Physicians and Nervous Patients, 1885–1910," *J. Soc. Hist.*, 20:251–268, 1986.

17. H. Ratnayake, "Doctors' House Calls Making a Comeback," *The New Journal* (Wilmington, DE), November 13, 2010 (http://usatoday30.usatoday .com/yourlife/health/healthcare/doctorsnurses/2010-11-13-house-calls_N .htm). One such house call program is at the University Hospitals of Case

Medical Center (https://casemed.case.edu/fammed/geriatrics/HCP%20 Brochure%2011.pdf). For a review of modern house call programs as of 2004, see A. U. Loengard & J. Boal, "Home Care of the Frail Elderly," *Clin. Geriatr. Med.*, 20:795–807, 2004.

18. M. A. Forciea & J. Yudin, "Home-Based Care of the Older Patient," in R. J. Pignolo, M. K. Crane, & M. A. Forciea, eds., *Classic Papers in Geriatric Medicine with Current Commentaries* (Totowa, NJ: Humana Press, 2008), 27–28; E. W. Campion, "New Hope for Home Care?, *N. Engl. J. Med.*, 333:1213–1214, 1995; E. W. Campion, "Can House Calls Survive?", *N. Engl. J. Med.*, 337:1840–1841, 1997.

19. G. S. Meyer & R. V. Gibbons, "House Calls to the Elderly—A Vanishing Practice Among Physicians," *N. Engl. J. Med.*, 337:1815–1820, 1997.

20. Campion, "Can House Calls Survive?", 1840.

21. Ibid.

22. G. Bayne, "Physician Housecalls: It Is Time for the Public to Act" (http://www.1800calldoc.com/press/timetoact).

CHAPTER 5—CAN WE TEACH DOCTORS TO CARE?

1. R. Pedersen's review article, "Empirical Research on Empathy in Medicine—A Critical Review," *Pat. Educ Couns.*, 76:307–322, 2009, covers 237 research articles.

2. E.g., "The physician should ask open-ended questions and reflect to the patient the way the patient seems to be feeling. The capacity to imagine oneself in the patient's world enhances empathic responsiveness. If the physician does not feel in good empathic contact with the patient, he or she must learn how to access the patient's deeper feelings. What is often useful is to recognize a feeling or thought that, by analogy, stimulates one's own imagination, memory, or experience." P. S. Bellet & M. J. Maloney, "The Importance of Empathy as an Interviewing Skill in Medicine," *JAMA*, 266:1831–1832, 1991, at 1831. The remark about "taking a few minutes to empathize" is at 1832.

3. F. W. Platt & V. F. Keller, "Empathic Communication: A Teachable and Learnable Skill," *J. Gen Intern. Med.*, 9:222–226, 1994; A. L. Suchmann, et al., "A Model of Empathic Communication in the Medical Interview," *JAMA*, 277:678–682, 1997; J. L. Coulehan, et al., "'Let Me See if I Have This Right . . .': Words That Help Build Empathy," *Ann. Intern. Med.*, 136:221–227, 2001; H. M. Adler, "Toward a Biopsychosocial Understanding of the Patient-Physician Relationship: An Emerging Dialogue,"

J. Gen. Intern. Med., 22:280–285, 2007; M. Neumann, et al., "Analyzing the 'Nature' and 'Specific Effectiveness' of Clinical Empathy: A Theoretical Overview and Contribution Towards a Theory-Based Research Agenda," *Patient Educ. Couns.*, 74:339–346, 2009; K. Treadway & N. Chatterjee, "Into the Water—The Clinical Clerkships," *New Engl. J. Med.*, 364:1190–1193, 2011.

4. Adler, "Biopsychosocial Understanding," 282.

5. Suchmann, et al., "Model of Empathic Communication, " op. cit; Neumann, "Analyzing 'Nature' and 'Specific Effectiveness'," 343; K. A. Stepien & A. Baernstein, "Educating for Empathy: A Review," *J. Gen. Intern. Med.*, 21:524–530, 2006; R. W. Squier, "A Model of Empathic Understanding and Adherence to Treatment Regimens in Practitioner-Patient Relationships," *Soc. Sci. Med.*, 30:325–339, 1990.

6. H. Spiro, "What Is Empathy and Can It Be Taught?", *Ann. Intern. Med.*, 116:843–846, 1992; W. Zinn, "The Empathic Physician," *Arch. Intern. Med.*, 153:306–312, 1993; H. Spiro, et al., *Empathy and the Practice of Medicine* (New Haven: Yale University Press, 1993); J. Shapiro & L. Hunt, "All the World's a Stage: The Use of Theatrical Performance in Medical Education," *Med. Educ.*, 37:922–927, 2003; J. Shapiro, et al., "Teaching Empathy to First Year Medical Students: Evaluation of an Elective Literature and Medicine Course," *Educ. Health*, 17:73–84, 2004; S. DasGupta & R. Charon, "Personal Illness Narratives: Using Reflective Writing to Teach Empathy," *Acad. Med.*, 79:351–356, 2004; J. Shapiro, D. Kasman, & A. Shafer, "Words and Wards: A Model of Reflective Writing and Its Uses in Medical Education," *J. Med. Humanit.*, 27:231–244, 2006; J. Halpern, "Empathy and Patient-Physician Conflicts," *J. Gen. Intern. Med.*, 22:696–700, 2007.

7. R. Charon, "Narrative Medicine: A Model for Empathy, Reflection, Profession, and Trust," *JAMA*, 286:1897–1902, 2001, at 1898.

8. Suchmann, et al., "Model of Empathic Communication," 681; Zinn, "Empathic Physician," 308; Halpern, "Empathy and Conflicts," 697.

9. On the constructed nature of patient stories, including the physician's role in their construction, see H. Brody, "'My Story Is Broken; Can You Help Me Fix It?' Medical Ethics and the Joint Construction of Narrative," *Lit. Med.*, 13:79–92, 1994; S. DasGupta, "Being John *Doe* Malkovich: Truth, Imagination, and Story in Medicine," *Lit. Med.*, 25:439–462, 2006; and R. Garden, "Telling Stories about Illness and Disability: The Limits and Lessons of Narrative," *Perspect. Biol. Med.*, 53:121–135, 2010. On the motivational biases and cultural metanarratives that shape patient stories, see J. Shapiro, "Illness Narratives: Reliability, Authenticity and the Empathic Witness," *Med. Humanit.*, 37:68–72, 2011. For probing discussions of the

methodological complexities of illness narratives, see L.-C. Hyden, "Illness and Narrative," *Sociol. Health Ill.*, 19:48–69, 1997 and M. Bury, "Illness Narratives: Fact or Fiction?", *Sociol. Health Ill.*, 23:263–285, 2001.

10. Halpern, "Empathy and Conflicts," 697; A. Smajdor, et al., "The Limits of Empathy: Problems in Medical Education and Practice," *J. Med. Ethics.*, 37:380–383, 2011, quoted at 381.

11. E. D. Pellegrino, *Humanism and the Physician* (Knoxville: University of Tennessee Press, 1979), 106.

12. V. Gallese, "The Roots of Empathy: The Shared Manifold Hypothesis and the Neural Basis of Intersubjectivity," *Psychopathology*, 36:171–180, 2003; L. Carr, et al., "Neural Mechanisms of Empathy in Humans: A Relay from Neural Systems for Imitation to Limbic Area," *P. Natl. Acad. Sci. USA*, 100:5497–5502, 2003; G. Rizzolatti & L. Craighero, "The Mirror-Neuron System," *Ann. Rev. Neurosci.*, 27:169–192, 2004; V. Gallese, et al., "Intentional Attunement: Mirror Neurons and the Neural Underpinnings of Interpersonal Relations," *J. Am. Psychoanal. Assn.*, 55:131–176, 2007.

13. P. E. Stepansky, "*Humanitas*: Nineteenth-Century Physicians and the Classics," presented to the Richardson History of Psychiatry Research Seminar, Weill Cornell Medical College, New York, NY, October 3, 2007. The "pivotal figures" discussed in this paper include T. Clifford Allbutt, Claude Bernard, Harvey Cushing, David Linn Edsall, Howard Kelly, René Laennec, Rudolph Matas, William Osler, and William Welch.

14. See P. E. Stepansky, *Psychoanalysis at the Margins* (New York: Other Press, 2009), 301–303 and the references cited therein.

15. Joseph Collins, "The Alienist in Court," *Harper's Monthly*, 150:280–286, 1924; Joseph Collins, "A Doctor Looks at Doctors," *Harper's Monthly*, 154:348–356, 1926; Joseph Collins, "Should Doctors Tell the Truth?", *Harper's Monthly*, 155:320–326, 1927; Joseph Collins, "Group Practice in Medicine," *Harper's Monthly*, 158:165–173, 1928; Joseph Collins, "The Patient's Dilemma," *Harper's Monthly*, 159:505–514, 1929. I have also consulted two of Collins's popular collections that make many of the same points: *Letters to a Neurologist*, 2nd series (New York: Wood, 1910) and *The Way with the Nerves: Letters to a Neurologist on Various Modern Nervous Ailments, Real and Fancied, with Replies Thereto Telling of Their Nature and Treatment* (New York: Putnam, 1911).

16. On the founding of the New York Neurological Institute, see H. A. Riley, "The Neurological Institute of New York," *Bull. N.Y. Acad. Med.*, 42:654–676, 1966.

17. Collins, *The Way with Nerves*, 268.

18. Collins's review of James Joyce's *Ulysses*, the first by an American, was published in *The New York Times* on May 28, 1922. His volume *The Doctor Looks at Literature: Psychological Studies of Life and Literature* (New York: Doran, 1923) appeared the following year.

19. Collins, "A Doctor Looks at Doctors," 356. Collins's injunction is exemplified in "The Healer's Art," a course developed by Dr. Rachel Naomi Remen over the past 22 years and currently taught annually in 71 American medical colleges as well as medical colleges in seven other countries. See David Bornstein, "Medicine's Search for Meaning," posted for *The New York Times/Opinionator* on September 18, 2013 (http://opinionator.blogs.nytimes.com/2013/09/18/medicines-search-for-meaning/).

CHAPTER 6—MEDICAL TOOLS AND MEDICAL TOUCH

1. I worked as Dr. Silen's editor in 2000–2001, during which time I was privileged to read his unpublished lectures, addresses, and general-interest medical essays as preparation for helping him organize his memoirs. Sadly, the memoirs project never materialized. I quote from these unpublished documents in my possession.

2. On the early use of x-rays in the American courtroom and the unhappiness it caused physicians, see T. Golan, "The Emergence of the Silent Witness: The Legal and Medical Reception of X-rays in the USA," *Soc. Stud. Sci.,* 34:469–499, 2004 and L. Daston & P. Galison, "The Image of Objectivity," *Representations*, 40:81–128, 1992, at 110.

3. In this paragraph, I am guided especially by two exemplary studies, C. Lawrence, "Incommunicable Knowledge: Science, Technology and the Clinical Art in Britain, 1850–1914," *J. Contemp. Hist.*, 20:503–520, 1985 and H. Evans, "Losing Touch: The Controversy Over the Introduction of Blood Pressure Instruments in Medicine," *Technol. Cult.*, 34:784–807, 1993. Broadbent and Steell are quoted in Lawrence, 516.

4. J. Mackenzie, "New Methods of Studying Affections of the Heart," *Brit. Med. J.*, 1:519–522, 587–589, 702–705, 759–762, 812–815, 1905.

5. R. McNair Wilson, *The Beloved Physician: Sir James Mackenzie* (New York: Macmillan, 1926), 103–104. A more recent, detailed account of Mackenzie's life and career is A. Mair, *Sir James Mackenzie, M.D., 1853–1925—General Practitioner* (London: Royal College of General Practitioners, 1986).

6. S. A. Levine, "Diagnostic Value of Cardiac Auscultation," *JAMA*, 141:589–593, 1949.

7. R. L. Rosenthal, "Throw the Stethoscope Away: A Historical Essay," *Am. J. Cardiol.*, 111:1823–1828, 2013, at 1824.

8. A. R. Feinstein, *Clinical Judgment* (Baltimore: Williams & Wilkins, 1967), 325, 326.

9. Spectral phonocardiography was a medical adaptation by Victor McKusick and his colleagues at Johns Hopkins of a method for displaying speech sound devised in the 1940s by Ralph Potter and his colleagues at Bell Laboratories. McKusick announced the breakthrough in a series of publications in 1954 and 1955, and by 1956, he could confidently assert that "Spectral phonocardiography can do, or at least can be made to do, all the ear can. It can exceed the performance of the ear because (1) resolution in the time dimension is better, (2) it is not wed to one particular frequency response curve, (3) it is not handicapped by psycho-acoustic phenomena such as masking, and (4) permanent, quantifiable records are produced." V. A. McKusick, et al., "Spectral Phonocardiographic Studies in Congenital Heart Disease," *Brit. Heart J.*, 18:403–416, 1956, at 403. For a review of his research of the 1950s and the superiority of spectral to oscilloscopic phonocardiography, see V. A. McKusick, "Spectral Phonocardiography," *Am. J. Cardiol.*, 4:200–206, 1959. For a contemporary appreciation of phonocardiography (which has evolved into "acoustic cardiography"), including recent advances in technology that permit continuous ambulatory monitoring of patients, see Yong-Na Wen, et al., "Beyond Auscultation: Acoustic Cardiography in Clinical Practice," *Int. J. Cardiol.*, 172:548–560, 2014.

10. Rosenthal, "Throw the Stethoscope Away," 1823.

11. Ibid.

12. Ibid.

13. See J. E. Schultz, "The Inhospitable Hospital: Gender and Professionalism in Civil War Medicine," *Signs*, 17:363–392, 1992.

14. Madelin Gleeson and Fiona Timmins provide a critical evaluation of the nursing literature on touch that focuses on the methodological shortcomings of research reports published through 2002. See M. Gleeson & F. Timmins, "A Review of the Use and Clinical Effectiveness of Touch as a Nursing Intervention," *Clin. Effective. Nurs.*, 9:69–77, 2005.

15. S. J. Weiss, "The Language of Touch," *Nurs. Res.*, 28:76–80, 1979; S. J. Weiss, "Psychophysiological Effects of Caregiver Touch on Incidence of Cardiac Dysrhythmia," *Heart Lung*, 15:494–505, 1986; C. A. Estabrooks, "Touch in Nursing Practice: A Historical Perspective: 1900–1920," *J. Nurs. Hist.*, 2:33–49, 1987; J. S. Mulaik, et al., "Patients' Perceptions of Nurses' Use of Touch," *Western. J. Nurs. Res.*, 13:306–323, 1991; J. L. Bottorff, *Nurse-Patient Interaction: Observations of Touch* (Unpublished Doctoral

Dissertation, University of Alberta, 1992), 54–67; C. A. Estabrooks & J. M. Morse, "Toward a Theory of Touch: The Touching Process and Acquiring a Touching Style," *J. Adv. Nurs.*, 17:448–456, 1992; A Carter & H. Sanderson, "The Use of Touch in Nursing Practice," *Nurs. Standard*, 9:31–35, 1995.

16. C. A. Estabrooks, "Touch: A Nursing Strategy in the Intensive Care Unit," *Heart and Lung*, 18:329–401, 1989; K. McCann & H. McKenna, "An Examination of Touch Between Nurses and Elderly Patients in a Continuing Care Setting in Northern Ireland," *J. Adv. Nurs.*, 18:838–846, 1993; R. Adomat & A. Killingworth, "Care of the Critically Ill Patient: The Impact of Stress on the Use of Touch in Intensive Therapy Units," *J. Adv. Nurs.*, 19:912–922, 1994 .

17. C. Green, "Philosophic Reflections on the Meaning of Touch in Nurse-Patient Interactions," *Nurs. Philos.*, 14:242–253, 2013, at 250–251.

18. Mulaik, "Patients' Perceptions of Nurses' Use of Touch," 317–318; S. C. Edwards, "An Anthropological Interpretation of Nurses' and Patients' Perceptions of the Use of Space and Touch," *J. Adv. Nurs.*, 28:809–817, 1998; C. A. Estabrooks & J. M. Morse, "Toward a Theory of Touch: The Touching Process and Acquiring a Touching Style," *J. Adv. Nurs.*, 17:448–456, 1992; R. Davidhizar & J. Newman, "When Touch Is *Not* the Best Approach," *J. Clin. Nurs.*, 6:203–206, 1997.

19. "Middle managers" is the characterization of the nursing historian Barbara Melosh, in "Doctors, Patients, and 'Big Nurse': Work and Gender in the Postwar Hospital," in E. C. Lagemann, ed., *Nursing History: New Perspective, New Possibilities* (New York: Teachers College Press, 1983), 157–179.

20. M. Sandelowski, *Devices and Desires: Gender, Technology, and American Nursing* (Chapel Hill: University of North Carolina Press, 2000), 166.

21. On the revalorization of the feminine in nursing in the Nursing Theory Movement of the 1970s and '80s, see Sandelowski, *Devices and Desires*, 131–134.

22. R. L. Pullen, et al., "Men, Caring, & Touch," *Men Nurs.*, 7:14–17, 2009. On the strategies (including the use of humor) that men nurses develop to combat stereotypes about masculine touch—a problem especially salient in obstetric nursing—see J. Evans, "Cautious Caregivers: Gender Stereotypes and the Sexualization of Men Nurses' Touch," *J. Adv. Nurs.*, 40:441–448, 2002.

23. The work of Regina Morantz-Sanchez is especially illuminating of this binary and the major protagonists at the two poles. See R. Morantz, "Feminism, Professionalism, and Germs: The Thought of Mary Putnam Jacobi and Elizabeth Blackwell," *Am. Quart.*, 34:459–478, 1982, with a slightly revised version of the paper in R. Morantz-Sanchez, *Sympathy and Science:*

Women Physicians in American Medicine (Chapel Hill: University of North Carolina Press, 2000 [1985]), 184–202.

24. I have discussed the "generalist gaze" in P. E. Stepansky, *The Last Family Doctor: Remembering My Father's Medicine* (Montclair, NJ: Keynote Books, 2011), 62–66 and P. E. Stepansky, "When Generalist Values Meant General Practice: Family Medicine in Post-WWII America" (precirculated paper, American Association for the History of Medicine, Atlanta, GA, May 16–19, 2013).

25. Therapeutic touch was devised and promulgated by the nursing educator Delores Krieger in publications of the 1970s and '80s, e.g., "Therapeutic Touch: The Imprimatur of Nursing," *Amer. J. Nurs.*, 75:785–787, 1975; *The Therapeutic Touch* (New York: Prentice Hall, 1985); and *Living the Therapeutic Touch* (New York: Dodd, Mead, 1987). I share the viewpoint of Therese Meehan, who sees the technique as a risk-free nursing intervention capable of potentiating a powerful placebo effect. See T. C. Meehan, "Therapeutic Touch as a Nursing Intervention," *J. Adv. Nurs.*, 1:117–125, 1998.

26. For a fairly recent examination of transgressive touch and its ramifications, see G. O. Gabbard & E. P. Lester, *Boundary Violations in Psychoanalysis* (Arlington, VA: Amer. Psychiat. Pub., 2002).

27. A. Wilson, *The Making of Man-Midwifery: Childbirth in England, 1660–1770* (Cambridge: Harvard University Press, 1995), 97–98, 127–128.

28. R. D. French, *Antivivisection and Medical Science in Victorian Society* (Princeton: Princeton University Press, 1975), 411.

29. See Mitchell's influential address to the Second Congress of American Physicians and Surgeons of 1891, S. W. Mitchell, *The Early History of Instrumental Precision in Medicine* (New Haven: Tuttle, Morehouse & Taylor, 1892). On the importance of the mechanization of measurement in nineteenth-century medicine, see T. M. Porter, *Trust in Numbers: The Pursuit of Objectivity in Science and Public Life* (Princeton: Princeton University Press, 1995), ch. 8, and P. E. Stepansky, *Psychoanalysis at the Margins* (New York: Other Press, 2009), 143–155.

30. J. P. Baker, "The Incubator Controversy: Pediatricians and the Origins of Premature Infant Technology in the United States, 1890 to 1910," *Pediatrics*, 87:654–662, 1991.

31. Quoted in E. H. Thomson, *Harvey Cushing: Surgeon, Author, Artist* (New York: Schuman, 1950), 244–245.

32. G. G. Stephens, *The Intellectual Basis of Family Practice* (Kansas City: Winter, 1982), 62, 56, 83–85, 135–139.

33. Ibid., 84, 191, 64, 39, 28.

34. E.g., ibid., 96, 194.

35. Ibid. In 1978, Stephens spoke of the incursion of family practice into the medical school curriculum of the early '70s as an assault on an entrenched power base: "The medical education establishment has proved to be a tough opponent, with weapons we never dreamed of. . . . We had to deal with strong emotions, hostility, anger, humiliation. Our very existence was a judgment on the schools, much in the same way that civil rights demonstrators were a judgment on the establishment. We identified ourselves with all the natural critics of the schools—students, underserved segments of the public, and their elected representatives—to bring pressure to bear on the schools to create academic units devoted to family practice" (184, 187).

36. Ibid., 69.

37. I. R. McWhinney, "Medical Knowledge and the Rise of Technology," *J. Med. Philos.,* 3:293–304, 1978.

38. During this same period, the Canadian family practice educator Walter Spitzer also struggled to formulate an intellectual foundation for family practice, and, like Stephens, he offered a distorted and deprecatory characterization of specialization to make his case. Whereas Stephens focused on technology, Spitzer went after specialization per se, reaching back to Ortega y Gasset's diatribe on "The Barbarism of Specialization" in *The Revolt of the Masses* (1930) to make his case. See W. O. Spitzer, "The Intellectual Worthiness of Family Medicine," *Pharos*, 40:2–12, 1977, at 6.

39. Stephens, *Intellectual Basis of Family Practice*, 94, 105, 120–123, 192.

40. McWhinney, "Medical Knowledge and the Rise of Technology," 299–300.

41. Evans, "Losing Touch," 797.

42. On trust in medical technology as a "mediated" encounter with several complementary dimensions (e.g., the provider's confidence in the technology; the patient's perception of how, and with what degree of confidence, the provider uses the technology), see the studies of Enid Montague and his colleagues, which include development of an instrument for measuring patients' trust in medical technology: E. N. H. Montague, W. W. Winchester, & B. M. Kleiner, "Trust in Medical Technology by Patients and Health Care Providers in Obstetric Work Systems," *Behav. Inform. Tech.*, 29:541–554, 2010; E. Montague, "Validation of a Trust in Medical Technology Instrument," *Appl. Ergon.*, 41:812–821, 2010; E. Montague & O. Asan, "Trust in Technology-Mediated Collaborative Health Encounters: Constructing Trust in Active and Passive User Interactions with Technologies," *Ergonomics*, 55:752–761, 2012.

43. I am appropriating for my own purpose the titles of the Danish philosopher Søren Kierkegaard's two most popular works, *Fear and Trembling*

(1843) and *Sickness Unto Death* (1849), both considered foundational to modern existentialist thought. Obviously, my secular use bears no relation whatsoever to Kierkegaard's Christian existentialism, in which total despair leads to the "ultimate resignation" that permits receptiveness, absent any act of will, to a Christian faith that is nonrational and unrelated to mundane human ethics.

44. Quoted in J. Duffin, *To See with a Better Eye: A Life of R. T. H. Laennec* (Princeton: Princeton University Press, 1998), 122.

45. R. A. Young, "The Stethoscope: Past and Present," *Lancet*, 216:883–888, 1930, at 885. On Broussais's eccentric "physiological medicine," which was discredited during his own lifetime, see J. D. Rolleston, "F. J. V. Broussais (1772–1838): His Life and Doctrines," *P. Roy. Soc. Med.*, 32:405–413, 1939.

46. Here are a few recent examples: O. Samuel, "On Hanging Up My Stethoscope," *Brit. Med. J.*, 312:1426, 1996; "Dr. Van Ausdal Hangs Up His Stethoscope," *YSNews.com*, September 26, 2013 (http://ysnews.com/news/2013/09/dr-van-ausdal-hangs-up-his-stethoscope); "At 90, Gardena Doctor Is Hanging Up His Stethoscope," *The Daily Breeze*, October 29, 2013 (http://www.dailybreeze.com/general-news/20131029/at-90-gardena-doctor-is-hanging-up-his-stethoscope); "Well-known Doctor Hangs Up His Stethoscope," *Bay Post*, February 8, 2014 (http://www.batemansbaypost.com.au/story/1849567/well-known-doctor-hangs-up-his-stethoscope).

47. D. Katz, "When Satan Wears a Stethoscope" [book review of K. V. Iverson, *Demon Doctors: Physicians as Serial Killers*], *Am. J. Bioethics*, 4:63–64, 2004.

48. C. Jackson, "Bronchoscopy and Esophagoscopy: Gleanings from Experience," *JAMA*, 53:1009–1013, 1909; C. Jackson, "A Fence Staple in the Lung: A New Method of Bronchoscopic Removal," *JAMA*, 64:1906–1908, 1915.

49. F. Zöllner, "Gustav Killian, Father of Bronchoscopy," *Arch. Otolaryngol.*, 82:656–659, 1965.

50. C. Jackson, "Bronchoscopy: Past, Present and Future," *New Engl. J. Med.*, 199:759–763, 1928, at 760.

51. A. Coolidge & D. A. Hefferman, "Recent Progress in Laryngology," *Bost. Med. Surg. J.*, 158:550–554, 1908, at 553; H. Dietrich & H. K. Berkley, "Foreign Bodies in the Bronchi in Children," *JAMA*, 81:1202–1204, 1923, at 1204.

52. C. Jackson, *The Life of Chevalier Jackson: An Autobiography* (New York: Macmillan, 1938), 105–106; Jackson, "Bronchoscopy: Past, Present and Future," 759.

53. J. P. Clark, "Strictures of the Esophagus Dilated Through the Esophagoscope. Report of a Case," *Bost. Med. Surg. J.*, 158:350–351, 1908, at 350.

54. See, for example, A. Barnard, "A Critical Review of the Belief that Technology Is a Neutral Object and Nurses Are Its Master," *J. Adv. Nurs.*, 26:126–131, 1997; J. Fairman & P. D'Antonio, "Virtual Power: Gendering the Nurse-Technology Relationship," *Nurs. Inq.*, 6:178–186, 1999; and B. J. Hoerst & J. Fairman, "Social and Professional Influences of the Technology of Electronic Fetal Monitoring on Obstetrical Nursing," *Western J. Nurs. Res.*, 22:475–491, 2000, at 481–482.

55. C. Crocker & S. Timmons, "The Role of Technology in Critical Care Nursing," *J. Adv. Nurs.*, 65:52–61, 2008.

56. M. McGrath, "The Challenges of Caring in a Technological Environment: Critical Care Nurses' Experiences," *J. Clin. Nurs.*, 17:1096–1104, 2008.

57. A. Bernardo, "Technology and True Presence in Nursing," *Holist. Nurs. Pract.*, 12:40–49, 1998; R. C. Locsin, *Technological Competency as Caring in Nursing: A Model for Practice* (Indianapolis: Centre Nursing Press, 2005); McGrath, "The Challenges of Caring," op. cit.

58. C. V. Little, "Technological Competence as a Fundamental Structure of Learning in Critical Care Nursing: A Phenomenological Study," *J. Clin. Nurs.*, 9:391–399, 2000, at 398, 396.

59. See E. A. McConnell, "The Impact of Machines on the Work of Critical Care Nurses," *Crit. Care Nurs. Q.*, 12:45–52, 1990, at 51; D. Pelletier, et al., "The Impact of the Technological Care Environment on the Nursing Role, *Int. J. Technol. Assess.*, 12:358–366, 1996.

CHAPTER 7—THE NEEDLE'S TOUCH

1. On the prehistory of hypodermic injection, see D. L. Macht, "The History of Intravenous and Subcutaneous Administration of Drugs," *JAMA*, 55:856–860, 1916; G. A. Mogey, "Centenary of Hypodermic Injection," *Brit. Med. J.*, 2:1180–1185, 1953; N. Howard-Jones, "A Critical Study of the Origins and Early Development of Hypodermic Medication," *J. Hist. Med.*, 2:201–249, 1947; N. Howard-Jones, "The Origins of Hypodermic Medication," *Scien. Amer.*, 224:96–102, 1971.

2. Macht, "History of Intravenous and Subcutaneous," 859; J. B. Blake, "Mr. Ferguson's Hypodermic Syringe," *J. Hist. Med.*, 15: 337–341, 1960.

3. A. Wood, "New Method of Treating Neuralgia by the Direct Application of Opiates to the Painful Points," *Edinb. Med. Surg. J.*, 82:265–281, 1855.

4. On Hunter's contribution and his subsequent vitriolic exchanges with Wood over priority, see Howard-Jones, "Critical Study of Development of Hypodermic Medication," op. cit. Patricia Rosales provides a contextually grounded discussion of the dispute and the committee investigation by Edinburgh's Royal Medical and Chirurgical Society to which it gave rise. See P. A. Rosales, *A History of the Hypodermic Syringe, 1850s–1920s.* Unpublished doctoral dissertation, Department of the History of Science, Harvard University, 1997, 21–30.

5. See Rosales, *History of Hypodermic Syringe*, ch. 3, on the early reception of hypodermic injections in America.

6. G. Lawrence, "The Hypodermic Syringe," *Lancet*, 359:1074, 2002; J. Calatayud & A. Gonsález, "History of the Development and Evolution of Local Anesthesia since the Coca Leaf," *Anesthesiology*, 98:1503–1508, 2003, at 1506; R. E. Kravetz, "Hypodermic Syringe," *Am. J. Gastroenterol.*, 100:2614–2615, 2005.

7. A. Kotwal, "Innovation, Diffusion and Safety of a Medical Technology: A Review of the Literature on Injection Practices," *Soc. Sci. Med.*, 60:1133–1147, 2005, at 1133.

8. K. E. Kassowitz, "Psychodynamic Reactions of Children to the Use of Hypodermic Needles," *Am. J. Dis. Child.*, 95:253–257, 1958, at 257.

9. Summaries of the various treatment approaches to needle phobia are given in J. G. Hamilton, "Needle Phobia: A Neglected Diagnosis," *J. Fam. Practice*, 41:169–175, 1995 and H. Willemsen, et al., "Needle Phobia in Children: A Discussion of Aetiology and Treatment Options, " *Clin. Child Psychol. Psychiatry*, 7:609–619, 2002.

10. Hamilton, "Needle Phobia," op. cit.; S. Torgersen, "The Nature and Origin of Common Phobic Fears," *Brit. J. Psychiat.*, 134:343–351, 1979; L.-G. Öst, et al., "Applied Tension, Exposure in vivo, and Tension-Only in the Treatment of Blood Phobia," *Behav. Res. Ther.*, 29:561–574, 1991; L.-G. Öst, "Blood and Injection Phobia: Background and Cognitive, Physiological, and Behavioral Variables," *J. Abnorm. Psychol.*, 101:68–74, 1992.

11. References to these surveys are provided by Hamilton, "Needle Phobia," op. cit.

12. On the University of Washington survey, see P. Milgrom, et al., "Four Dimensions of Fear of Dental Injections," *J. Am. Dent. Assoc.*, 128:756–766, 1997 and T. Kaakko, et al., "Dental Fear Among University Students: Implications for Pharmacological Research," *Anesth. Prog.*, 45:62–67, 1998. Lawrence Prouix reported the results of the survey in the *Washington Post* under the heading "Who's Afraid of the Big Bad Needle?" July 1, 1997, p. 5.

13. R. M. Kennedy, et al., "Clinical Implications of Unmanaged Needle-Insertion Pain and Distress in Children," *Pediatrics*, 122:S130–S133, 2008.

14. See Kotwal, "Innovation, Diffusion and Safety," at 1136 for references.

15. S. R. Whyte & S. van der Geest, "Injections: Issues and Methods for Anthropological Research," in N. L. Etkin & M. L. Tan, eds., *Medicine, Meanings and Contexts* (Quezon City, Philippines: Health Action Information Network, 1994), 137–138.

16. C. MacDowall, "Intra-Peritoneal Injections in Cholera," *Lancet*, 122:658–659, 1883, at 658.

17. T. L. Leavitt, "The Hypodermic Injection of Morphia in Gout and Pleurisy," *Am. J. Med. Sci.*, 55:109, 1868.

18. W. Hardman, "Treatment of Choleraic Diarrhea by the Hypodermic Injection of Morphia," *Lancet*, 116:538–39, 1880, at 539.

19. P. E. Hill, "Morphia Poisoning by Hypodermic Injection; Recovery," *Lancet*, 120:527–528, 1882, at 527.

20. Leavitt, "Hypodermic Injection of Morphia in Gout and Pleurisy," op. cit.

21. On the ingestion and injection of glandular extracts in the 1890s and their allegedly rejuvenating and/or curative effects, see especially the papers of Merriley Borell: "Setting the Standards for a New Science: Edward Schäfer and Endocrinology," *Med. Hist.*, 22:282–290, 1978; "Brown-Séquard's Organotherapy and Its Appearance in America at the End of the Nineteenth Century," *Bull. Hist. Med.*, 50:309–320, 1976; "Organotherapy, British Physiology, and Discovery of the Internal Secretions," *J. Hist. Biol.*, 9:235–268, 1976; and "Organotherapy and the Emergence of Reproductive Endocrinology," *J. Hist. Biol.*, 18:1–30, 1985.

22. F. C. Shattuck, "Multiple Sarcoma of the Skin: Treatment by Hypodermic Injections of Fowler's Solution; Recovery," *Bost. Med. Surg. J.*, 112:618–619, 1885; N.A., "Treatment of Neurasthenia by Transfusion (Hypodermic Injection) of Nervous Substance," *Bost. Med. Surg. J.*, 126:273–274, 1892, at 274; T. Churton, "Cases of Acute Maniacal Delirium Treated by Inhalation of Chloroform and Hypodermic Injection of Morphia," *Lancet*, 141:861–862, 1893.

23. R. White, "Hypodermic Injection of Medicine, with a Case," *Bost. Med. Surg. J.*, 61:289–292, 1859, at 290.

24. N. B. Kennedy, "Carbolic Acid Injections in Hemorrhoids and Carbuncles," *JAMA*, 6:529–530, 1886.

25. E. Andrews, "The Latest Methods of Treating Carcinoma by Hypodermic Injection," *JAMA*, 26:1159–1160, 1897, at 1159.

26. For one such example, see N.A., "The Hypodermic Injection of Mercurials in the Treatment of Syphilis," *Bost. Med. Surg. J.*, 131:246, 1894.

27. H. H. Kane, *The Hypodermic Injection of Morphia: Its History, Advantages and Danger* (New York: Birmingham, 1880), 273, 277, 303, 307.

28. S. Maberly-Smith, "On the Treatment of Puerperal Convulsions by Hypodermic Injection of Morphia," *Lancet*, 118:86–87, 1881; J. D. Eggleston, quoted in "The Treatment of Puerperal Convulsions," *JAMA*, 8:295–296, 1887, at 295.

29. D. H. Cullumore, "Case of Traumatic Tetanus, Treated with the Hypodermic Injection of Atropia; Amputation of Great Toe; Recovery," *Lancet*, 114:42–43, 1897.

30. Hardman, "Treatment of Choleraic Diarrhea," op. cit.; C. MacDowall, "Hypodermic Injections of Morphia in Cholera," *Lancet*, 116:636, 1880.

31. Kane, *Hypodermic Injection of Morphia*, 244–266, 309.

32. On the "heroic surgery" of the final decades of the nineteenth century and the exalted status of late-nineteenth-century surgeons, see P. E. Stepansky, *Freud, Surgery, and the Surgeons* (New York: Routledge, 1999), 23–34 and passim.

33. J. Travell, "Factors Affecting Pain of Injection," *JAMA*, 58:368–371, 1955, at 368.

34. J. Travell, "Factors Affecting Pain of Injection," op. cit.; L. C. Miller, "Control of Pain of Injection," *Bull. Parenter. Drug Assoc.*, 7:9–13,1953; E. P. MacKenzie, "Painless Injections in Pediatric Practice," *J. Pediatr.*, 44:421, 1954; O. F. Thomas & G. Penrhyn Jones, "A Note on Injection Pain with Streptomycin," *Tubercle*, 36:157–159, 1955; F. H. J. Figge & V. M. Gelhaus, "A New Injector Designed to Minimize Pain and Apprehension of Parenteral Therapy," *JAMA*, 160:1308–1310, 1956. There were also needle innovations in the realm of intravenous therapy, e.g., L. I. Gardner & J. T. Murphy, "New Needle for Pediatric Scalp Vein Infusions," *Am. J. Dis. Child.*, 80:303–304, 1950.

35. My thanks to Kathie Bischoff, archivist of Becton, Dickinson, for sending me copies of the new product information that accompanied the release of the B-D Hypak in 1954.

36. D. M. Oshinsky, *Polio: An American Story* (New York: Oxford, 2005), 191, 197.

37. S. Fraiberg, "A Critical Neurosis in a Two-and-a-Half-Year Girl," *Psychoanal. Stud. Child*, 7:173–215, 1952, at 180; S. Fraiberg, "Tales of the Discovery of the Secret Treasure," *Psychoanal. Stud. Child*, 9:218–241, 1954, at 236.

38. I. D. Buckingham, "The Effect of Hysterectomy on the Subjective Experience of Orgasm," *J. Clin. Psychoanal.*, 3:607–12, 1994.

39. D. Weston, "Response," *Int. J. Psychoanal.*, 78:1218–1219, 1997, at 1219; C. Troupp, "Clinical Commentary," *J. Child Psychother.*, 36:179–182, 2010.

40. There is ample documentation of needle anxiety among present-day diabetics, e.g., A. Zambanini, et al., "Injection Related Anxiety in Insulin-Treated Diabetes," *Diabetes Res. Clin. Pr.,* 46:239–246, 1999 and A. B. Hauber, et al., "Risking Health to Avoid Injections: Preferences of Canadians with Type 2 Diabetes," *Diabetes Care*, 28:2243–2245, 2005.

41. S. Stearns, "Some Emotional Aspects of the Treatment of Diabetes Mellitus and the Role of the Physician," *N. Engl. J. Med.,* 249:471–476, 1953, at 473.

42. Ibid., 474.

43. Ibid.

44. P. E. Stepansky, *Psychoanalysis at the Margins* (New York: Other Press, 2009), 287–313; G. S. Moran, "Psychoanalytic Treatment of Diabetic Children," *Psychoanal. Stud. Child*, 39:407–447, at 413, 440.

45. W. C. Menninger, "Interrelationships of Mental Disorders and Diabetes Mellitus," *J. Ment. Sci.,* 81:332–357, 1935; W. C. Menninger, "Psychological Factors in Etiology of Diabetes," *J. Nerv. Ment. Dis.,* 81:1–13, 1935; G. E. Daniels, "Analysis of a Case of Neurosis with Diabetes Mellitus, *Psychoanal. Quart.,* 5:413–547, 1936, quoted at 536–537; G. E. Daniels, "Brief Psychotherapy in Diabetes Mellitus," *Psychoanal. Quart.,* 7:121–128, 1944. In the published discussion that followed Daniels's paper of 1936, his viewpoint received supportive elaboration by Bertram Lewin, Robert Fliess, Abraham Kardiner, and Smith Ely Jelliffe.

46. J. Miller, "Heroin Addiction: The Needle as Transitional Object," *J. Am. Acad. Psychoanal.,* 30:293–304, 2002.

CHAPTER 8—MY DOCTOR, MY FRIEND

1. H. Brownell Wheeler, "Healing and Heroism," *N. Engl. J. Med.,* 322:1540–1548, 1990, at 1540, 1543.

2. T. S. Cullen, "The Gay of Heart," *Arch. Intern. Med.,* 84:41–45, 1949, at 45.

3. J. M. T. Finney, *A Surgeon's Life* (New York: Putnam's, 1940), 109–110.

4. S. W. Mitchell, *Doctor and Patient*, 2nd ed. (Philadelphia: Lippincott, 1888), 28.

5. R. C. Cabot, *Training and Rewards of the Physician* (Philadelphia: Lippincott, 1918), 52–53.

6. A. E. Hertzler, *The Horse and Buggy Doctor* (New York: Harper, 1938); W. C. Williams, *The Doctor Stories* (New York: New Directions, 1984 [1932–1962]).

7. W. Osler, "Medicine in the Nineteenth Century" (1901), in *Aequanimitas, with other Addresses to Medical Students, Nurses, and Practitioners of Medicine*, 3rd ed. (New York: McGraw-Hill, 1932 [1904]), 219–262, at 259.

8. A. G. Gerster, *Recollections of a New York Surgeon* (New York: Hoeber, 1917), e.g., 177–180; M. Thorek, *A Surgeon's World* (Philadelphia: Lippincott, 1943), e.g., 95–106, 125–133. On Gerster's and Thorek's contributions to surgical training and practice in America, see R. M. Langer, "Arpad Gerster and Max Thorek: Contributions to American Surgery," *J. Invest. Surg.*, 22:162–166, 2009.

9. Thorek, *Surgeon's World*, 133.

10. On the circumstances leading up to passage of the Patient's Bill of Rights in the early '70s, see especially D. J. Rothman, *Strangers at the Bedside: A History of How Law and Bioethics Transformed Medical Decision Making* (New York: Basic Books, 1991), 143–147.

11. R. Veatch, "The Physician as Stranger: The Ethics of the Anonymous Patient-Physician Relationship," in E. E. Shelp, ed., *The Clinical Encounter: The Moral Fabric of the Patient-Physician Relationship* (New York: Springer, 1983), 187–207; P. M. L. Illingworth, "The Friendship Model of Physician/ Patient Relationship and Patient Autonomy," *Bioethics*, 2:22–36, 1988.

12. Illingworth, "Friendship Model," 29. Illingworth takes her definition of "psychological oppression" from the feminist philosopher Sandra Bartky, "On Psychological Oppression," in S. Bishop & M. Weinzweig, eds., *Philosophy and Women* (Belmont, CA: Wadsworth, 1979), at 34. The paper is reprinted in S. Bartky, ed., *Femininity and Domination: Studies in the Phenomenology of Oppression* (New York: Routledge, 1990), 22–32.

13. According to Veatch, the physician does not even retain the *prerogative* to care for the patient in traditionally caring ways, since in all but a few situations (nonspecified by Veatch), medical care and the recommendations to which it leads are inherently value-laden and, as such, antithetical to the *patient's* prerogative to make health care decisions on the basis of his or her own values alone. See R. Veatch, *Patient, Heal Thyself: How the New Medicine Puts the Patient in Charge* (New York: Oxford University Press, 2008). His admission that "There surely are at least a few situations in which the doctor really does know best" is at 49.

14. P. E. Stepansky, *The Last Family Doctor: Remembering My Father's Medicine* (Montclair, NJ: Keynote Books, 2011).

15. E.g., M. DeCamp, T. W. Koenig, & M. S. Chisolm, "Social Media and Physicians' Online Identity Crisis," *JAMA*, 310:581–582, 2013. Indeed, these authors claim, the very attempt of physicians to separate professional and personal identities online "may be inadvertently harmful," saddling them

with "the psychological or physical burden of trying to maintain two identities" (581). Happily, I find nothing in the literature bearing out this dire possibility. The fact that identities cannot be rigidly separated in some ultimate existential sense obscures the pragmatic fact that we all go through life with multiple identities (just like we all have different kinds of friends), and reasonable efforts to keep them separate does not propel us into Eriksonian "identity crises"; rather, it seems to be, more often than not, in everyone's best interest.

16. Regarding Facebook, see, for example, L. A. Thompson, et al., "The Intersection of Online Social Networking with Medical Professionalism," *J. Gen. Intern. Med.*, 23:954–957, 2008; S. H. Jain, "Practicing Medicine in the Age of Facebook," *N. Engl. J. Med.*, 361:649–651, 2009; J. S. Guseh, R. W. Brendel, & D. H. Brendel, "Medical Professionalism in the Age of Online Social Networking," *J. Med. Ethics*, 35:584–586, 2009; and A. Mostaghimi & B. H. Crotty, "Professionalism in the Digital Age," *Ann. Intern. Med.*, 154:560–562, 2011. Regarding Twitter, see K. C. Chretien, "Research Letter: Physicians on Twitter," *JAMA*, 305:566–568, 2011; A. Brynolf, et al., "Virtual Colleagues, Virtually Colleagues—Physicians' Use of Twitter: A Population-Based Observational Study," *BMJ Open*, 3:1–5, 2013; and E. K. Choo, "Twitter as a Tool for Communication and Knowledge Exchange in Academic Medicine: A Guide for Skeptics and Novices," *Med. Teach.*, December 19, 2014, 1–6 [Epub ahead of print].

17. R. Collier, "Professionalism: Social Media Mishaps," *Can. Med. Assoc. J.*, 184:E627–E628, 2012.

18. Thompson, et al. found that only one-third of Facebook accounts of University of Florida medical students had been made private. As one goes up the hierarchy of medical training, the percentage who use privacy settings increases. Two small-scale overseas studies in France and New Zealand, respectively, found that just over 60% of young medical graduates had changed the default privacy setting of their Facebook accounts. Finally, Clyde and his colleagues remind us that even the use of Facebook privacy settings does not keep a profile private: it remains open to, on average, an additional 45,000 "friends of friends." See Thompson, et al., "Intersection of Online Social Networking," 256; A. Moubarak, et al., "Facebook Activity of Residents and Fellows and Its Impact on the Doctor-Patient Relationship," *J. Med. Ethics*, 37:101–104, 2011; J. MacDonald, S. Sohn, & P. Ellis, "Privacy, Professionalism and Facebook: A Dilemma for Young Doctors," *Med. Educ.*, 44:805–813, 2010; J. W. Clyde, M. M. Rodriguez, & C. Geiser, "Medical Professionalism: An Experimental Look at Physicians' Facebook Profiles," *Med. Educ. Online*, 19:1–7, 2014, at 1.

19. A. Jain, "What Is Appropriate to Post on Social Media? Ratings from Students, Faculty Members and the Public," *Med. Educ.*, 48:157–169, 2014.

20. A. Jain, "What Is Appropriate to Post," 167.

21. S. J. Langenfeld, et al., "An Assessment of Unprofessional Behavior Among Surgical Residents on Facebook: A Warning of the Dangers of Social Media," *J. Surg. Educ.*, 71:e28–e32, 2014.

22. See "Photos of drinking, grinning aid mission doctors cause uproar" (http://www.cnn.com/2010/WORLD/americas/01/29/haiti.puerto.rico .doctors). The incident is mentioned, for example, by S. Ryan Greysen, T. Kind, & K. C. Chretien, "Online Professionalism and the Mirror of Social Media," *J. Gen. Intern. Med.*, 25:1227–1229, 2010, and Collier, "Professionalism," op. cit.

23. Decamp, "Social Media and Physicians' Online Identity Crisis," 582.

24. Greyson, "Mirror of Social Media," 1229; S. R. Greyson, et al., "Online Professionalism Investigations by State Medical Boards: First, Do No Harm," *Ann. Intern. Med.*, 158:124–130, 2013.

25. Mostaghimi & Crotty, "Professionalism in the Digital Age," op. cit.; Thompson, "Intersection of Online Social Networking," op. cit; and G. T. Bosslet, et al., "The Patient-Doctor Relationship and Online Social Networks: Results of a National Survey," *J. Gen. Intern. Med.*, 27:1168–1174, 2012.

26. AMA, "Opinion 9.124 - Professionalism in the Use of Social Media" (http://www.ama-assn.org/ama/pub/physician-resources/medical-ethics /code-medical-ethics/opinion9124.page); FSMB, "Model Policy Guidelines for the Appropriate Use of Social Media and Social Networking in Medical Practice" (http://www.fsmb.org/Media/Default/PDF/FSMB/Advocacy /pub-social-media-guidelines.pdf).

27. Greyson, "Online Professionalism Investigations," 127.

28. Brynolf, "Virtual Colleagues, Virtually Colleagues," 4.

29. A. Jain, "What Is Appropriate to Post?", 167; Gusch, "Medical Professionalism," 585.

30. Gusch, "Medical Professionalism," 585.

31. Ibid., 584.

32. Langenfeld, "Assessment of Unprofessional Behavior," op. cit.

33. T. Kind, S. R. Greysen, & K. C. Chretien, "Advantages and Challenges of Social Media in Pediatrics," *Pediatr. Ann.*, 40:430–434, 2011, at 433.

34. R. Maghnezi, L. C. Bergman, & S. Urotitz, "Would Your Patient Prefer to Be Considered Your Friend? Patient Preferences in Physician Relationships," *Health Educ. Behav.*, 42:210–219, 2015, at 217. These Israeli researchers found that as many surveyed patients preferred the term "friend" to characterize their relationship to their family doctors as preferred all three designations of a more businesslike relationship (consumer, client, insured) combined (217).

35. J. M. Kelly, G. Kraft-Todd, L. Schapira, et al., "The Influence of the Patient-Clinician Relationship on Healthcare Outcomes: A Systematic Review and Meta-Analysis of Randomized Controlled Trials," *PLoS ONE* 9(6): e101191. doi:10.1371/journal.pone.0101191.

36. Nancy Tomes provides an astute analysis of these and other developments (e.g., the emergence of computer-assisted information technology, health services research, and health services marketing) related to the "rapid commercialization of the report card concept" in American health care in "The 'Information Rx'," in D. J. Rothman & D. Blumenthal, eds., *Medical Professionalism in the New Information Age* (New Brunswick: Rutgers University Press, 2010), 40–65, quoted at 55.

37. ZocDoc, founded in 2007, differs from other rating services. It requires registration by patients and physicians alike, and provides online scheduling of appointments along with physician reviews. But ZocDoc, unlike Healthgrades, et al., only allows reviews from patients who have actually seen a physician through ZocDoc. As such, it is a "closed loop" review system. See O. Kharraz, "Providers Should Think Seriously About Leveraging Online Reviews," March 12, 2013 (http://www.thedoctorblog.com /providers-should-think-seriously-about-leveraging-online-reviews).

38. S. Jain, "Googling Ourselves—What Physicians Can Learn from Online Rating Sites," *N. Engl. J. Med.*, 362:6–7, 2010.

39. G. Gao, et al., "A Changing Landscape of Physician Quality Reporting: Analysis of Patients' Online Ratings of Their Physicians Over a 5-Year Period," *J. Med. Internet Res.*, 14:e38, 2012.

40. R. Reitman, "Medical Justice: Stifling Speech of Patients with a Touch of 'Privacy Blackmail'," May 4, 2011 (https://www.eff.org/deeplinks/2011 /05/medical-justice-stifling-speech-patients-touch); E. Goldman, "Medical Justice Capitulates by 'Retiring' Its Anti-Patient Review Contracts," December 1, 2011 (http://blog.ericgoldman.org/archives/2011/12/medical _justice.htm); R. Lieber, "The Web Is Awash in Reviews, but Not for Doctors. Here's Why," *New York Times*, March 9, 2012 (http://www.nytimes .com/2012/03/10/your-money/why-the-web-lacks-authoritative-reviews-of -doctors.html?_r=0&pagewanted=print).

41. S. Reddy, "Doctors Check Online Ratings from Patients and Make Change," *Wall Street Journal*, May 14, 2014. Cf. C. Ellimootil, et al., "Online Reviews of 500 Urologists," *J. Urology*, 189:2269–2273, 2013 and D. B. Bumpass & J. B. Samora, "Understanding Online Physician Ratings," AAOS Now [American Academy of Orthopedic Surgeons], September 2013 (http://www.aaos.org/news/aaosnow/sep13/advocacy4.asp).

42. Lieber, "The Web Is Awash in Reviews," op. cit.

43. W. N. Espeland & M. Sauder, "Rankings and Reactivities: How Public Measures Recreate Social Worlds," *Am. J. Sociol.*, 113:1–40, 2007. Gaming the system can go far beyond "leading" the patient to give positive feedback. It can result in both unnecessary treatment (e.g., overprescribing pain medications) and the withholding of treatment. As to the latter, consider the interventional cardiologists surveyed by the New York State Department of Health between 1998 and 2000, as reported by Craig R. Narins and his colleagues in 2005. Almost 80% of the cardiologists agreed they might refuse to perform angioplasty on high-risk patients lest bad outcomes, in the form of physician-specific procedural mortality rates, affect their report cards. See C. R. Narins, et al., "The Influence of Public Reporting of Outcome Data on Medical Decision Making by Physicians," *Arch. Intern. Med.*, 165:83–87, 2005 and R. M. Werner & D. A. Asch, "The Unintended Consequences of Publicly Reporting Quality Information," *JAMA*, 293:1239–1244, 2005.

44. J. Hyatt, "Responding to Negative Online Comments," *MCMS Physician* (Official Publication of the Montgomery County Medical Society of Pennsylvania), Summer 2014, 6–8.

45. See J. A. Barondess, "Is Osler Dead?" *Perspect. Biol. Med.*, 45:65–84, at 82.

46. An online survey of over 700 ER doctors by *Emergency Physicians Monthly* found that 59% admitted increasing the number of tests they ordered because of patient satisfaction surveys. When the South Carolina Medical Association asked its members whether they ever ordered a test they felt was inappropriate because of such pressure, 55% said "yes," and nearly half of the 131 respondents admitted improperly prescribing antibiotics and narcotics in direct response to patient satisfaction surveys. These studies are cited by Kai Falkenberg in "Why Rating Your Doctor Is Bad for Your Health," *Forbes*, January 21, 2013 (http://www.forbes.com/sites/kaifalkenberg/2013/01/02/why-rating-your-doctor-is-bad-for-your-health/).

47. J. J. Fenton, et al., "The Cost of Satisfaction: A National Study of Patient Satisfaction, Health Care Utilization, Expenditures, and Mortality," *Arch. Intern. Med.*, 172:405–411, 2012.

48. J. T. Chang, et al., "Patients' Global Ratings of Their Health Care Are Not Associated with the Technical Quality of Their Care," *Ann. Intern. Med.*, 144:665–672, 2006; D. S. Lee, et al., "Patient Satisfaction and Its Relationship with Quality and Outcomes of Care after Acute Myocardial Infarction," *Circulation*, 118:1938–1945, 2008; A. Zgierska, M. Miller, & D. Rabago, "Patient Satisfaction, Prescription Drug Abuse, and Potential Unintended Consequences," *JAMA*, 307:1377–1378, 2012, quoted at 1378; A. Lembke, "Why Doctors Prescribe Opioids to Known Opioid Abusers," *N. Engl. J. Med.*, 367:1580–1581, 2012.

49. A. Zgierska, D. Rabago, & M. M. Miller, "Impact of Patient Satisfaction Ratings on Physicians and Clinical Care," *Patient Prefer. Adherence*, 8:437–446, 2014.

50. See, for example, L. S. Dugdale, "Friendship with Patients," *J. Gen. Intern. Med.*, 30:265–266, 2014; D. M. Boyd, "A Matter of Respect: A Friendship with an Unusual Patient Changes How a Young Doctor Approaches the Practice of Medicine," *Med. Econ.*, 88:79–81. For an especially powerful contemporary account of personal transformation arising from doctor-patient friendship, see L. M. Ramondetta & D. R. Stills, *The Light Within: The Extraordinary Friendship of a Doctor and Patient Brought Together by Cancer* (New York: William Morrow, 2008).

51. P. D. White, "Shattuck Lecture: La Médecine du Coeur," *New Engl. J. Med.*, 240:825–830, 1949, at 826. For a contemporary instance of a doctor-patient relationship that developed into friendship and, ultimately, into love and marriage, see David Goldblatt's exquisite brief essay, "Light of My Life," *Am. J. Med.*, 118:1454, 2005.

52. W. C. Alvarez, "Doctors Should Show Friendship to Patients," *Los Angeles Times*, September 5, 1955, 16. Alvarez's remark followed his reading of the marketing expert Ernest Dichter's report on the doctor-patient relationship commissioned by the Committee on Medical Economics of the California Medical Association and published as *A Psychological Study of the Doctor-Patient Relationship, Submitted to the California Medical Association, Alameda County Medical Association, May 1950* (Los Angeles: California Medical Association, 1950).

53. White, "La Médecine du Coeur," 826.

54. O. W. Holmes, "The Young Practitioner" (1871), in *Medical Essays, 1842–1882* (Boston: Houghton Mifflin, 1895), 370–395; W. S. Thayer, "Duties and Problems of the Physician" (1928), in *Osler and Other Papers* (Baltimore: Johns Hopkins, 1931), 347–370; White, "La Médecine du Coeur," op. cit.

55. This point is stressed especially by the eminent cardiologist Paul Dudley White, the son of a small-town family doctor, in "La Médecine du Coeur," 826–827.

56. D. H. Murray, "The Family Doctor," *JAMA*, 161:671–672, 1956, at 671.

57. Holmes, "The Young Practitioner," 383.

58. J. Jackson, *Letters to a Young Physician Just Entering Upon Practice* (Boston: Phillips, Samuel, 1855), 16 (emphasis in original).

59. Jackson, *Letters to a Young Physician*, 22–23.

60. M. de Montaigne, *Essays*, trans. J. M. Cohen (Baltimore: Penguin, 1958), 94.

CHAPTER 9—GENERAL PRACTICE
AND ITS DISCONTENTS

1. A. H. Smith, "The Family Physician," *Harper's Magazine*, 78:722–729, 1888, at 724.

2. A. Jacobi, "Commercialized Medicine," *The Independent*, 69:413–416, 1910, at 415.

3. A. F. Van Bibber, "The Swan Song of the Country Doctor," *N. Am. Rev.*, 227:89–94, 1929, at 92.

4. P. Dufault, "Medicinae Doctor, 1950," *N. Engl. J. Med.*, 242:429–436, 1950, at 430.

5. D. D. Rutstein, "Do You Really Want a Family Doctor?", *The Crisis in American Medicine* (Harper's Supplement), 221:144–150, 1960, at 150.

6. T. Bodenheimer, "Primary Care—Will It Survive?", *New Engl. J. Med.*, 355:861–864, 2006, at 863.

7. J. Brown, *Rab and His Friends and Other Essays* (1858–1861) (London: Dent, n.d.), 18, quoted in I. Loudon, "The Concept of the Family Doctor," *Bull. Hist. Med.*, 58:347–362, 1982, at 348.

8. My remarks on the early history of internal medicine in America draw on W. L. Bierring, "The American Board of Internal Medicine," in W. G. Morgan, ed., *The American College of Physicians: Its First Quarter Century* (Philadelphia: American College of Physicians, 1940), 87–102; P. B. Beeson, "One Hundred Years of American Internal Medicine: A View from the Inside," *Ann. Intern. Med.*, 1986, 105:436–444; R. Stevens, "Issues for American Internal Medicine Through the Last Century," *Ann. Int. Med.*, 105:592–602, 1986; P. B. Beeson & R. C. Maulitz, "The Inner History of Internal Medicine," in R. C. Maulitz & D. E. Long, eds., *Grand Rounds: One Hundred Years of Internal Medicine* (Philadelphia: University of Pennsylvania Press, 1988), 15–54; and J. D. Howell, "The Invention and Development of American Internal Medicine," *J. Gen. Intern. Med.*, 4:127–133, 1989.

9. W. Osler, "Internal Medicine as a Vocation" (1897), in *Aequanimitas, With other Addresses to Medical Students, Nurses and Practitioners of Medicine*, 3rd ed. (New York: McGraw-Hill, 1932 [1904]), 133–145.

10. Howell, "Invention and Development of American Internal Medicine," 129.

11. Sharon R. Kaufman, *The Healer's Tale: Transforming Medicine and Culture* (Madison: University of Wisconsin Press, 1993), 235, 245.

12. D. Funkenstein, *Medical Students, Medical Schools and Society during Five Eras* (Cambridge: Cambridge University Press, 1968), 12; R. Stevens, *American Medicine and the Public Interest: A History of Specialization*, updated ed. (Berkeley: University of California Press, 1998 [1971]), 312.

13. M. P. Jacoby, "Specialism in Medicine," *Arch. Med.*, 7:87, 1882.

14. W. Osler, "Remarks on Specialism," *Bost. Med. Surg. J.*, 126:457–459, 1892, at 458.

15. E.g., F. H. Davenport, "Specialism in Medical Practice: Its Present Status and Tendencies," *Bost. Med. Surg. J.*, 145:81–86, 1901, at 83; R. W. Taylor, "The Widening Sphere of Medicine," *Bost. Med. Surg. J.*, 61:39–47, 1909, at 41, 42; R. Fitz, "The Rise of the Practice of Internal Medicine as a Specialty," *N. Engl. J. Med.*, 242:569–574, 1950, at 574.

16. H. G. Weiskotten, "I. The Future of Family Practice: The Present Scene—Trends in Medical Practice," *JAMA*, 176:895–897, 1961, at 895.

17. H. G. Weiskotten, "Trends in Specialization," *JAMA* 160:1303–1305, 1956, Table 1 at 1304.

18. Stevens, *American Medicine and the Public Interest*, 299.

19. J. A. Curran, "Internships and Residencies: Historical Backgrounds and Current Trends," *J. Med. Educ.*, 34:873–884, 1959.

20. W. B. Fye, "Ventricular Fibrillation and Defibrillation: Historical Perspectives with Emphasis on the Contributions of Jon MacWilliam, Carl Wiggers, and William Kouwenhoven," *Circulation*, 71:858–865, 1985, at 864.

21. J. Fairman & J. E. Lynaugh, *Critical Care Nursing: A History* (Philadelphia: University of Pennsylvania Press, 1998), 12–20.

22. W. B. Fye, *American Cardiology: The History of a Specialty and Its College* (Baltimore: Johns Hopkins University Press, 1996), 100–101, 118ff.

23. D. J. Rothman, *Beginnings Count: The Technological Imperative in American Health Care* (New York: Oxford University Press, 1997), 89.

24. Ibid., 96–109.

25. M. Epstein, "John P. Merrill: The Father of Nephrology as a Specialty," *Clin. J. Am. Soc. Nephrol.*, 4:2–8, 2009.

26. Rothman, *Beginnings Count*, 24–26.

27. R. Cunningham III & R. M. Cunningham Jr., *The Blues: A History of the Blue Cross and Blue Shield System* (Dekalb, IL: Northern Illinois University Press, 1997), 58–60, 90.

28. Weiskotten, "Trends in Specialization," 1304.

29. S. A. Truman, *The History of the Founding of the American Academy of General Practice* (St. Louis: Green, 1969), 16.

30. P. A. Davis, "The American Academy of General Practice," *Southern Med. J.*, 41:651–55, 1948, at 654; W. C. Allen & S. A. Garlan, "Educational Motivation in the Field of General Practice," *New York State J. Med.*, 53:1243–1245, 1953, at 1243; E. A. Royston, "The American Academy of General Practice: Its Origin, Objectives, Growth and Outlook," *S. Afr. Med. J.*, 30:298–99, 1956.

31. The AAGP had well over 2,000 members by the end of 1947, the year of its founding, and reached 25,000 members by the end of 1959. Between 1960 and 1968, membership increased only incrementally to 30,000. Truman, *History of Founding of AAGP*, 54, 60 and S. A. Garlan, "Rebirth of General Practice," *JAMA*, 171:1937–1940, 1959, at 1938.

32. American Academy of Family Physicians, *Family Practice: Creation of a Specialty* (Kansas City, MO: American Academy of Family Physicians, 1980), 34; Truman, *History of Founding of AAGP*, 43.

33. J. Dunbar Shields, "Any Kind of Work," in S. R. Kaufman, *The Healer's Tale: Transforming Medicine and Culture* (Madison: University of Wisconsin Press, 1993), 151–157, at 153.

34. Editorial, "General Practitioners and Hospitals," *JAMA*, 144:766, 1950.

35. J. O. Boyd, "General Practice" [Letter], *JAMA*, 146:1151–1152, 1951, at 1151.

36. Ibid., 1152.

37. D. P. Adams, "Community and Professionalization: General Practitioners and Ear, Nose, and Throat Specialists in Cincinnati, 1945–1947," *Bull. Hist. Med.*, 68:664–684, 1994.

38. *Family Practice: Creation of a Specialty*, op. cit., 12, 20.

39. On the early history and meaning of the internship in America, see R. Stevens, *American Medicine and the Public Interest: A History of Specialization*, updated ed. (Berkeley: University of California Press, 1998 [1971]), 116–120.

40. Editorial, "Preparation for General Practice," *JAMA*, 156:178–179, 1954; E. G. Dimond, "The Generalist and the Internist," *JAMA*, 64:1306–1309, 1957, at 1306–1307.

41. Garlan, "Rebirth of General Practice," 1939.

42. Dimond, "Generalist and Internist," 1307.

43. L. F. Ritelmeyer, "Essentials of a Residency Program in General Practice," *JAMA*, 162:19–22, 1956.

44. I have written at length about my father's multispecialty reach, unusual even among the competent generalists of his generation, in P. E. Stepansky, *The Last Family Doctor: Remembering My Father's Medicine* (Montclair, NJ: Keynote Books, 2011).

45. S. Rushmore, "Some Aims of Medical Education," *N. Engl. J. Med.*, 204:314–318, 1931, at 316.

46. These data from the AMA Council on Medical Education and Hospitals' annual reports on internships and residencies are given by C. Wesley Eisele, "Essentials of a Residency in General Practice," *JAMA*, 164:384–388, 1957, at 385.

47. E. H. Leveroos, A. N. Springall, & C T. Heinze, "Approved Internships and Residencies in the United States," *JAMA*, 159:251–260, 1955, at 258 (Table 8).

48. C. W. Eisele, "Essentials of a Residency in General Practice," *JAMA*, 164:384–388, 1957, at 385.

49. See for example Deborah Sweaney's account of her GP father, Frank Sweaney, who, from 1953 until his untimely death in1960, joined several other rural generalists at a 37-bed community hospital in tiny Oregon, Missouri, where they performed all the surgery. D. Sweaney, *Unpacking Memories: The Story of a Suitcase, a Country Doctor and a Community* (Tarentum, PA: Word Association, 2013).

50. Quoted in Dimond, "Generalist and the Internist," 1307.

51. *Family Practice: Creation of a Specialty*, 37–38.

52. Ibid., 42.

53. Eisele, "Essentials of a Residency in General Practice," 387.

54. G. G. Stephens, *The Intellectual Basis of Family Practice* (Kansas City: Winter, 1982), 22–23, 38.

55. W. S. Biggs, et al., "Entry of US Medical School Graduates into Family Medicine Residencies: 2011–2012," *Fam. Med.*, 44:620–626, 2012.

56. S. Tavernise, "Emergency Visits Seen Increasing with Health Law," *New York Times*, January 3, 2014, A1 (http://www.nytimes.com/2014/01/03/health/access-to-health-care-may-increase-er-visits-study-suggests.html); R. Calandra, "With Health Law, ERs Still Packed," *Philadelphia Inquirer*, August 15, 2014 (http://kaiserhealthnews.org/news/with-health-law-er-still-packed).

CHAPTER 10—A NEW KIND OF DOCTOR

1. S. M. Petterson, et al., "Projecting US Primary Care Physician Workforce Needs: 2010–2025," *Ann. Fam. Med.*, 10:503–509, 2012.

2. Quoted in N. Nathan, "Doc Shortage Could Crash Health Care," November 13, 2012 (http://abcnews.go.com/Health/doctor-shortage-healthcare-crash/story?id=17708473).

3. D. R. Rittenhouse & S. M. Shortell, "The Patient-Centered Medical Home: Will It Stand the Test of Health Reform?", *JAMA*, 301:2038–2040, 2009, at 2039. Among recent commentaries, see further D. M. Berwick, "Making Good on ACOs' Promise—The Final Rule for the Medicare Shared Savings Program," *New Engl. J. Med.*, 365:1753–1756, 2011; D. R. Rittenhouse, et al., "Primary Care and Accountable Care—Two Essential Elements of Delivery-System Reform," *New Engl. J. Med.*, 361:2301–2303, 2009, and

E. Carrier, et al., "Medical Homes: Challenges in Translating Theory into Practice," *Med. Care*, 47:714–722, 2009.

4. The "Joint Principles of the Patient-Centered Medical Home" were set forth in 2007 (http://www.acponline.org/newsroom/pcmh.htm) and revised in 2011 (http://www.acponline.org/running_practice/delivery_and _payment_models/pcmh/understanding/guidelines_pcmh.pdf).

5. See the comments of PCPs and health care managers gathered in T. Hoff, *Practice Under Pressure: Primary Care Physicians and Their Medicine in the Twenty-First Century* (New Brunswick: Rutgers University Press, 2010), 173–193.

6. On the provisions of the HITECH Act, especially its financial incentives for rewarding hospitals and physicians who make "meaningful use" of certified EHR (Electronic Health Records) systems, see D. Blumenthal, "Launching HITECH," *N. Engl. J. Med.*, 362:382–385, 2010.

7. I am grateful to my brother, David Stepansky, M.D., whose former medical group participated in both PCMH and ACO entities, for these insights on the impact of participation on PCPs who are not part of relatively large health systems.

8. Hoff, *Practice Under Pressure*, 180–181, 183.

9. Petterson, et al., "Projecting US Primary Care Physician Workforce Needs," op. cit.

10. E.g., R. G. Petersdorf, "Financing Medical Education: A Universal 'Berry Plan' for Medical Students," *New Engl. J. Med.*, 328, 651, 1993; K. M. Byrnes, "Is There a Primary Care Doctor in the House? The Legislation Needed to Address a National Shortage," *Rutgers Law Rev.*, 25: 799, 806–808, 1994. On the Medicare Incentive Payment Program for physicians practicing in designated HPSAs—and the inadequacy of the 10% bonus system now in place—see L. R. Shugarman & D. O. Farley, "Shortcomings in Medicare Bonus Payments for Physicians in Underserved Areas," *Health Affairs*, 22:173–178, 2003, at 177 (http://content.healthaffairs.org/content /22/4/173.full.pdf+html) and S. Gunselman, "The Conrad 'State-30' Program: A Temporary Relief to the U.S. Shortage of Physicians or a Contributor to the Brain Drain," *J. Health Biomed. Law*, 5:91–115, 2009, at 107–108.

11. G. Cheng, "The National Residency Exchange: A Proposal to Restore Primary Care in an Age of Microspecialization," *Am. J. Law Med.*, 38:158–195, 2012.

12. The NHSC, founded in 1970, provides full scholarship support for medical students who agree to serve as PCPs in high-need, underserved locales, with one year of service for each year of support provided by the government. For medical school graduates who have already accrued debt,

the program provides student loan payment for physicians who commit to at least two years of service at an approved site. Descriptions of the scholarship and loan repayment program are available at http://nhsc.hrsa.gov.

13. See the rationale for rural training programs set forth in a document of the Association of American Medical Colleges, "Rural Medicine Programs Aim to Reverse Physician Shortage in Outlying Regions," online at http://www.aamc.org/newsroom/reporter/nov04/rural.htm. One of the best such programs, Jefferson Medical College's Physician Shortage Area Program, is described and its graduates profiled in H. K. Rabinowitz, *Caring for the Country: Family Doctors in Small Rural Towns* (New York: Springer, 2004).

14. Hoff, *Practice Under Pressure*, 86–91 and passim.

15. See especially the 2003 white paper by the AMA's taskforce on student debt (http://www.ama-assn.org/ama1/pub/upload/mm/15/debt_report.pdf) and, more recently, P. A. Pugno, et al., "Results of the 2009 National Resident Matching Program: Family Medicine," *Fam. Med.*, 41:567–577, 2009 and H. S. Teitelbaum, et al., "Factors Affecting Specialty Choice Among Osteopathic Medical Students, *Acad. Med.*, 84:718–723, 2009.

16. The testimonies gathered by Hoff about the devaluation of primary care in medical school are striking and unsettling. See, for example, the remarks of a third-year medical student planning to become a family physician: "If you're interested in primary care, you feel left out. There's so much emphasis on surgery and other medical specialties. We have a class advisor that goes over our program every year, reviews our classes, asks us how we are doing academically and she always asks, 'What do [you] intend to do moving forward?' And when you say primary care it's like, 'OK, fine, we don't have to keep track of you anymore.' Like we can do anything we want and no one needs to keep track of us. And so we don't have to be competitive or have an actual plan for the future. It's like getting tossed off." Hoff, *Practice Under Pressure*, 112–122, quoted at 121.

17. D. Hogberg, "The Next Exodus: Primary-Care Physicians and Medicare," National Policy Analysis #640 (http://www.nationalcenter.org/NPA640.html); C. S. Weissert & S. L. Silberman, "Sending a Policy Signal: State Legislatures, Medical Schools, and Primary Care Mandates," *J. Health Polit. Policy Law*, 23:743–770, 1998.

18. G. G. Stephens, "The Family Physician as Focus of Care in the United States" (1967), in *The Intellectual Basis of Family Practice* (Tucson, AZ: Winter Publishing, 1982), 77.

19. A. Feinstein, *Clinical Judgment* (Baltimore: Williams & Wilkins, 1967), 362.

20. See E. S. More, *Restoring the Balance: Women Physicians and the Profession of Medicine, 1850–1995* (Cambridge: Harvard University Press, 1999), 170–172. Edith Dunham, Martha Eliot, Helen Taussig, Edith Banfield Jackson, and Virginia Apgar stand out among the pioneer pediatricians who were true generalist-specialists.

21. See W. J. Stephen, *An Analysis of Primary Care: An International Study* (Cambridge: Cambridge University Press, 1979) and B. S. Starfield, *Primary Care: Concept, Evaluation and Policy* (Oxford: Oxford University Press, 1992).

22. The percentile range denotes the different protocols employed by researchers. See M. J. Dill & E. S. Salsberg, "The Complexities of Physician Supply and Demand: Projections Through 2025," Association of American Medical College, 2008 (http://www.innovationlabs.com/pa_future/1 /background_docs/AAMC%20Complexities%20of%20physician%20 demand,%202008.pdf); J. M. Colwill, et al., "Will Generalist Physician Supply Meet Demands of an Increasing and Aging Population?", *Health Affairs*, 27:w232–w241, 2008; and "Who Will Provide Primary Care and How Will They Be Trained?" Proceedings of a conference chaired by L. Cronenwett & V. J. Dzau, transcript edited by B. J. Culliton & S. Russell (New York: Josiah Macy, Jr. Foundation, 2010), 140n.

23. See the Federal Office of Rural Health Policy, "Facts About . . . Rural Physicians" (http://www.shepscenter.unc.edu/rural/pubs/finding_brief /phy.html) and J. D. Gazewood, et al., "Beyond the Horizon: The Role of Academic Health Centers in Improving the Health of Rural Communities," *Acad. Med.*, 81:793–797, 2006. In all, the federal government has designated 5,848 geographical areas HPSAs in need of primary medical care (http://datawarehouse.hrsa.gov/factSheetNation.aspx).

24. These non-immigrant visa waivers, authorized since 1994 by the Physicians for Underserved Areas Act (the "Conrad State 30" Program), allow foreign-trained physicians who provide primary care in underserved communities for at least three years to waive the two-year home residence requirement. That is, these physicians do not have to return to their native countries for at least two years prior to applying for permanent residence or an immigration visa. On the negative impact of this program on health equity and, inter alia, the global fight against HIV and AIDS, see V. Patel, "Recruiting Doctors from Poor Countries: The Great Brain Robbery?" *Brit. Med. J.*, 327:926–928, 2003; F. Mullan, "The Metrics of the Physician Brain Drain," *New Engl. J. Med.*, 353:1810–1818, 2005; and N. Eyal & S. A. Hurst, "Physician Brain Drain: Can Nothing Be Done?" *Public Health Ethics*, 1:180–192, 2008.

25. See H. K. Rabinowitz, et al., "Medical School Programs to Increase the Rural Physician Supply: A Systematic Review and Projected Impact of Widespread Replication," *Acad. Med.*, 83:235–243, 2008, at 242: "It is, therefore, unlikely that the graduation of rural physicians will be a high priority for most medical schools, unless specific regulations require this, or unless adequate financial resources are provided as incentives to support this mission."

26. U. Lehmann, "Mid-level Health Workers: The State of Evidence on Programmes, Activities, Costs and Impact on Health Outcomes," World Health Organization, 2008 (http://www.who.int/hrh/MLHW_review_2008.pdf).

27. R. S. Hooker, "Federally Employed Physician Assistants," *Mil. Med.*, 173:895–899, 2008.

28. J. F. Cawley & R. S. Hooker, "Physician Assistant Role Flexibility and Career Mobility," *J. Am. Acad. Physician Assist.*, 23:10, 2010.

29. D. M. Brock, et al., "The Physician Assistant Profession and Military Veterans," *Mil. Med.*, 176:197–203, 2011.

30. N. Holt, "'Confusion's Masterpiece': The Development of the Physician Assistant Profession," *Bull. Hist. Med.*, 72:246–278, 1998; Brock, "Physician Assistant Profession," 197.

31. H. K. Rabinowitz, et al., "Critical Factors for Designing Programs to Increase the Supply and Retention of Rural Primary Care Physicians," *JAMA*, 286:1041–1048, 2001; H. K. Rabinowitz, et al., "The Relationship Between Entering Medical Students' Backgrounds and Career Plans and Their Rural Practice Outcomes Three Decades Later," *Acad. Med.*, 87:493–497, 2012; H. K. Rabinowitz, et al., "The Relationship Between Matriculating Medical Students' Planned Specialties and Eventual Rural Practice Outcomes," *Acad. Med.*, 87:1086–1090, 2012.

32. D. P. Olson & K. E. Roth, "Diagnostic Tools and the Hands-On Physical Exam," *AMA J. Ethics*, 9:113–118, 2007.

33. The prerogative to develop specialized knowledge and treatment skills within certain areas has always been part of general practice, and it was explicitly recommended in the Report of the AMA Ad Hoc Committee on Education for Family Practice (the Willard Committee) of 1966 that paved the way for establishment of the American Board of Family Practice in 1969. See American Academy of Family Physicians, *Family Practice: Creation of a Specialty* (Kansas City, MO: American Academy of Family Physicians, 1980), 41.

34. C. G. Morris & F. M. Chen, "Training Residents in Community Health Centers: Facilitators and Barriers," *Ann. Fam. Med.*, 7:488–494, 2009; C. G. Morris, et al., "Training Family Physicians in Community Health Centers," *Fam. Med.*, 40:271–276, 2008; E. M. Mazur, et al., "Collaboration

Between an Internal Medicine Residency Program and a Federally Qualified Health Center: Norwalk Hospital and the Norwalk Community Health
Center," *Acad. Med.*, 76: 1159–1164, 2001.

35. http://m.mlb.com/news/article/79082538/2014-draft-signingbonus
-tracker.

36. "Specialty and Geographic Distribution of the Physician Workforce:
What Influences Medical Student and Resident Choices?" A publication
of the Robert Graham Center, funded by the Josiah Macy, Jr. Foundation
(2009), at 5, 47; Culliton & Russell, "Who Will Provide Primary Care and
How Will They Be Trained?" 140n.

37. "Who Will Provide Primary Care and How Will They Be Trained?",
147, 148.

38. Ibid., 151.

39. J. Winakur, *Memory Lessons: A Doctor's Story* (New York: Hyperion,
2009), 68.

40. J. D. Goodman, "Unintended Consequences of Resource-Based Value
Scale Reimbursement," *JAMA*, 298:2308–2310, 2007.

41. William Hsiao is quoted by Scott Baltic in "How RUC Determines
the Value of Health Care," *Ophthalmology Times*, October 1, 2013, 44. On
the AMA's Relative Value Scale Update Committee (RUC) and its primary
care critics, see further M. E. Schneider, "Primary Care Is Ready to Rumble
Over RUC," *Fam. Pract. News*, 41:1, 2011; J. F. Sweeney, "AAFP Wants
Change in RUC Composition," *Med. Econ.*, July 25, 2011, 21; B. Klepper
(interview), "How the RUC Harms PCPs—and What You Can Do About
It," *Med. Econ.*, May 25, 2013, 65–66; S. Baltic, "Uncovering the Myster-
ies of RUC," *Med. Econ.*, October 10, 2013, 35–40; and B. Gatty, "Expect
Federal Scrutiny of RUC to Intensify," *Urology Times*, 42:49, 2014.

42. Hoff, *Practice Under Pressure*, 189.

43. There is, sadly, a growing literature on burnout among primary care
physicians. See, e.g., T. D. Shanafelt, S. Booner, L. Tan, et al., "Burnout and
Satisfaction with Work-Life Balance Among U.S. Physicians Relative to the
General U.S. Population," *Arch. Intern. Med.*, 172:1377–1385, 2012; L. N.
Dyrbye & T. D. Shanafelt, "Physician Burnout: A Potential Threat to Suc-
cessful Health Care Reform," *JAMA*, 305:2009–2010, 2011; and S. Okie,
"Innovation in Primary Care—Staying One Step Ahead of Burnout," *New
Engl. J. Med.*, 359:2305–2309, 2008.

44. D. L. Roter, J. A. Hall, & Y. Aoki, "Physician Gender Effects in
Medical Communication: A Meta-Analytic Review," *JAMA*, 288:756–764,
2002; D. L. Roter & J. A. Hall, "Physician Gender and Patient-Centered
Communication: A Critical Review of Empirical Research," *Annu. Rev.
Publ. Health*, 25:497–519, 2004, quoted at 510.

45. Hoff, *Practice Under Pressure*, 153.

46. S. Freud, "The Ego and the Id" (1923) in J. Strachey, ed., *Standard Edition of the Complete Psychological Works of Sigmund Freud*, 19:3–66 (London: Hogarth Press, 1961), 26, 26n.

47. G. Majno, *The Healing Hand: Man and Wound in the Ancient World* (Cambridge: Harvard University Press, 1975), 104–105; C. O'Keefe Aptowicz, *Dr. Mütter's Marvels* (New York: Avery, 2014), 94–95, 103; W. T. Longcope, "Random Recollections of William Osler, 1899–1918," *Arch. Intern. Med.*, 84:93–103, 1949, at 95.

48. For an introduction to these and other fascinating topics in contemporary "touch" research, see T. Field, *Touch* (Cambridge: MIT Press, 2014), 87–118.

49. J. Lawick-Goodall, *In the Shadow of Man* (London: Collins, 1971), 240.

50. M. Prigg, "A Tender Touch of the Trunk: Researchers Reveal for the First Time Elephants DO Console Each Other," DailyMail.com, February 18, 2014 (http://www.dailymail.co.uk/sciencetech/article-2562259 /Elephants-really-DO-console-putting-tongue-animals-mouth-equivalent -hug.html).

51. Winakur, *Memory Lessons*, 181, 97–98.

52. S. S. Barold, "Willem Einthoven and the Birth of Clinical Electrocardiography a Hundred Years Ago," *Card. Electrophysiol. Rev.*, 7:99–104, 2003.

53. My father retained letters from many patients over the course of his 40-year practice, a number of which are quoted in my memoir, P. E. Stepansky, *The Last Family Doctor: Remembering My Father's Medicine* (Montclair, NJ: Keynote Books, 2011). This one is at 59–60.

CHAPTER 11—WHAT DO NURSE PRACTITIONERS PRACTICE?

1. American Association of Nurse Practitioners, NP Fact Sheet (http:// www.aanp.org/all-about-nps/np-fact-sheet).

2. J. Spetz, S. T. Parente, R. J. Town, et al., "Scope-of-Practice Laws for Nurse Practitioners Limit Cost Savings That Can Be Achieved in Retail Clinics," *Health Affairs*, 32:1977–1984, 2013; C. K. Cassel, "Retail Clinics and Drugstore Medicine," *JAMA*, 307:2151–2152, 2012; A. Mehrotra, H. Liu, J. L. Adams, et al., "Comparing Costs and Quality of Care at Retail Clinics with That of Other Medical Settings for Common Illnesses," *Ann. Intern. Med.*, 151:321–328, 2009.

3. M. Evans, "Data-Sharing Between Retail Clinics, Health Systems Hits Hurdles," *Modern Healthcare*, February 14, 2014 (http://www.modern healthcare.com/article/20140215/MAGAZINE/302159939); Health Capital Consultants, "Retail Clinics and Health Systems Coordinate Care," *Health Capital Topics*, 7:1–2, 2014.

4. T. Bodenheimer, A. Ghorob, R. Willard-Grace, et al., "The 10 Building Blocks of High-Performing Primary Care," *Ann. Fam. Med.*, 12:166–171, 2014, at 168.

5. Bodenheimer, "10 Building Blocks," 168–169; A. Ghorob & T. Bodenheimer, "Sharing the Care to Improve Access to Primary Care," *New Engl. J. Med.*, 366:1955–1957, 2012.

6. These numbers are drawn from federal census data, as compiled by P. D'Antonio & J. C. Whelan, "Counting Nurses: The Power of Historical Census Data," *J. Clin. Nurs.*, 18:2717–2724, 2009, Table 1 ("Individual Women and Men Self-Identifying as Professional Nurses, by Gender and Race, 1900–2006").

7. "By replacing graduate nurses who already have gone into the military, the U.S. Cadet Nurse Corps has prevented a collapse of nursing care in civilian hospitals. Moreover, the increasing number of graduates constitute a reservoir of nurse power which if effectively distributed would in my opinion meet both the military and minimum civilian needs." "The Cadet Nurse Corps: Testimony of Thomas Parran, Surgeon General, U.S. Public Health Service, Before the House Committee on Military Affairs, February 6," *JAMA*, 127:995, 1945. The history of the cadet nurses and the stories of those who served are recounted by former cadet nurse Thelma Robinson in T. M. Robinson & P. M. Perry, *Cadet Nurse Stories: The Call for and Response of Women During World War II* (N.P.: Sigma Theta Tau International, Center for Nursing, 2001) and P. Ruston, L. C. Callister, & M. K. Wilson, compilers, *Latter-day Saint Nurses at War: A Story of Caring and Sacrifice* (Provo, UT: Brigham Young University, 2005), 115–154.

8. P. D'Antonio, *American Nursing: A History of Knowledge, Authority, and the Meaning of Work* (Baltimore: Johns Hopkins University Press, 2010), 165; D. C. Hine, *Black Women in White: Racial Conflict and Cooperation in the Nursing Profession, 1890–1950* (Bloomington: Indiana University Press, 1989), 151–153.

9. P. A. Kalisch & B. Kalisch, *The Advance of American Nursing*, 3rd ed., (Philadelphia: Lippincott, 1995), 504, 370.

10. H. E. Peplau, "Some Reflections on Earlier Days in Psychiatric Nursing," *J. Psychosoc. Nurs. Ment. Health Serv.*, 20:17–24, 1982, at 23; H. E. Peplau, "Future Directions in Psychiatric Nursing from the Perspective of History," *J. Psychosoc. Nurs. Ment. Health Serv.*, 27:18–28, 1989, at 20.

11. K. Dawley, "Doubling Back Over Roads Once Traveled: Creating a National Organization for Nurse-Midwifery," *J. Midwifery Women's Health*, 50:71–82, 2005, at 75–78.

12. Patricia D'Antonio provides a rich account of one such segregated nurse training program, that affiliated with Atlanta's Grady Memorial Hospital, in *American Nursing*, 106–130.

13. U.S. Department of Labor, Bureau of Labor Statistics, *The Economic Status of Registered Professional Nurses: 1946–1947* (Bulletin No. 931), Washington, DC: U.S. Government Printing Office.

14. D. Deming, "Why Practical Nurses, Part II," *RN J.*, 11:43–45, 64, 66, 1948 and American Nurses' Association, "The American Nurses' Association and Nonprofessional Workers in Nursing," *Am. J. Nurs*, 55:43–45, 1955, both cited by V. T. Grando, "Making Do with Fewer Nurses in the United States, 1945–1965," *Image J. Nurs. Sch.*, 30:147–149, 1998.

15. C. M. Silverstein, "From the Front Line to the Home Front: A History of the Development of Psychiatric Nursing in the U.S. During the World War II Era," *Issues Ment. Health Nurs.*, 29:719–737, 2008, at 732–733.

16. J. E. Lynaugh, "Nursing the Great Society: The Impact of the Nurse Training Act of 1964," *Nurs. Hist. Rev.*, 16:13–28, 2008, at 16.

17. J. Fairman & J. E. Lynaugh, *Critical Care Nursing: A History* (Philadelphia: University of Pennsylvania Press, 1998), 28–32.

18. Lynaugh, "Nursing the Great Society," 23.

19. J. Fairman, *Making Room in the Clinic: Nurse Practitioners and the Evolution of Modern Health Care* (New Brunswick: Rutgers University Press, 2008), 119–121.

20. L. Freitas, "Historical Roots and Future Perspectives Related to Nursing Ethics," *J. Prof. Nurs.*, 197–205, 1990, at 202.

21. M. Sandelowski, *Devices and Desires: Gender, Technology, and American Nursing* (Chapel Hill: University of North Carolina Press, 2000), 127–128.

22. Fairman, *Making Room in the Clinic*, 91.

23. J. Fairman, "Delegated by Default or Negotiated by Need? Physicians, Nurse Practitioners, and the Process of Clinical Thinking," in E. D. Baer, et al., *Enduring Issues in American Nursing* (New York: Springer Pub., 2002), 309–333, at 323.

24. Fairman, *Making Room in the Clinic*, 95ff.

25. N.B. I do not understand "clinical judgment," with its reliance on mentoring and tacit knowing, in the same way Fairman understands "clinical thinking," viz., as a process or skill set. See Fairman, "Delegated by Default," 311–312 and *Making Room in the Clinic*, 187.

26. For a wonderful popular exposition of Nightingale's vision of the nurse transposed to the Bellevue Hospital Training School in the early 1880s, see F. H. North, "A New Profession for Women," *The Century Magazine*, 25:30–37, 1882.

27. I. H. Robb, *Nursing Ethics* (Cleveland: Koeckert, 1900), 34, 40.

28. Fairman, "Delegated by Default," 323.

29. These brief remarks allude to, without doing justice to, the brilliant analysis of Thomas Haskell on the emergence of modern professions in post-bellum America. See T. L. Haskell, *The Emergence of Professional Social Science: The American Social Science Association and the Nineteenth-Century Crisis of Authority* (Baltimore: Johns Hopkins University Press, 2000 [1977]), 68–74, 91–121, and passim.

30. K. Koch, "Agatha Hodgins, Lakeside Alumnae Association, and the Founding of the AANA," *AANA Journal*, 73:259–262, 2005; L. E. Ettinger, *Nurse Midwifery: The Birth of a New American Profession* (Columbus: Ohio State University Press, 2006), 174–175; K. Dawley, "Doubling Back Over Roads Once Traveled: Creating a National Organization for Nurse-Midwifery," *J. Midwifery Womens Health*, 50:71–82, 2005.

31. Fairman, *Making Room in the Clinic*, 175–180.

32. A dissociation of primary care nursing from primary care medicine has been explicitly made, e.g., "A common question was 'Are you a nurse, or are you a mini-doc?' My answer was, is, and will always be: 'I am a nurse with primary care skills. I take care of my patients within a nursing framework. . . . my values lie in nursing, not in the medical model. I care for my patients as a fully prepared, primary care provider of women." J. A. Berg & M. E. Roberts, "Recognition, Regulation, Scope of Practice: Nurse Practitioners' Growing Pains," *J. Am. Acad. Nurse Pract.*, 24:121–123, 2012, at 121.

33. On Peplau's graduate training at Teachers College and the William Alanson White Institute, see B. J. Callaway, *Hildegard Peplau: Psychiatric Nurse of the Century* (New York: Springer Pub., 2002), 167–191.

34. Dominique Tobbell documents the perceived deficiencies of 1960s graduates of the UCLA and University of Minnesota nursing schools, where the new curriculum was implemented, in "'Coming to Grips with the Nursing Question': The Politics of Nursing Education Reform in 1960s America," *Nurs. Hist. Rev.*, 22:37–60, 2014.

35. This paragraph is culled from my memoir of my father's life and career, P. E. Stepansky, *The Last Family Doctor: Remembering My Father's Medicine* (Montclair, NJ: Keynote Books, 2011).

36. Stepansky, *Last Family Doctor*, 3–7.

37. E. M. Norman, *We Band of Angels: The Untold Story of American Nurses Trapped on Bataan by the Japanese* (New York: Random House,

1999); D. B. Silver, *Refuge in Hell: How Berlin's Jewish Hospital Outlasted the Nazis* (Boston: Houghton Mifflin, 2003).

38. J. A. Fairman, et al., "Broadening the Scope of Nursing Practice," *New Engl. J. Med.*, 364:193–196, 2011, at 193.

39. As quoted in J. A. Fairman & S. M. Okoye, "Nursing for the Future, From the Past: Two Reports on Nursing from the Institute of Medicine," *J. Nurs. Educ.*, 50:305–311, 2011, at 309.

40. Quoted in J. K. Iglehart, "Expanding the Role of Advanced Nurse Practitioners—Risks and Rewards," *New Engl. J. Med.*, 368:1935–1941, 2013, at 1940.

41. L. Poghosyan, D. Boyd, & A. R. Knutson, "Nurse Practitioner Role, Independent Practice, and Teamwork in Primary Care," *J. Nurse Practitioners*, 10:472–479, 2014, at 477.

42. M. D. Naylor & E. T. Kurtzman, "The Role of Nurse Practitioners in Reinventing Primary Care," *Health Affairs*, 29:893–899, 2010.

43. S. Isaacs & P. Jellinek, *Accept No Substitute: A Report on Scope of Practice.* White paper for The Physicians Foundation, November 2012 (http://www.khi.org/documents/2014/aug/26/accept-no-substitute-report-scope -practice), 1, 2, 3, 6.

44. S. M. Petterson, et al., "Projecting US Primary Care Physician Workforce Needs: 2010–2025," *Ann. Fam. Med.*, 10:503–509, 2012.

45. Isaacs & Jellinek, *Accept No Substitute*, 8–13.

46. G. C. Richardson, et al., "Nurse Practitioner Management of Type 2 Diabetes," *Perm. J.*, 18:e134–140, 2014; M. J. Goolsby, "2006 American Academy of Nurse Practitioners Diabetes Management Survey," *J. Am. Acad. Nurse Pract.*, 19:496–498, 2007; Fairman, et al., "Broadening the Scope of Nursing Practice," 193.

47. Richardson, "Nurse Practitioner Management of Type 2 Diabetes," op. cit.; K. G. Shojania, et al., "Effects of Quality Improvement Strategies for Type 2 Diabetes on Glycemic Control: A Meta-Regression Analysis," *JAMA*, 296: 427–440, 2006; S. Ingersoll, et al., "Nurse Care Coordination for Diabetes: A Literature Review and Synthesis," *J. Nurs. Care Qual.*, 20:208–214, 2005.

48. C. Feudtner, *Bittersweet: Diabetes, Insulin, and the Transformation of Illness* (Chapel Hill: University of North Carolina Press, 2003), 36.

49. C. Fletcher, L. A. Copeland, J. C. Lowery, et al., "Nurse Practitioners as Primary Care Providers Within the VA," *Mil. Med.*, 176:791–797, 2011.

50. C. Rosenberg, "The Art of Medicine: Managed Fear," *Lancet*, 373:802–803, 2009, at 803.

51. R. E. G. Upshur & S. Tracy, "Chronicity and Complexity: Is What's Good for the Diseases Always Good for the Patients?" *Can. Fam. Physician*, 54:1655–1657, 2008.

52. Spetz, "Scope-of-Practice Laws for Nurse Practitioners," 1982.

53. R. E. Upshur, "Looking for Rules in a World of Exceptions: Reflections on Evidence-Based Practice," *Perspect. Biol. Med.*, 48:477–489, 2005.

54. R. E. Becker, "Remembering Sir William Osler 100 Years After His Death: What Can We Learn from His Legacy?", *Lancet*, 384: 2260–2263, 2014, at 2262. The lessons of variational biology, as they pertain, for example, to "the power of positive numbers," are learned anew by contemporary physicians. See J. Groopman, *How Doctors Think* (Boston: Houghton Mifflin, 2007), 150. The infectious diseases specialist Philip Lerner was an Oslerian proponent of variational biology at the bedside in the 1970s and '80s. As his son Barron Lerner writes: "More provocatively, he thought that doctors could use their clinical acumen, experience, and even empathy to reach conclusions about how specific illnesses acted or were likely to act in specific patients. Without scientific proof, of course, these claims could always be contested. But for my father and those trained in a similar manner, such insights needed to be considered at patients' bedsides." B. H. Lerner, *The Good Doctor: A Father, a Son, and the Evolution of Medical Ethics* (Boston: Beacon Press, 2014), 28.

55. On the notion of clinical competence as acquisition of a "skill set," see, e.g., Fairman, "Delegated by Default," 311–312 and Fairman, *Making Room in the Clinic*, 187, 190.

56. Feudtner terms it a "cyclical transmuted disease" in *Bittersweet*, 36.

57. Upshur & Tracy, "Chronicity and Complexity," 1656. For exemplary instances of how clinical judgment—and not a clinical "skill set"—enters into the prioritizing of treatment interventions among concurrent chronic diseases, see K. C. Stange, et al., "The Value of a Family Physician," *J. Fam. Practice*, 46:363–369, 1998; K. C. Stange, "The Generalist Approach," *Ann. Fam. Med.*, 7:198–203, 2009, and E. J. Cassell, *Doctoring: The Nature of Primary Care Medicine* (New York: Oxford University Press, 1997).

58. Of course, the issue of levels of prescriptive authority pertains not only to physicians and NPs, but also to physician assistants, dentists, optometrists, osteopaths, pharmacists, and podiatrists. For the concrete manner in which the state of Florida spells out prescriptive levels for each of these professions, see http://www.thehealthlawfirm.com/resources/health-law-articles-and-documents/prescribing-in-florida.html.

59. M. Crane, "Malpractice Risks with NPs and PAs in Your Practice," *Medscape*, January 3, 2013 (http://www.medscape.com/viewarticle/775746).

60. E.g., C. Buppert, "Scope of Practice," *J. Nurse Pract.*, 1:11–13, 2005.

61. C. D. DeAngelis, "Nurse Practitioner Redux," *JAMA*, 271:868–871, 1994. The studies DeAngelis cites are: P. Repicky, et al., "Professional

Activities of Nurse Practitioners in Adult Ambulatory Care Settings," *Nurse Pract.*, 4:27–40, 1980; D. Munroe, et al., "Prescribing Patterns of Nurse Practitioners," *Amer. J. Nurs.*, 82:1538–1540, 1982; and J. Resenaur, "Prescribing Behavior of Primary Care Nurse Practitioners," *Am. J. Public Health*, 74:10–13, 1984.

62. "Nurse Practitioner Prescribing Authority and Physician Supervision Requirements for Diagnosis and Treatment" (http://kff.org/other /state-indicator/nurse-practitioner-autonomy).

63. D. M. Keepnews, "Scope of Practice Redux?," *Policy Polit. Nurs. Pract.*, 7:84–86, 2006, at 84.

64. AAFP, "Patient Perceptions Regarding Health Care Providers," March 2012 (http://www.aafp.org/dam/AAFP/documents/about_us /initiatives/PatientPerceptions.pdf). Physician concern with the growing number of nurse "doctors" received media attention following the AMA's "truth in advertising campaign" of 2010. See, e.g., G. Harris, "Calling More Nurses 'Doctors,' A Title Physicians Begrudge," *New York Times*, October 2, 2011, A1, and M. Beck, "Battles Erupt Over Filling Doctors' Shoes," *Wall Street Journal*, February 4, 2013, A3.

65. D. Marbury, "Scope of Practice Debate," *Med. Econ.*, September 10, 2013, 26–30, at 27 (http://medicaleconomics.modernmedicine.com /medical-economics/news/scope-practice-debate).

66. An extensive literature explores the tacit dimension of clinical understanding, which is especially integral to the daily work of generalist physicians. High points of this literature include: H. D. Brande, "Clinical Intuition versus Statistics: Different Modes of Tacit Knowledge in Clinical Epidemiology and Evidence-Based Medicine," *Theor. Med. Bioeth.*, 30:181–198, 2009; S. G. Henry, "Recognizing Tacit Knowledge in Medical Epistemology," *Theor. Med. Bioeth.*, 27:187–213, 2006; J. Gabbay & Andrée le May, "Evidence-Based Guidelines or Collectively Constructed 'Mindlines'? Ethnographic Study of Knowledge Management in Primary Care," *Brit. Med. J.*, 329:1013–1016, 2004; K. Malterud, "The Art and Science of Clinical Knowledge: Evidence Beyond Measures and Numbers," *Lancet*, 358:397–400, 2001; S. R. Jha, "The Tacit-Explicit Connection: Polanyian Integrative Philosophy and a Neo-Polanyian Medical Epistemology," *Theor. Med. Bioeth.*, 19:547–568, 1998; K. Malterud, "The Legitimacy of Clinical Knowledge: Towards a Medical Epistemology Embracing the Art of Medicine," *Theor. Med. Bioeth.*, 16:183–198, 1995; G. M. Goldman, "The Tacit Dimension of Clinical Judgment," *Yale J. Biol. Med.*, 63, 47–61, 1990.

67. Naylor & Kurtzman, "Reinventing Primary Care," 896.

68. J. Stanik-Hutt, R. P. Newhouse, K. M. White, et al., "The Quality and Effectiveness of Care Provided by Nurse Practitioners," *J. Nurse Pract.*, 9:492–500.e13, 2013. This metastudy compiled data from 37 articles published from 1990–2009 and summarized their respective findings in 11 aggregated outcomes of care by NPs and physicians, respectively. While taking the findings of such metastudies seriously, one must note that this particular study all but collapses under the weight of its own methodological shortcomings, which include: "Heterogeneity of study designs and measures, multiple time points for measuring outcomes, limited number of randomized designs, and inadequate statistical data for meta-analysis" (497).

69. A. R. Feinstein, *Clinical Judgment* (Baltimore: Williams & Wilkins, 1967), 80, 332.

70. J. Spetz, St. T. Parente, R. J. Town, et al., "Scope-of-Practice Laws for Nurse Practitioners Limit Cost Savings That Can Be Achieved in Retail Clinics," *Health Affairs*, 32:1977–1984, 2013; C. K. Cassel, "Retail Clinics and Drugstore Medicine," *JAMA*, 307:2151–2152, 2012; R. Rudavsky, C. E. Pollack, & A. Mehrotra, "The Geographic Distribution, Ownership, Prices, and Scope of Practice at Retail Clinics," *Ann. Intern. Med.*, 151:315–320, 2009; A. Mehrotra, H. Liu, J. L. Adams, et al., "Comparing Costs and Quality of Care at Retail Clinics with That of Other Medical Settings for Common Illnesses," *Ann. Intern. Med.*, 151:321–328, 2009.

71. "Virginia Law Promotes Team-Based Care by Doctors and Nurse Practitioners" (http://www.amednews.com/article/20120423/profession /304239960/4/); "Virginia Academy Helps Craft State Legislation Clarifying Physician, NP Roles" (http://www.aafp.org/news/chapter-of-the -month/20121130virginiachapter.html).

72. N. Sciamanna, K. Alvarez, J. Miller, et al., "Attitudes Toward Nurse Practitioner-Led Chronic Disease Management to Improve Outpatient Quality of Care," *Am. J. Med. Qual.*, 21:375–381, 2006.

EPILOGUE— HOME IS WHERE OUR HEALTH IS

1. "Guidelines for Patient-Centered Medical Home (PCMH) Recognition and Accreditation Programs," jointly issued by the American Academy of Family Physicians, American Academy of Pediatrics, American College of Physicians, and American Osteopathic Association, February 2011, criterion #2: "Address the Complete Scope of Primary Care Services."

2. C. Sia, et al., "History of the Medical Home Concept," *Pediatrics*, 113:1473–1478, 2004.

3. E. Carrier, M. N. Gourevitch, & N. R. Shah, "Medical Homes: Challenges in Translating Theory into Practice," *Med. Care*, 47:714–722, 2009.

4. G. Gayle Stephens, "The Horse and Buggy Doctor—1980 Style" (1973) in *The Intellectual Basis of Family Practice* (Tucson: Winter, 1982), 27–33, at 29.

5. G. C. Robinson, *The Patient as a Person: A Study of the Social Aspects of Illness* (New York: Commonwealth Fund, 1939). Robinson's book grew out of his Rockefeller-funded "Study of the Accessory Factors on Health" that analyzed a series of 174 new patients admitted to Johns Hopkins Hospital during 1936 and 1937. On Robinson and the Hopkins study, see T. M. Brown, "George Canby Robinson and 'The Patient as a Person'," in C. Lawrence & G. Weisz, eds., *Greater Than the Parts: Holism in Biomedicine, 1920–1950* (New York: Oxford University Press, 1998), 135–160 and S. W. Tracy, "George Draper and American Constitutional Medicine, 1916–1946: Reinventing the Sick Man," *Bull. Hist. Med.*, 66:53–89, 1992, at 64.

6. On the child guidance movement and the child guidance team, see K. W. Jones, *Taming the Troublesome Child: American Families, Child Guidance, and the Limits of Psychiatric Authority* (Cambridge: Harvard University Press, 1999). Cabot set forth the essential role of the medical social worker in carrying out treatment in *Social Service and the Art of Healing* (New York: Moffat, Yard, 1909). See R. Lubove, *The Professional Altruist: The Emergence of Social Work as a Career, 1880–1930* (New York: Macmillan, 1969), 24ff. and for a general appreciation of Cabot's role in the professionalization of social work, T. F. Williams, "Cabot, Peabody, and the Care of the Patient," *Bull. Hist. Med.*, 24:462–481, 1950.

7. T. Hoff, *Practice Under Pressure: Primary Care Physicians and Their Medicine in the Twenty-First Century* (New Brunswick: Rutgers University Press, 2010), 174.

8. Such concerns about the tenability of patient-centered medical homes were voiced by Hoff's PCP interviewees in *Practice Under Pressure*, 175–193. It is no small irony that one successful implementation of Patient-Centered Medical Home values has been in the private sector, where Iora Health, a corporation of primary care practices, contracts with employers and private Medicare plans to provide comprehensive care for a flat payment for each patient. Profits accrue to the corporation because it also receives a percentage of client savings on overall health spending, most of which is realized by keeping at-risk patients out of the hospital through easy access (absent any copays), preventive care, and early intervention. In effect, the Iora model reframes the provision of a "home" environment as the corporate obligation to provide "customer satisfaction," to which end it makes staff available to patients

around the clock via email and phone and also relies on the proactive role of "health coaches" assigned to each patient. See M. Sanger-Katz, "Company Thinks It Has Answer for Lower Health Costs: Customer Service," *New York Times*, March 27, 2015 (http://www.nytimes.com/2015/03/29/upshot /small-company-has-plan-to-provide-primary-care-for-the-masses.html). The piece appeared in the print edition of the Sunday Business Section of the *Times* on March 29, 2015, as "A Starbucks for Medicine" (1, 4–5).

9. The founding of many such "homes" in the 1850s and thereafter was part of the turn of female reformers away from moral suasion, rooted in norms of womanly virtue and Christian benevolence, and toward legislative and political action. See L. D. Ginzberg, *Women and the Work of Benevolence: Morality, Politics, and Class in the 19th-Century United States* (New Haven: Yale University Press, 1990), 98–132, from which my examples of the various homes are drawn.

10. For an illuminating study of these various homes and the people who lived in them, see J. W. Trent, *Inventing the Feeble Mind: A History of Mental Retardation in the United States* (Berkeley: University of California Press, 1994).

11. On ZocDoc, see O. Kharraz, "Providers Should Think Seriously About Leveraging Online Reviews," March 12, 2013 (http://www.thedoctorblog .com/providers-should-think-seriously-about-leveraging-online-reviews/).

12. The first quoted passage is reprinted in P. E. Stepansky, *The Last Family Doctor: Remembering My Father's Medicine* (Montclair, NJ: Keynote Books, 2011), 123. The second passage is not in the book and is among my father's personal effects.

13. L. Macmillan & M. Pringle, "Practice Managers and Practice Management," *Brit. Med. J.*, 304:1672–1674, 1992; L. S. Hill, "Telephone Techniques and Etiquette: A Medical Practice Staff Training Tool," *J. Med. Pract. Manage.*, 3:166–170, 2007; M. Gallagher, et al., "Managing Patient Demand: A Qualitative Study of Appointment Making in General Practice," *Br. J. Gen. Pract.*, 51:280–285, 2001.

14. S. Arber & L. Sawyer, "The Role of the Receptionist in General Practice: A 'Dragon Behind the Desk'?" *Soc. Sci. Med.*, 20:911–921, 1985; P. M. Neuwelt, R. A. Kearns, & A. J. Browne, "The Place of Receptionists in Access to Primary Care: Challenges in the Space Between Community and Consultation," *Soc. Sci. Med.*, 133:287–295, 2015.

15. R. G. Fielding, *Telephone Apprehension: A Study of Individual Differences in Attitudes to and Usage of the Telephone*. Doctoral Dissertation, Sheffield City Polytechnic [now Sheffield Hallam University], 1990.

16. Of course, "Marge speaking" is gendered and, among Foucaultians, may also be interpreted as the "slave" identity of the powerless receptionist alongside the all-powerful physician, who is always identified as "Doctor" followed by surname or, more imposingly still, as "The Doctor." It would no doubt be more politically correct for phone receptionists to refer to themselves by first name and surname. But in point of fact one rarely if ever hears nonphysician staff members in an office setting identify themselves over the phone by first and last names, and I find it hard to believe that most of them feel depreciated by the friendly outreach conveyed by use of first name only. This could be the subject of another essay at another time and place.

17. See J. L. Austin, *How to Do Things with Words* (Cambridge: Harvard University Press, 1962) and the work of his student, J. R. Searle, *Speech Acts: An Essay in the Philosophy of Language* (Cambridge: Cambridge University Press, 1970).

18. Ainsworth's typology of mother-infant attachment states grew out of her observational research on mother-infant pairs in Uganda, gathered in her *Infancy in Uganda* (Baltimore: Johns Hopkins University Press, 1967). On the nature of secure attachments, see especially J. Bowlby, *A Secure Base: Parent-Child Attachment and Healthy Human Development* (New York: Basic Books, 1988) and I. Bretherton, "The Origins of Attachment Theory: John Bowlby and Mary Ainsworth," *Dev. Psychol.,* 28:759–775, 1992.

Index

About the Author

A Yale-trained historian of ideas specializing in the history of American medicine and psychiatry, Paul E. Stepansky, Ph.D., enjoyed a 30-year career as a consulting editor and mental health publisher. Long sought out by physician-writers seeking high-level help developing book projects, Stepansky has worked collaboratively with senior writers in fields as diverse as psychiatry, psychoanalysis, medical sociology, psychopharmacology, surgery, and architecture. He was Managing Director of The Analytic Press from 1984 to 2006.

Stepansky's scholarship has taken him from early articles on the role of psychiatry in family medicine; to history of psychoanalysis (*A History of Aggression in Freud* [1977]; *In Freud's Shadow: Adler in Context* [1983]); to interdisciplinary studies in medicine and psychiatry (*Freud, Surgery, and the Surgeons* [1999]); to historical critiques of psychiatry and psychoanalysis in relation to scientific medicine as it evolved in the late-nineteenth and twentieth centuries (*Psychoanalysis at the Margins* [2009]). He has taught seminars in history of medicine and women's studies at Montclair State University and retains an appointment at Weill-Cornell Medical College, where he is interdisciplinary research faculty at the DeWitt Wallace Institute of the History of Psychiatry. His blog, "Medicine, Health, and History" (www.adoseofhistory.com) explores the impact of medical history on contemporary health care.